A
WRITER'S GUIDE
TO
MEDICINE

VOLUME 2: ILLNESS & INJURY

NATALIE DALE, MD

TABLE OF CONTENTS

For my dad,
who gave me the courage
to take the leap.

Thank you for reading *Volume 2: Illness & Injury* of the "Writer's Guide to Medicine" series. I think you'll enjoy it. If so, I'm hoping you'll write a brief review on Amazon or Goodreads. Authors like me rely on reviews to increase visibility and open doors to new audiences. Writing a review is one of the best and easiest ways you can help up-and-coming authors succeed. A few words can make a big difference. Thank you in advance!

Please subscribe to my **newsletter** for infrequent announcements about upcoming publications, bonus content, freebies, lectures, book signings, and more: https://nataliedaleauthor.com/

LIKE me on Facebook:
https://www.facebook.com/NatalieDaleAuthorMD

FOLLOW me on Instagram:
https://www.instagram.com/natalierose6627/

FOLLOW me on Twitter:
@DaleNatalie

ADD me on Goodreads:
https://www.goodreads.com/author/show/15282031.Natalie_Dale

PART I: MEDICAL EMERGENCIES

1. CHEST PAIN

Amna is on her morning walk with her friend, Alice. It's their first walk since Amna's hip surgery, so she's using her walker at the approximate pace of a leisurely snail. While walking up the short hill to the house, Amna suddenly can't catch her breath. She feels lightheaded, and her left shoulder hurts something fierce. Alice asks if she's feeling ok, is she having a heart attack? Amna is now having shooting chest pain every time she tries to breathe in and is terrified that Alice is right. What if this is a heart attack? Her chest tightens and she sways on her feet, abruptly dizzy. She clutches Alice and begs her to drive to the hospital.

CHEST PAIN IS ONE OF the most common reasons for trips to the emergency department, and a common ploy for killing off characters. But chest pain is not necessarily synonymous with a heart attack; there are lots of reasons your character could develop chest pain. This chapter will cover some of the reasons your character might develop chest pain, organized by the organ system causing the pain.

BACKGROUND

The chest contains two primary organ systems: the heart and great vessels, and the lungs. The **heart** is a four-chambered organ that uses electricity to generate a rhythm that allows it to pump blood out through the arteries, through the capillaries, and back via the veins in a complex organ system called the **cardiovascular** system. There are lots of things that can go wrong with the heart—insufficient blood flow to the heart muscle, valve disease, holes between the chambers, damage to the electrical system, stretching or overgrowth of muscles, insufficient pumping—but in this chapter, I'm only going to focus on the issues that cause chest *pain*.

The heart is made up of four chambers. The left and right atria are on top, and the left and right ventricles are on the bottom. The ventricles are the muscular workhorses of the heart, responsible for most of what it takes to pump blood. Blood enters the right atria from the *vena cava* and passes through the *tricuspid valve* into the right ventricle, where it is pumped out through the pulmonary artery into the lungs.

The **lungs** are the other major organ in the chest. Their main function is to provide oxygen to the blood, a process known as gas exchange; this process occurs in tiny air pockets, called *alveoli*. In the alveoli, waste products (like carbon dioxide) are pulled out of the blood and replaced with oxygen. The lungs are a big organ with lots of redundancies, meaning your character might have severe lung disease but show minimal symptoms, such as cough or feeling a bit short of breath while exercising.

> The heart's contraction is choreographed by a series of electrical signals. Unlike every other muscle, the heart does not need input from the brain to contract.

Once the blood has been oxygenated, it returns to the heart through the *pulmonary veins*. Blood enters the left atrium and then passes through the mitral valve into the muscular left ventricle. As the left ventricle contracts, blood is pumped through the aortic valve and out into the aorta.

The great vessels—the vena cava and the aorta—are the blood vessels that carry blood to and from the heart, respectively. The **aorta** has three important sections: the *ascending aorta*, where it first leaves the heart, the *aortic arch*, with three main branches to the upper body, and the *descending aorta*, which carries blood to the lower body.

There are also several organs that run through the chest: the **esophagus** conveys contents from the mouth to the stomach, while the **trachea** connects the mouth and nose to the lungs. The **diaphragm** is the large muscle that separates the thoracic cavity from the abdominal cavity. Innervated by the phrenic nerve, contraction of the diaphragm is required to initiate breathing. Finally, a small organ of the immune system, called the **thymus,** sits at the center of the thoracic cavity, nestled between the lungs.

You will notice this chapter has sections on organs that are *not* located in the chest, such as the GI tract. That's because our body doesn't have good pain sensors inside the chest and abdominal cavities. Because of this, our body sometimes interprets pain from one location (such as the stomach) as coming from another region (such as the chest). This is also why people with an acute heart problem will often experience pain in their shoulder, back, jaw, or left arm—the body just isn't very good at pinpointing the exact source of pain from within these body cavities.

CARDIOVASCULAR (HEART & GREAT VESSELS) CAUSES

At the hospital, Amna is seen by triage, then immediately wheeled back to a room. There, she's surrounded by nurses and technicians who help her change into a hospital gown and start an IV in the crook of her arm. The nurse puts a plastic mask over her face that blows cold air into Amna's mouth and nostrils, while someone else applies sticky pads to her chest and under her left breast, attaching the wires to what Amna recognizes as an EKG machine. A third person draws blood into little vials, then leaves. The nurse takes her blood pressure and puts a white sticker on the tip of her finger to monitor her blood oxygen level, which he says is a bit low. Then, a technician comes into the room to take a chest x-ray.

> Everyone coming to the ED with chest pain will get a barrage of tests and interventions before they ever see a doctor. These include supplemental oxygen, an IV, a blood draw for labs, an EKG, and a chest x-ray.

If you're writing about chest pain caused by the cardiovascular system, you're probably thinking of giving your character a "heart attack." But it turns out that "heart attack" isn't actually a diagnosis. Several different cardiovascular diagnoses can cause chest pain and lead to your character's untimely demise. Let's start with the medical equivalent of a heart attack: ischemic heart disease.

ISCHEMIC HEART DISEASE

Minutes later, the doctor arrives. He asks a few curt questions about her symptoms and her recent hospitalization, then listens to Amna's heart and lungs. He tells her that there are several possible diagnoses.

Ischemic heart disease is a range of different conditions caused by decreased blood flow in the coronary arteries—the arteries that deliver blood to the heart. This reduced blood flow means that the heart muscle isn't getting the oxygen it needs. Without enough oxygen, the heart muscle can become damaged and even die.

> **Ischemia** is the medical term for inadequate blood flow leading to lack of oxygen in the tissue.

Most of the time, the decreased blood flow is due to atherosclerotic lesions—plaque buildup in the coronary arteries due to high cholesterol levels in the blood. There are three main subtypes of ischemic heart disease: stable angina, unstable angina, and myocardial infarction.

Angina is chest pain due to the gradual narrowing of the coronary arteries over years to decades. When the heart beats faster, it requires more oxygen, but if the arteries are narrowed, the blood supply can't keep up. Angina can be separated into two subtypes: stable angina and unstable angina.

If your character has **stable angina**, they will have chest pain on exertion—running, doing yard work, even just walking—but the pain will go away with rest.

Stable angina can be scary, but it is usually not an emergency—it can be treated on an outpatient basis.

Unstable angina occurs when the coronary arteries are so narrow that they can't supply adequate blood flow, even at rest. There are two ways your character might present with unstable angina. First, they might start having chest pain while walking or exerting themselves, but the pain will not go away when they stop to rest. Or second, they may start having chest pain without any exertion at all. While stable angina can be treated outpatient, unstable angina requires a trip to the hospital.

> The main difference between unstable angina and an MI is that an MI will have damaged heart tissue, evidenced by the presence of troponins in their blood.

A **myocardial infarction** (MI) occurs when a coronary vessel is suddenly blocked. The heart tissue isn't getting any blood flow, so it dies. Dead heart muscle spews out specific proteins (called *troponins*) into the blood. Doctors test for these proteins to see if your character has had any damage to their heart tissue.

Myocardial infarctions come in two flavors: STEMI (ST-Elevation MI) and NSTEMI (Non-ST-Elevation MI); doctors can tell the difference based on patterns seen on the EKG. STEMIs are generally considered more serious.

> While only 30% of MIs are fatal, complete blockages of the left anterior descending artery (**LAD**) are notorious for causing sudden death. Hence the artery's nickname: **The Widowmaker**.

<u>Symptoms</u>

- Chest pain, pressure, or squeezing
  - Can range from mild to severe
  - Chest pressure is more common than pain
  - Sometimes described as 'crushing' or 'an elephant sitting on my chest'
  - Pain may move down the arm (usually left) or shoulder, or up to the neck and jaw
- Mid-back, neck, left arm, or jaw pain with or without significant chest pain
- Trouble catching their breath (*dyspnea*)
- Profuse sweating (*diaphoresis*)
- Nausea and vomiting
- Fainting or lightheadedness

- Anxiety or a feeling of impending doom

- Weakness and fatigue

- Symptoms made worse with exertion

Diagnosis

The doctor looks at her EKG and smiles—it shows sinus tachycardia—a normal rhythm, just a little fast. This is encouraging, as a myocardial infarction would usually show changes on the EKG. He logs into the in-room computer and notes that her labs are back—her troponins were negative. Whatever is causing her chest pain, it is not a myocardial infarction.

Ischemic heart disease can't be diagnosed with a history and physical alone—the doctor needs tests and imaging to confirm not only the cardiac etiology but also what type of heart disease your character is experiencing. These include:

Electrocardiogram (EKG/ECG): Measures the electrical current of the heart. If heart tissue has died (myocardial infarction) or is not getting enough oxygen (angina), the EKG will change in predictable ways. An EKG has 10 sticky nodes placed in a specific pattern along the chest, arms, and legs. Doctors can use the EKG to determine which area of the heart is affected and therefore which artery is blocked.

Cardiac Enzymes: When the heart muscle dies, the cells release troponins. The presence of troponins in the blood indicates a myocardial infarction.

Risk Factors

Anyone can have ischemic heart disease; I have personally seen otherwise healthy 40-year-olds laid low by this condition. However, because ischemic heart disease is usually caused by clogged arteries, there are some frequently shared characteristics:

- Older men (>45) and post-menopausal women

- Family history of heart disease

Women tend to have less stereotypical presentations of MI. They may not have chest pain at all, and are more likely to experience anxiety, shortness of breath, sweating, or neck/arm pain than their male counterparts. Because of this, they are more often misdiagnosed.

EKG comes from the German "Elektrokardiogram." Technically, since we're speaking English, we should call it an ECG. But old habits die hard, and EKG is well established in popular culture.

Genetics is more important than lifestyle factors when it comes to cardiac disease. You can use this to subvert expectations in your writing; no one expects a 45-year-old ultramarathoner to die of a heart attack.

- People who are obese or sedentary

- Smokers

- Diabetics

- Cocaine use

Treatment

Myocardial infarctions and unstable angina are treated by opening the blocked artery as quickly as possible. Your character will be prescribed a host of medications that work together to increase blood flow to the heart. While medications might be enough to treat stable angina, unstable angina and myocardial infarctions almost always require that doctors go in and physically open up the coronary arteries. There are two ways to do this: percutaneous intervention or surgery.

> Med students remember the medications for MI and unstable angina using the mnemonic MONA BEACH: **M**orphine, **O**xygen, **N**itrates, **A**spirin, **B**eta-blockers, **E**noxaparin, **A**CE-inhibitors, **C**lopidogrel, **H**eparin.

Percutaneous intervention (PCI), also called cardiac catheterization, is a minimally invasive procedure. A cardiologist threads a wire from the groin up into the heart to manually unclog the artery. The whole procedure can take less than 30 minutes.[1] The goal is to perform catheterization within 90 minutes of arrival at the hospital.[2]

The second option is coronary artery bypass grafting (CABG), a surgical procedure that restores blood flow to dying heart tissue. It's the most common type of open-heart surgery. Your character will need a CABG if they have significant blockages in their biggest coronary arteries, or if multiple vessels are involved. It's a big, scary procedure, that takes 3-4 hours to complete. It is a gut-wrenching time for family, with lots of tension and story potential. However, recent studies have shown that people have lower mortality after CABG than after PCI.[3]

> The saying amongst cardiologists is "Time is Tissue." The faster the procedure is performed, the better the outcome.

AORTIC DISSECTION

The aorta is the giant, muscular blood vessel that carries blood out of the heart to the rest of the body. An aortic dissection occurs when there's a tear in the inner layer of the aorta, allowing blood to flow in between the layers of the aorta. It is a medical emergency; even with timely treatment and surgery, 20-30% of people with the condition will die.[4]

Symptoms

- Sudden, severe chest pain (tearing, ripping, stabbing)

- Sudden severe stomach pain

- Trouble breathing, shortness of breath, and/or dizziness

- Fainting

- Profuse Sweating

- Can cause stroke-like symptoms, such as weakness or paralysis in one half of the body, trouble talking, and vision changes

- Leg pain and difficulty walking

Signs are what your character feels.

Symptoms are what an observer would notice.

Stroke-like symptoms are due to a lack of blood flow to the brain and spinal cord.

Signs

When doctors evaluate your character for aortic dissection, they will look for an asymmetrical pulse and blood pressure, meaning that the pulse and blood pressure are stronger in certain limbs than in others. For example, if your character has strong pulses and high blood pressure in their arms, but low blood pressure in both legs, the aortic dissection is likely located in an area of the aorta called the *descending aorta*.

Risk Factors

- A long history of high blood pressure (*hypertension*)
  - o This is the most common cause

- Cocaine use
  - o Causes severe and abrupt high blood pressure

- Pregnancy
  - o Particularly in the third trimester

- Genetic conditions that affect connective tissue, such as Marfan Syndrome and Ehlers-Danlos syndrome

- Aortic aneurysm (a bulge in their aorta)

  - o Particularly if the aneurysm is large (>5cm)

- High cholesterol

- History of syphilis or other diseases that cause inflammation of the blood vessels

<u>Testing</u>

A chest X-ray is usually the first step. They might see a widening of the area containing the heart and aorta (called *widened mediastinum*), but it usually isn't enough to definitively diagnose aortic dissection. Instead, your character will be given a CT scan of their chest with IV contrast injected into their veins. This will allow the doctors to visualize the dissection directly.

<u>Treatment</u>

The first step is to control your character's heart rate and blood pressure using IV antihypertensive medications. Pain control is also an important aspect of treatment. Depending on where in the aorta the dissection is located, your character may be taken for emergency surgical repair.

OTHER CARDIOVASCULAR CAUSES OF CHEST PAIN

Pericarditis: Inflammation of the sac surrounding the heart (*pericardium*) causes chest pain that shoots to the back and shoulder. It is worse with breathing in (*inspiration*) and lying down, and improves with sitting up and leaning forward. Pericarditis can be caused by a variety of issues, from viral infections to lupus and cancer. The first step in treatment is to figure out the underlying cause and fix that. If a cause can't be found, pericarditis is treated with anti-inflammatory medications like ibuprofen or aspirin.

Pericardial effusion: Fluid or blood trapped in the space between the heart and the pericardium. If there is enough fluid that it is pressing down on the heart and restricting its motion, it is called *cardiac tamponade*. Symptoms of pericardial effusion differ depending on how quickly the fluid accumulated. Quick accumulation, usually due to blood, may cause cardiogenic shock, while slower accumulation leads to trouble breathing and heart failure. Your character may have chest pain, low blood pressure, and bulging neck veins. Treatment is to pull out the fluid using a big needle inserted through the chest wall and into the space between the pericardium and the heart.

LUNGS

The doctor asks if her pain has gotten any better, but Amna just shakes her head. If anything, it's gotten worse; every time she breathes in, it's like being stabbed in the shoulder. Even with the oxygen, she's still having trouble speaking in complete sentences, and she's developed a cough.

The lungs are a lot bigger than the heart and just as important—pumping blood is completely useless if that blood doesn't have oxygen in it—but writers seem to forget about them. That's not fair to anyone; the lungs are a fascinating organ and there are so many things that can go wrong with them! Since Chapter 2 is dedicated to diseases that can cause trouble breathing, I'll stick to lung issues that cause chest pain here.

PULMONARY EMBOLISM

If a character has sudden, severe chest pain, they could be experiencing a pulmonary embolism or PE. This is a common and life-threatening diagnosis. It is estimated that about 100,000 people in the US die of PE every year.[5]

A pulmonary embolism is a blood clot that lodges itself in the blood vessels of the lungs, blocking blood flow to that area of the lung. Even a small clot can wreak havoc on your character's lungs, decreasing their ability to get oxygen into their blood and backing up the blood flow. A big pulmonary embolism—one that blocks off a major pulmonary blood vessel—can cause sudden death.

But why would your character have a blood clot in the first place? Most of the time, the clot in the lungs is a dislodged piece of a larger clot hidden deep in the veins of the calf, called a *deep vein thrombosis*, or DVT. If your character has a DVT, they might have a red, swollen, or painful calf. Or, they might have no symptoms at all. Sometimes, the source clot is never found.

Low blood oxygen levels—called **hypoxemia**—are a sign of pulmonary embolism that doctors might find on exam.

<u>Symptoms</u>

The symptoms of a pulmonary embolism are very similar to those of ischemic heart disease: chest pain, trouble breathing, racing pulse, and lightheadedness or fainting. However, there are some differences that you can use to clue in your readers that this might not be a "heart attack" after all. These include:

- **Chest pain:** Pain that is worse with breathing in (*pleuritic chest pain)*, is a sign of inflammation of the lungs' lining. Note that pericarditis (inflammation of the heart's lining) has a similar effect.

- **Cough**: Though a cough is present in less than half of people with PE, it is a good way to signal that the problem is in the lungs, rather than the heart. Rarely, they may even cough up blood (called *hemoptysis*).

- **Swollen or painful calf**: A swollen or painful calf is a reliable sign that they have a DVT. While not everyone with PE will have a swollen or painful calf, its presence makes the diagnosis of PE much more likely.

- **Lightheadedness or fainting:** Usually seen with very large pulmonary embolisms.

Risk Factors

Pulmonary embolisms only occur if there is a clot somewhere in the body. For that reason, most PEs happen if your character has a condition that makes them susceptible to blood clots. These include:

- Pregnant women

- Women on birth control pills

- Someone who has been recently immobile (recently hospitalized, on bed rest, or even just off a long flight)

- Older age (over 60)

- Cancer

- Recently had extensive surgery (particularly orthopedic surgery), or major trauma

- History of clots or clotting diseases

- Injection drug user

> Cancer significantly increases the risk of blood clots. Unexplained blood clots and PE can be a unique and heartbreaking way for your character to find out they have cancer.

Most clots come from the legs. But in injection drug users, they can come from the arm instead.

Tests

The doctor tells Amna that, given her recent surgery, he's worried she might have a pulmonary embolism, so he wants an ultrasound of the veins in her calf to look for potential clots. He leaves, returning a few minutes later with a computer-like machine on wheels. He rubs the gel onto the probe, then runs it along her calf muscle. When he gets to her left leg, she's surprised to find that the mild pressure of the ultrasound probe is quite painful. Seconds later, he's found it—a small clot in the deep veins of her leg.

- **D-dimer:** This is a blood test that is used to rule out PE. If it's negative, your character doesn't have a PE. If it's positive, they need more tests.

- **Calf ultrasound:** Looks for a clot in the leg veins (DVT). Again, the presence or absence of a DVT isn't diagnostic; many people with PE have no discernable DVT. But if there is a clot, your character will be prescribed blood thinners (*anticoagulants*) either way.

  NATALIE DALE, MD

- **Chest CT (CT angiogram):** A special type of chest CT with IV contrast will allow doctors to visualize the pulmonary blood vessels and any clots wherein, making the definitive diagnosis.

Treatment

The doctor tells Amna that he's going to put her on a blood thinner called heparin to prevent the formation of more clots. And because she's still having so much trouble breathing, even with the oxygen mask, he's going to give her a clot-busting medication called tPA to hopefully break up the blood clot in her lungs. He's also going to get a special CT of her chest and visualize the clots within the pulmonary vasculature.

Treatment of pulmonary embolism includes giving oxygen through a face mask and starting your character on anticoagulation medications, such as heparin. These medications prevent the formation of another clot. If the clot is small and your character's vital signs are stable, they may be able to be treated at home. But if their blood oxygen is dropping precipitously, or they are having significant trouble breathing, they may need to be admitted to the hospital. In some instances, they'll be given clot-busting medications, called tPA.

If the clot in the lungs is particularly large, or if your character is very ill, they may even need to be put on a ventilator.

SPONTANEOUS PNEUMOTHORAX

A pneumothorax is a collapsed lung. In Chapter 14, we'll go into detail about traumatic pneumothorax, but there are also non-traumatic causes. Spontaneous pneumothorax occurs when the lung just collapses for no discernable reason. It primarily affects tall, thin young males (ages 10-30) with no other known lung conditions. However, smoking and exposure to environmental chemicals can increase your character's risk for pneumothorax.

Signs & Symptoms

If your character has a spontaneous pneumothorax, they'll have sudden and severe pain on one side of their chest *(ipsilateral chest pain),* possibly accompanied by trouble breathing. I say possibly because the people who get spontaneous pneumothorax are usually young and healthy, so they don't have as much trouble breathing as you might expect. In fact, they might only have some mild, persistent chest pain and a cough. When the doctor examines your character, they'll immediately notice that they can't hear "breath sounds"—the sound of air whooshing in and out of the lungs—on the affected side.

Diagnosis & Treatment

Spontaneous pneumothorax is diagnosed with a chest x-ray; it'll be patently clear that part of the lung has collapsed. Not all spontaneous pneumothoraxes need treatment—some will resolve on their own. But if your character is in significant pain or is having trouble breathing, the pneumothorax will be treated with the placement of a chest tube—a small tube inserted into the chest space to remove excess air and re-expand the lung. A second chest X-ray, taken a few days later, can confirm that the lung has successfully re-expanded.

OTHER PULMONARY CAUSES OF CHEST PAIN

Pleuritis is inflammation of the fibrous lining of the lungs. It causes pleuritic chest pain that can be severe enough that your character will try to only breathe very shallowly. It is often caused by infections (particularly viral) and autoimmune diseases (such as lupus), though there are many possible causes, including tuberculosis and cancer. Treatment focuses on the underlying cause, along with anti-inflammatory drugs such as ibuprofen.

Pneumonia can sometimes cause chest pain. However, we'll cover pneumonia in-depth in Chapter 2.

GASTROINTESTINAL

The gastrointestinal (GI) system runs from the mouth to the anus and is primarily involved in the breakdown, digestion, and absorption of nutrients. Organs of the GI system include the mouth, esophagus, stomach, small intestine, large intestine, rectum, anus, pancreas, liver, and gallbladder.

GASTROESOPHAGEAL REFLUX DISEASE (GERD)

I can guess what you're thinking. What is acid reflux doing on here? No one in their right mind would confuse a little heartburn with a heart attack. Right? Wrong!

Unfortunately (or perhaps, fortunately), mistaking GERD for a heart attack is much more common than you think. Over half of people admitted to EDs for chest pain are eventually found to have a non-cardiac cause; of those, nearly 60% are ultimately diagnosed with GERD instead of a heart attack.[6] That means 30% of people presenting to the ED with chest pain have—you guessed it—heartburn.

Imagine how mortified your character would feel when she finds out she went to the ED for something as silly as heartburn. Will she blame whoever made her go to the hospital? Will she refuse to go to the ED the next time she feels chest pain?

GERD may seem like a boring let-down of a diagnosis, but there's a lot of story potential there.

Symptoms

GERD can feel almost exactly like cardiac pain: chest tightness, pressure, even nausea, and vomiting. But there are a few clinical pearls you can use to give your reader hints that this "heart attack" may not be what it seems.

- Can sometimes feel like a burning behind the chest—hence the name, "heartburn"

- Pain worse after meals or laying down (remember, angina feels better at rest!)

- May be triggered by certain foods (tomatoes, coffee, citrus)

- May be accompanied by regurgitation or salivation

- Cough (usually after eating)

- Sore throat

- Hoarse voice

GERD is not the only food-related cause of chest pain. **Holiday Heart Syndrome** (also known as alcohol-induced atrial arrhythmias) is an irregular heartbeat caused by heavy drinking, most often seen around the holidays.

Risk Factors

- Overweight

- Someone who drinks a lot of coffee, alcohol, or orange juice

- Though anyone can have GERD (even small children), it tends to get worse with age

Tests

Endoscopy—a procedure where the doctor places a scope down the patient's throat to look at the esophagus and stomach—is considered diagnostic but is usually not necessary. Most doctors diagnose GERD with a good history and physical. The key is the physical exam: a character with GERD will feel pain when the doctor presses on the middle of their stomach, right beneath the sternum.

Treatment

Treatment for GERD is pretty simple: lifestyle changes and medication to decrease the stomach's acid production. Lifestyle changes include cutting down on alcohol and coffee, eating smaller meals, and sleeping with the head propped up. Nothing is hurt but your character's pride.

DIFFUSE ESOPHAGEAL SPASM

An esophageal spasm occurs when the muscles surrounding the esophagus contract painfully. Since the majority of the esophagus is in the chest, the symptoms of esophageal spasm can mimic that of ischemic heart disease.

Symptoms

The primary symptom of esophageal spasms is sudden, severe chest pain that can almost perfectly mimic pain caused by the heart. The pain is described as a squeezing feeling or pressure on the chest that may move to the jaw, back, and arms. Sound familiar?

There is, however, one symptom that you can use to clue in your readers that this isn't a heart attack: trouble swallowing. If your character has difficulty swallowing or feels like there's something stuck in their throat while they're having chest pain, there's a good chance that they're experiencing an esophageal spasm and not a heart attack.

> The medical term for trouble swallowing is **dysphagia**.

Diagnosis & Treatment

Esophageal spasm is diagnosed with a special test called *esophageal manometry* that measures the contraction strength of the muscles around the esophagus. Your character might also need a barium swallow—a procedure in which they swallow a drink of thick, chalky fluid (barium)—before getting an X-ray of their neck and chest. This allows doctors to see the shape of the esophagus.

Unfortunately, there isn't a whole lot that can be done to treat esophageal spasms. There are a few medications that can help with the symptoms, but there is no real cure.

ESOPHAGEAL TEAR

If the esophagus is torn, your character will not only feel pain from the tear itself, but also from the contents of the esophagus spilling out into the chest cavity. While there are a lot of things that can cause a torn esophagus—blunt trauma, medical procedures, etc.—forceful vomiting is the most typical cause. For this reason, if your character has bulimia or struggles with binge drinking and/or alcoholism, an esophageal tear is a very realistic cause of their chest pain.

Symptoms

- Sudden, severe chest pain, usually during vomiting
- Racing heart, trouble breathing, and dizziness
- Fever and chills
- Trouble swallowing

<u>**Diagnosis & Treatment**</u>

The first imaging test for chest pain—a chest x-ray—will show free air in the chest, a bad sign that something has been perforated. However, for a definitive diagnosis, your character might have to swallow a different solution (called *gastrografin*) and get another x-ray to prove the esophagus has been punctured.

If your character's symptoms are mild, they'll be admitted to the hospital and put on IV fluids, antibiotics, and acid blockers. They also won't be allowed to eat or drink anything. If they are very ill, they'll need urgent surgery to repair the damage.

> Gastrografin is used when esophageal tear is suspected, because it won't irritate the chest cavity should there be a leak.

OTHER GI CAUSES OF CHEST PAIN

- **Pancreatitis:** Inflammation of the pancreas usually causes abdominal pain (see *Ch. 2: Trouble Breathing*), but the pain can sometimes mimic the chest/back pain of ischemic heart disease.

- **Esophageal hematoma**: A collection of blood within the walls of the esophagus. Symptoms include chest pain, trouble swallowing, and vomiting blood.

MUSCULOSKELETAL & NERVE

You would think that people would be able to tell the difference between a bone or muscle pain and a heart attack, but you would be mistaken. One small study found that 30% of the patients who came to the ED for chest pain had **costochondritis**.[7]

COSTOCHONDRITIS

Costochondritis is the inflammation of the cartilage connecting the ribs to the sternum. Generally described as aching or pressure, the pain is usually worse with deep breathing, arm movement, and exertion. Often, it is associated with a recent viral illness or strenuous upper body exercise.

If someone presses on your character's chest wall at the spot where the ribs meet the breastbone, they'll feel the pain. Most of the time, that's enough to diagnose costochondritis, though the doctor may get an EKG just to be safe. There isn't much to do in the way of treatment, other than pain relief with ibuprofen or Tylenol, minimizing activity, and heating pads.

SHINGLES (HERPES ZOSTER)

Also known as shingles, herpes zoster causes severe pain and rash in a line along the left or right half of your character's body. Caused by the reactivation of the chickenpox virus, Shingles can cause severe chest pain. But, given the presence of the bright red rash, it's unlikely to be confused for cardiac pain.

PSYCHIATRIC

ANXIETY

Anxiety and panic attacks can mimic angina or even myocardial infarction. Chest pain, nausea, sweating, trouble breathing, anxiety, feelings of impending doom—it's all there. However, there are some clues that might point to a panic attack over an ACS event. These include:

- Feeling a loss of control, or as if they are going crazy

- Feeling detached from their body, an experience called depersonalization

If you give your character these symptoms, you are signaling that they are likely to be having a panic attack, rather than an acute coronary event. However, it's just a signal. That's because it simply isn't possible to differentiate a panic attack from an acute coronary event just by talking to the patient. They need labs and imaging to make sure that it isn't one of the potentially lethal causes of chest pain that we already talked about. At the very least, your character should get an ECG, chest x-ray, and cardiac laboratory studies.

Immediate treatment of anxiety and panic attacks may include medications to help the patient calm down, called benzodiazepines, like Xanax or Valium. The long-term treatment, however, includes psychotherapy and long-term anti-anxiety medications.

REAL TALK: THE "ANXIOUS FEMALE"

Doctors (like nurses and lawyers and carpenters) aren't perfect. They have their own personal biases, as well as biases cultivated by the culture of medicine. One of those biases is the "anxious female." Women, in general, are less likely to be taken seriously and more likely to experience delays in diagnosis and treatment.[8] The phrase "it's all in your head," is one most women have heard uttered by a healthcare provider at some point in their life. Once you add a diagnosis of anxiety into the mix, it can be very difficult for a female patient to be taken seriously. Anxiety can be a catch-all diagnosis for everything from headaches to abdominal pain to—you guessed it—chest pain.

 NATALIE DALE, MD

An old man is going about his business when he suddenly clutches his chest and gasps in pain. Then he staggers around a bit until he finally falls to the floor, dead.

A myocardial infarction—the medical term for what most people consider a "heart attack"—is a specific condition diagnosed by a combination of imaging and bloodwork, along with the history and physical. Caused by blockages in the coronary arteries, a myocardial infarction causes chest pain, trouble breathing, and dizziness or lightheadedness.

But myocardial infarctions don't usually cause the heart to stop beating immediately. Instead, the damaged heart muscle causes electrical problems (*arrhythmias*) that are potentially fatal.

One such problem is called ventricular fibrillation. Without the appropriate electrical signals, the heart can't coordinate its beats, leading to a fast rhythm that can't pump blood effectively. This type of arrhythmia can potentially lead to death. The treatment for ventricular fibrillation is a medical-grade electrical shock, called *defibrillation.*

However, the heart *can* suddenly stop beating, a phenomenon called **sudden cardiac arrest** or SCA. Like ventricular fibrillation, SCAs are often due to a problem with the heart's electrical system that causes the heart to stop beating. Myocardial infarctions, particularly those caused by multiple blockages or a complete blockage of the left anterior descending artery (LAD), are one potential cause of sudden cardiac arrests. But SCA has lots of different causes—extra electrical pathways, *arrhythmias*, structural changes to the heart, low levels of potassium or magnesium in the blood, even blood loss, and lack of oxygen.

If your character has a sudden cardiac arrest, they need CPR and a defibrillator immediately (see <u>Volume 1: Setting & Character</u>, *Ch. 15: CPR*).

2. TROUBLE BREATHING

TROUBLE BREATHING COMES IN MANY forms. *Dyspnea*, also called shortness of breath (SOB), is usually described as an inability to catch one's breath, though it can also be described as a feeling of choking, asphyxiation, or hunger for air. Trouble breathing can also mean your character is breathing too fast, too slow, or that something is blocking their airway. It can present acutely—meaning it comes on suddenly—or the feeling can be chronic Often, dyspnea is associated with chest pain, but since the previous chapter covered chest pain in detail, this chapter will focus on causes of dyspnea that do not generally cause severe chest pain.

BACKGROUND

Brayden's lungs have never been strong—he was born prematurely and spent the first few weeks of his life in the neonatal ICU (NICU)—but he hasn't let that prevent him from reaching his goals. Now, he is on the varsity baseball team, preparing to pitch for a game watched by no less than six college scouts.

If your character is having trouble breathing, it means they aren't getting oxygen to the tissues that need it. And while the lungs may seem the obvious culprit, many organ systems contribute to the oxygenation of blood and tissues.

The **trachea** conducts air from the mouth down the neck and through the **larynx**, or voice box, and into the lungs. This airflow occurs because of a large muscle called the **diaphragm**, which contracts and pulls air down into the lungs. For the diaphragm to do its job, it needs input from the brain telling it to contract; a signal is sent down the spinal cord and out to the diaphragm in a bundle of motor neurons called the **phrenic nerve.**

> **Motor neurons** are cells that conduct signals from the brain through the spinal cord out to the muscles.

Once the air reaches the **lungs**, it's pulled into tiny air sacs called *alveoli*, wherein carbon dioxide (CO_2)—the primary waste product of cellular processes—is removed from the blood and replaced with oxygen in a process called *gas exchange*. The **heart** pumps this newly oxygenated blood out through the **arteries** and into

NATALIE DALE, MD

the tiny **capillaries**, where the body's cells exchange waste products in return for oxygen. Then, the blood (laden with carbon dioxide and other waste products) returns to the heart via the veins, where it is pumped back into the lungs, and the process begins all over again. A problem with any of these organs—the trachea, the diaphragm, the brain, the nerves, the lungs, the heart—can cause trouble breathing.

RESPIRATORY FAILURE

Brayden was born very early—at only 28 weeks. His dad loves telling the story of how Brayden had been doing well, then took a turn for the worse a few days after he was born. His expression darkens as he describes how scary it was, to watch his newborn son's nostrils flare, listening to him grunt with each breath as his skin turned a grayish blue. He always says that when Brendan was diagnosed with respiratory failure and put on the ventilator, it was the worst day of his life. But then he smiles and tells Brayden that he was a fighter, even then. So many things went wrong he fought, and he overcame. Brayden loves this story, because it reminds him that he came into this world fighting—and winning.

Respiratory failure means that your character either has too little oxygen or too much carbon dioxide in their blood—often both. Lots of conditions can cause respiratory failure, from smoke inhalation to pneumonia. It's a medical emergency that can be fatal if not treated promptly. If your character is having trouble speaking in complete sentences, they are on the verge of respiratory failure.

Symptoms of respiratory failure include trouble breathing, fast heart rate and breathing rate, fatigue, blue-tinged lips, and fingers (called cyanosis), and trouble speaking in complete sentences.

Treatment is to give oxygen and provide breathing support. If your character is conscious, that could mean a breathing device such as BiPAP or CPAP, but if they are really struggling, they may need to be intubated and put on a ventilator. However, the most important step in treatment is to figure out why your character has developed respiratory failure in the first place and treat the underlying cause.

CPAP (Continuous Positive Airway Pressure) and **BiPAP** (Bilevel Positive Airway Pressure) machines use pressure gradients to force air into the lungs. They do not require intubation.

VENTILATORS

Volume 1 devoted an entire chapter to ventilators (see <u>Volume 1: Setting &</u>

<u>Character</u>, *Ch. 20: Ventilators*), so I'm not going to go into too much detail here. However, it's an important enough topic that we'll touch briefly on it.

Ventilators are machines that breathe for your character. They deliver "breaths" of air directly into your character's lungs. In order to be on a ventilator, your character needs to be intubated, meaning a tube (called an *endotracheal,* or *ET tube*) is threaded from their mouth or nose down their trachea and into the lungs. The ET tube is connected to the ventilator that gives breaths at a specific volume, rate, and level of humidity and oxygen. Being intubated is extremely uncomfortable—your character won't be able to eat, drink, or talk while on the vent—so they'll probably be lightly sedated. They'll probably sleep most of the time, though they may be awake enough to write notes and communicate non-verbally. Being on a ventilator absolutely does not mean your character is in a coma (though if your character is in a coma, they might be on a ventilator).

If you're thinking of having a character sneak in and kill the victim by unplugging the ventilator, think again. Ventilators are loud, with tons of different alarms. If your character were to unplug the machine or disconnect any of the tubing, the machine will alarm loudly and abrasively, alerting the entire ICU of what is going on. To avoid triggering the alarms, your character would have to understand how to work the ventilator machine to turn off the breaths.

> Most modern ventilators have a battery backup system, so unplugging it won't stop the alarms.

RESPIRATORY EMERGENCIES

Sudden difficulty breathing comes in many forms. Your character may be breathing too fast, too slow, or feel like they are having trouble catching their breath. While there are many different reasons your character might be having trouble breathing, acute onset breathing troubles are almost always a medical emergency.

ALLERGIC REACTION (ANAPHYLAXIS)

Anaphylaxis is a severe allergic reaction characterized by a rash and swelling of the airways. Without treatment, it can be fatal. For more on anaphylaxis, see *Ch. 4: Allergy & Anaphylaxis.*

ACUTE RESPIRATORY DISTRESS SYNDROME (ARDS)

If you're looking to suddenly kill off a character that is already in the hospital, ARDS might fit the bill. It occurs when fluid fills the tiny air sacs in the lungs, preventing the exchange of gases. The primary symptom of ARDS is severe shortness of breath, often accompanied by fast and labored breathing, low blood pressure, and extreme fatigue. Your character will look sick—really sick—and will be having so much

 NATALIE DALE, MD

trouble breathing they won't be able to speak more than a word or two at a time if they can speak at all.

Though anyone in the hospital can get ARDS, you can put your character at increased risk by giving them specific underlying diseases. These include:

- Burns

- COVID-19

- Infection that has reached the bloodstream (*sepsis*)

- Pneumonia

- Recent major trauma, particularly head and chest injuries

- Recently had a major blood transfusion

Sepsis is a potentially life-threatening condition caused by bacteria that have entered the bloodstream. Symptoms include fever, fast breathing rate, fast heat rate, and increased white blood cell count.

ARDS is often fatal and your character's chances of dying from it increase if they're older or severely ill.

Treatment of ARDS requires close management of IV fluids, prevention of blood clots and infection, and supplemental oxygen. If your character has ARDS, they may need to be put on a ventilator.

ASTHMA ATTACK

Brayden was diagnosed with asthma when he was in kindergarten. He always had a cough during the dry Wisconsin winters, and he seemed to get colds more often than his friends. But one day, while he and his best friend were "jousting" with icicles they'd found broken off from the school's roof, his chest started feeling tight and filled with air, like he could breathe in, but couldn't breathe out. By the time he got to the nurse's office, his breath sounded like a high-pitched wheeze. The nurse called an ambulance, and Brayden was whisked away. After that, he had to take daily inhalers, as well as carry a "rescue inhaler" with him at all times. At first, the other kids made fun of his inhaler, but they stopped laughing once they realized he could still kick their butts at every sport in recess.

An asthma attack can be life-threatening. Asthma is an intermittent disease that causes inflammation of the airways, resulting in coughing, wheezing, chest tightness, and shortness of breath. It is usually—though not always—provoked by certain triggers, ranging from exercise or
viral infections to environmental triggers like pet dander or pollens. These

symptoms are usually within 30 minutes of exposure. Asthma exacerbations can range from mild to life-threatening.

Symptoms: Wheezing (most common), cough, and chest tightness.

Signs: Audible wheezing, visibly struggling for breath

Treatment: Rescue inhaler (Albuterol) + Inhaled steroids

- If the asthma attack is severe enough that they need to be admitted to the hospital, they'll also be put on oxygen, given IV steroids, and given albuterol via a nebulizer (a device that aerosolizes liquid medications so the meds can be breathed in through a face mask) rather than an inhaler. If things get really bad, they'll be started on IV magnesium.

- If your character goes into respiratory failure, they will need to be intubated and put on a ventilator that will breathe for them.

CHOKING (AIRWAY OBSTRUCTION)

For his first date, Brayden took his crush, Bella to a drive-in movie. They were laughing and throwing peanuts at the image in the car window when Bella stopped laughing. Her mouth opened and closed, but no sound came out. Brayden kept asking what was wrong, but she just kept staring forward and touching her throat. Finally, Brayden realized what was going on, and he raced to the other side of the car and pulled her out. Wrapping his hands around her stomach, he thrust his fist into her stomach and up, over, and over, until Bella began to cough, then spit out a peanut. They've been inseparable ever since.

Choking occurs when food or small object get caught in the airway, preventing the flow of air. Obstruction can be complete, or incomplete. Signs of partial airway obstruction include difficulty speaking, noisy breathing, choking or squeaking sounds, cough, or a suddenly hoarse voice. If your character is visibly fighting to breathe but not making any sounds, they probably have complete airway obstruction. Other signs of complete obstruction include *cyanosis* (turning blue around the lips and fingernail beds), uncontrolled drooling, and a lack of chest movement. Your character may even lose consciousness.

Treatment is to clear the airway. Current Red Cross recommendations are to use the "five and five" approach (five back blows followed by five abdominal thrusts, also known as the Heimlich Maneuver) though other organizations recommend jumping straight to abdominal thrusts.[1] Either way, the goal is to remove the blockage.

If the victim is unconscious, your character should lay them on their back with their jaw thrust forward. If there is something visibly blocking the airway, they should pull it out—ideally with a tool like tweezers, if they don't want to risk getting their fingers chomped off.

If your character is the one choking, they can perform the Heimlich on themselves! Have them make a fist, then settle it in the space between the belly button and the bottom of the ribs. Then grab the fist with the other hand and force it in and up. If that doesn't work, they can position the fist and then fall onto a hard surface at an angle, forcing the fist in and up.[2]

If your character is performing the Heimlich—on themselves or others—they should continue doing abdominal thrusts until the foreign body is removed or until they lose consciousness. While your character is performing the Heimlich, someone else should call 911.

Once the victim is unconscious, the next step in treatment depends on your character. If they're just a layperson, the next step is to start CPR. But if your character has some medical knowledge, and the right equipment, they can do more. Intubation (threading a tube down the airway and providing breaths through a bag-valve-mask (BVM) or ventilator) is the ideal next step if your character is choking and unconscious. However, if intubation fails, or your character doesn't have the proper equipment, they might still be able to save a life using a procedure called a *cricothyroidotomy*.

In a cricothyroidotomy, a knife or needle is inserted between the thin cartilage rings of the trachea. This allows your character to bypass the above blockage and deliver air straight into the lungs. TV shows love this procedure, but in reality, it is rarely performed outside the controlled setting of the operating room (OR). However, it is a very exciting procedure, so I don't blame you for wanting to use it. To perform a cricothyroidotomy your character should:

- Stabilize the trachea with the non-dominant hand

- Identify the "Adam's apple"—the cartilage that protects the trachea

- Make a small incision just below, but above the second, smaller bump (*cricotracheal cartilage*)

- Ignore the blood—and there will be a lot of blood—use fingers to find the soft membrane (*cricothyroid membrane*) between the two cartilage rings

- Cut through the membrane

- Insert a tube through the membrane and into the windpipe. An endotracheal tube is best, but you can let your character get creative. Anything hollow and rigid—a straw or plastic tubing—will work.

- Give breaths. Ideally using a bag valve mask (BVM); this can also be accomplished by manually blowing into the tube.

- Then get the character to the ED, fast! This is absolutely not a stable situation.

CHEST INJURIES

Trauma to the chest can make it hard for your character to breathe. Broken ribs can make it difficult to breathe deeply—or they can puncture a lung, causing bruising, bleeding, or even a collapsed lung. Chapter 14 focuses on chest trauma in more detail.

COLLAPSED LUNG (PNEUMOTHORAX)

Pneumothorax occurs when there's air in the space between the lung tissue and the lung lining (*pleura*), causing the lung tissue to collapse. Symptoms include sudden and severe one-sided chest pain, trouble breathing, and cough (See Ch: 1: Chest Pain).

DRUGS & TOXINS

Certain drugs—illicit or prescribed—and toxins can cause acute changes in your character's breathing.

Aspirin overdose causes rapid, shallow breathing. It is treated with decontamination, such as activated charcoal to soak up any remaining toxin, along with IV fluids, electrolytes, and glucose. If the poisoning is severe, your character may require hemodialysis—a procedure that uses a machine to filter blood—to correct pH and electrolyte imbalances.

Botulinum toxin is a neurotoxin used in Botox treatments. It can also be found in raw honey, dirty wounds, and improperly canned foods. Young children (< 2 years) are more likely to get botulism from raw honey, while adults are more likely to be exposed via improperly canned foods. It shuts down the motor neurons' ability to communicate with the muscles by disturbing the exchange of chemicals at the *neuromuscular junction*. This disturbance causes full-body paralysis—including the diaphragm. Since the diaphragm can't contract, your character can't initiate breathing and will suffocate without immediate treatment. Treatment is supportive; keep your character alive using intubation/ventilation until the antidote can be administered.

Aerosolized botulinum toxin is considered a potential weapon of bioterrorism.

Carbon monoxide is a naturally occurring gas that binds tightly to your character's red blood cells, displacing the oxygen that their body's cells need to survive. Carbon monoxide is a product of incomplete combustion reactions, so it can be found anywhere gas is being burned. Common sources of carbon monoxide include boilers, water heaters, gas fires, and central heating systems. Historically, gas appliances (such as Sylvia Plath's oven) were also a source. Running a car in a garage to cause carbon monoxide poisoning is another historical way of using CO to commit suicide. However, with the widespread use of catalytic converters, this method has become much more difficult. Open fires—such as house fires or indoor fireplaces without a flue)—are also a good way to get carbon monoxide poisoning (See *Ch. 17: Burns* for more on CO poisoning after a house fire).

> Carbon monoxide is of particular concern when your character is sleeping or inebriated, or if they recently survived a fire.

Your character won't have any trouble breathing—they'll still be able to breathe in and out—but their red blood cells won't be able to carry oxygen to their brain. They'll start breathing faster and faster, feeling dizzy, weak, and confused, until they finally pass out. Carbon monoxide poisoning is treated by breathing pure oxygen. If your character is very sick, they may need to be placed in a pressure chamber with oxygen, called *hyperbaric oxygen therapy*.

Curare is a neurotoxin that, like Botox, disrupts the neuromuscular junction. It prevents the nerve from communicating with the diaphragm and causes acute respiratory failure. *Neostigmine* and *Physostigmine* are antidotes for curare poisoning.

Opioids, like heroin and codeine, can cause your character's breathing to slow. An overdose could cause them to stop breathing entirely. *Naloxone* is a medication that reverses the effects and can save your character's life. Volume 1 covers opioid use and overdose in much greater detail (see <u>Volume 1: Setting & Character</u>, *Ch. 17: Drugs & Addiction*).

Organophosphates are toxins found in certain insecticides, herbicides, and nerve gases. They cause respiratory failure, along with other symptoms like muscle weakness and twitching, convulsions, runny nose and eyes, excess salivation, headache,

> Sarin gas is a famous organophosphate.

nausea/vomiting and diarrhea, blurry vision, confusion, and constricted pupils. Organophosphate poisoning is treated by removing all potential sources of contamination and giving IV medications to reverse the effects. Your character may need to be put on a ventilator.

HEART FAILURE (ACUTE DECOMPENSATED CONGESTIVE HEART FAILURE)

Heart failure occurs when the heart is unable to pump blood adequately to supply to the body (See *Ch. 20: Chronic Breathlessness*). Usually, heart failure is a chronic disease; as the heart slowly fails to keep up, the body has time to use other mechanisms to compensate. But sometimes, something happens that causes the heart to fail quickly. When that happens, the body suddenly isn't getting the blood it needs, and things go downhill rapidly. Blood backs up into the lungs, causing them to fill with fluid (*pulmonary edema*) and give your character a cough and trouble breathing. Low blood flow to the brain may cause confusion and poor memory. As the fluid continues to back up, your character will develop swelling in their feet and ankles.

If your character comes to be the ED, they'll be given a chest x-ray plus EKG and bloodwork. But the important diagnostic test is an echocardiogram (a detailed ultrasound of the heart) that provides more detail about the type of heart failure and how the heart is performing.

Acute decompensated heart failure is treated with admission to the hospital, along with oxygen and breathing assistance—ranging from face masks to intubation and mechanical ventilation. They'll also be given medications to decrease the fluid in their lungs (called *diuretics*) and, if they're very sick, may need medications to help the heart to beat more strongly (called *inotropic agents)*.

INHALATION INJURIES

We'll talk more about inhalation injuries in *Ch. 17: Burns*. If your character has been exposed to smoke, extreme heat, or other inhaled irritants it can cause the airway to swell up and make breathing difficult.

NEUROMUSCULAR DISEASE

Diseases that affect the nerves' ability to communicate with muscles can cause trouble breathing; if the nerves can't tell the diaphragm to contract, your character can't breathe in no matter how hard they try. There are several nerve and muscle diseases that can cause acute diaphragmatic paralysis. They include:

Guillain-Barré syndrome (GBS) is a rare autoimmune disease in which the immune system attacks your character's nerves, resulting in muscle weakness and paralysis. Usually, the symptoms start in the hands and feet, moving upwards over the course of a few weeks, until your character is completely paralyzed—including the diaphragm. If this happens, your character will need to be on a ventilator until they recover the use of their diaphragm. Full

Though GBS usually occurs after a bacterial infection causing diarrhea, it can also be caused by viral infections. Rarely, GBS is a side effect of certain vaccines.

NATALIE DALE, MD

recovery usually takes around 6-12 months, though your character shouldn't need to be on a ventilator that whole time. If you're looking for a reason to put your young, otherwise healthy character on a ventilator, Guillain-Barré is a great option.

If it wasn't for baseball, Brayden wouldn't have noticed the weakness right away. But his hand couldn't hold the ball quite right. At first, he thought it was nothing—just nerves. There were so many scouts in the bleachers watching him intently. But at practice the next day, his grip is weaker, and his hand feels numb—he can barely toss the ball, never mind pitch. The next morning, his legs give out beneath him when he tries to get out of bed. His dad drives him to the ED, where doctors measure the electrical output of his nerves and diagnose him with Guillain-Barré Syndrome. Twenty-four hours later, Brayden is paralyzed from the neck down and can't breathe on his own. To his parent's horror, he's placed on a ventilator and the doctors can't say for sure if he'll ever be able to breathe on his own, never mind walk again.

Myasthenia gravis (See *Ch. 21: Autoimmune Diseases*) is an autoimmune disease that causes your character's muscles to get progressively weaker with repeated use. This weakness usually affects voluntary muscles—the muscles your character uses to control their eyes, face, throat, and limbs—and improves with rest. However, in a *myasthenic crisis*, the diaphragm itself becomes weak, making it difficult to breathe. Since your character can't rest their diaphragm without suffocating, the only treatment is to intubate them and put them on a ventilator, allowing the diaphragm to rest and regain its strength. Like many autoimmune diseases, myasthenia gravis predominantly affects young women (ages 20-40), so it's a good option for causing a breathing crisis if your character falls into this demographic.

Polio is another rare disease that can cause ascending paralysis severe enough to cause trouble breathing. Children under 5 years old are particularly susceptible. However, since polio has an effective vaccine and has been eradicated in the US since 1979, it isn't a great option unless you're writing historical fiction, or your character is unvaccinated and living in one of the few countries where polio is still an endemic.[3]

PNEUMONIA

After a month on the ventilator, Brayden develops a severe cough and a fever. He's diagnosed with pneumonia and put on special antibiotics. Brayden's dad freaks out—first the Guillain-Barré, now pneumonia?—but the doctors comfort him by telling him that Brayden is young and otherwise healthy. They caught the pneumonia early, so they expect him to fully recover.

Pneumonia is an infection of the lungs that causes inflammation in the tiny alveoli responsible for gas exchange in the lungs. Pneumonia is usually caused by bacteria, but it can also be caused by viruses and even fungi. COVID-19 causes a type of viral pneumonia. Symptoms of pneumonia include fever and chills, cough, trouble breathing, fatigue, and chest pain when coughing. Nausea, vomiting, and diarrhea can also be seen with certain types of pneumonia.

Pneumonia is diagnosed with a chest x-ray that shows fluffy white spots on one or both lungs, called "infiltrates." A sputum test uses the gunk your character is coughing up to look for bacteria and determine which antibiotic to give. They'll also be given blood tests to check the levels of white blood cells.

While anyone can get pneumonia, if your character is elderly, has a pre-existing lung disease, or has a weakened immune system, they'll be at a higher risk. Additionally, if your character has been on a ventilator, they are at risk of ventilator-associated pneumonia (VAP), a particularly nasty variant that requires slightly different antibiotics. Finally, if your character is immunosuppressed—particularly if they have HIV/AIDS or if they're undergoing chemotherapy for cancer—they are at higher risk of fungal pneumonia.

Human immunodeficiency virus (HIV): A viral infection that attacks white blood cells and causes a compromised immune system.

Autoimmune deficiency syndrome (AIDS): Condition caused by severe HIV infection.

Treatment for bacterial pneumonia is with antibiotics. Fungal pneumonias are treated with antifungals, while viral pneumonias usually only need supportive treatment—rest, fluids, anti-fever drugs (antipyretics), and cough suppressants—though severe cases are sometimes given antivirals. If your character is sick enough to need admission to the hospital, they may also be given oxygen, IV fluids, and inhaled medications, like steroids and/or albuterol, to decrease inflammation and open up the airways.

Though pulmonary embolisms often cause pleuritic chest pain, sudden shortness of breath is the most common symptom.

PULMONARY EMBOLISM (PE)

As discussed in *Ch. 1: Chest Pain,* a pulmonary embolism occurs when a clot breaks off from somewhere in the body (usually a deep vein in the calf, called a *deep venous thrombosis* or *DVT*) and lodges itself in the blood vessels of the lungs. Symptoms include sudden shortness of breath, chest pain while breathing in (*pleuritic chest pain*), dizziness or lightheadedness, and an irregular or racing heartbeat (*palpitations*). Your character may start to sweat and cough—sometimes even coughing up blood. Their blood pressure will drop, as will the oxygen levels in their blood. They may also notice swelling and redness in their calf—a sign that they have a DVT.

See *Ch. 1: Chest Pain,* for more on the diagnosis and treatment of PE.

BREAKING DOWN THE CLICHÉ: THE HELPFUL HEIMLICH

"She's choking!"

Grabs victim and begins abdominal thrusts

Peanut flies from the victim's mouth and hits a bystander on the head

Every time I've seen abdominal thrusts (the "Heimlich maneuver") performed on tv; the victim's airway is always cleared. Usually, with just a few thrusts. But the crazy thing is that's not unrealistic. Abdominal thrusts, when done properly, are extremely effective at clearing the airway. In fact, one study found that abdominal thrusts alone had over a 70% success rate.[3] Compare that to CPR, which has a success rate of closer to 3%.[4]

Of course, there are devices and techniques that can increase the chances of a choking victim's survival even more. Lifevac and Dechoker are kits that use suction to remove foreign objects from an airway; the success rates with these devices range from 75-99%.[5] However, your character would need to carry these devices with her, making them a less realistic option.

If you have a character that is choking, it is totally reasonable for your main character (or another character) to save their life with abdominal thrusts alone.

3. ABDOMINAL PAIN

After her divorce, Celine moves back to her hometown to take over her aging Aunt Charlotte's horse farm, dragging her two teenage children along with her. They aren't happy about the prospect of living in a town so small it doesn't even have a proper traffic light but having all of the horses around almost makes up for it. One day, while brushing down the horses after a long ride, Celine feels a cramping pain in her belly, strong enough to double her over. It lasts for a few minutes, then disappears as quickly as it came.

ABDOMINAL PAIN IS A COMMON medical complaint, making up 5–10% of all Emergency Department visits.[1] Severity ranges from mild to life-threatening. In this section, I'll focus on medical emergencies that present with abdominal pain.

BACKGROUND

The abdomen is a soft body cavity beneath the chest cavity, or thorax, and above the pelvis. It holds a wealth of internal organs, ranging from the small intestines and colon to the liver, spleen, the tail of the pancreas, appendix, and gallbladder. It is also home to several large blood vessels, including the abdominal aorta and renal arteries. The abdominal cavity is lined by a sack called the peritoneum.

> What about the kidneys? The kidneys—along with the aorta, the inferior vena cava, and most of the pancreas—are located behind the peritoneal lining, and thus are considered 'retroperitoneal' organs, rather than abdominal ones.

The gastrointestinal tract (GI tract) runs all the way from the mouth to the anus. Involved organs are—in order—the mouth, esophagus, stomach, small intestine, colon, rectum, and anus. Organs like the pancreas and the gallbladder contribute to the functioning of the GI tract but are not considered part of it. The appendix is a tiny, non-functioning organ that dangles off the ascending colon, an evolutionary hold-over whose main purpose now is to get clogged and infected, causing appendicitis.

Anatomically, the abdomen is split up into four quadrants: left upper quadrant (LUQ), right upper quadrant (RUQ), left lower quadrant (LLQ), and right lower quadrant (RLQ). Epigastric—translating to "above stomach"—means located in the middle of the abdomen, just below the bone where the ribs meet.

Abdominal pain is notorious for *radiating*—pain moving to an area not directly impacted by the pathology. This happens because the abdomen doesn't have many nerve receptors inside it, so the body generalizes pain to a nearby area. In the abdomen (and the chest cavity) pain often radiates to the back and shoulder. Lower abdominal pain may radiate to the groin.

Celine's mysterious belly pain worsens over the next few weeks. After a few months, it's happening almost every day. The only pattern Celine notices is that it tends to happen after meals. Her father suffered from heartburn, and she wonders if this is the same thing.

CONDITIONS CAUSING ABDOMINAL PAIN

Disease	Organ	Location	Symptoms	Who Gets it
Appendicitis	Appendix	RLQ	Fever, pain, nausea/ vomiting, anorexia	Young (10-30) and old (< 70)
Bowel Obstruction	Small intestines	Diffuse	Cramping pain, n/v, abdominal bloating, inability to pass gas	History of surgery, opiates, older adults, colon cancer
Cholecystitis	Gallbladder	RUQ	Cramping pain, n/v, anorexia	5Fs—female, fat, fertile, fair, 40+
Diverticulitis	Large Intestine	LLQ	Cramping pain, fever, diarrhea/ constipation	Older adult, chronic constipation
Pancreatitis	Pancreas	Epigastric	Severe pain, fever, fast heart rate	Alcoholics, history of gallbladder disease or stomach cancer
Peptic Ulcer Disease	Stomach, small intestine	Epigastric	Gnawing pain, worse at night, n/v, weight loss, early satiety	Alcohol or tobacco use, anxious personality, NSAID use

APPENDICITIS

Just before Christmas, Celine's youngest daughter, Clara, wakes her in the middle of the night. She's fourteen, and far past the age when she wakes up her mom because of nightmares. Crying, she says that her tummy hurts. She's clutching her right side, bent over by the pain. Celine takes her temperature and finds that she has a fever, so she takes Clara straight to the hospital.

> Recent studies suggest the appendix may play a role in in promoting "good" bacteria within the gut biome.[7]

Appendicitis occurs when the appendix is obstructed and subsequently, infected. Appendicitis is the most common surgical emergency in the world.[2] And while anyone, child, or adult, can get appendicitis, most people with appendicitis are between the ages of 10 and 30.[3]

The stereotypical presentation of appendicitis is sudden-onset epigastric pain that moves over time down towards the belly button (*umbilicus*) until finally settling in the right lower quadrant (RLQ). The other cardinal feature of appendicitis is a loss of appetite.

> The medical term for loss of appetite is **anorexia**. The eating disorder is called **anorexia nervosa**.

Your character may or may not experience nausea and vomiting, but if they're hungry, they probably don't have appendicitis. They may also have some fatigue and a mild fever.

> The **speed bump sign** is when your character's abdomen is so tender that jostling it—such as speedbumps on the road—cause intense pain.

As they drive to the hospital, Clara cries out in pain every time they go over a speedbump or take a curve too quickly. Celine berates herself for not noticing the signs earlier; Clara barely touched her dinner and went to bed early. Is she a bad mother for not paying attention?

Appendicitis is usually diagnosed clinically—no need for labs or imaging, particularly if they need to be rolled back for emergency surgery. The caveat is that if your character could possibly be pregnant—any person who menstruates and is sexually active could fall into this category—and then they'll need to run a blood pregnancy test to rule out ectopic pregnancy (see *Ch. 8: Childbirth*). If your character is stable

> Laparoscopic surgery uses cameras and surgical tools inserted into small cuts to visualize and operate on the organs. Recovery times for laparoscopic surgeries are usually shorter.

enough, they'll get further labs and an abdominal CT—providing the pregnancy test is negative.

Appendicitis is treated with an urgent surgery called an *appendectomy*. Though open appendectomies were the gold standard for centuries, most appendectomies are now laparoscopic. If the appendicitis is not treated promptly, it can lead to a perforation—literal sh*t spilling into the abdominal cavity. It is a life-threatening, extremely painful emergency (See "Perforation" below).

At the ED, Clara is promptly diagnosed with appendicitis. After a few blood tests, she's given pain meds and a CT scan of her stomach. The doctors tell Celine that Clara's appendix has not ruptured but is very inflamed. They start her on IV antibiotics and make her NPO. Twelve hours later, she's wheeled into the OR for laparoscopic appendectomy or, as the surgeons call it, a "Lap Appy." The whole thing takes less than an hour.

> NPO = nil per os
> (nothing by mouth)

BOWEL OBSTRUCTION

A bowel obstruction occurs when the lumen of the intestine is blocked; either partially or completely. Small bowel obstructions (SBOs) are more common than large bowel obstructions and can be more dangerous. The most common causes of an SBO are hernias, tumors, and adhesions—a thick, string-like substance that forms in the abdominal cavity after surgery.

> **Obstipation** = complete inability to pass gas or fecal matter.
>
> **Feculent vomitus** = regurgitation of fecal matter.

If your character has an SBO, they'll have cramping, abdominal pain, and bloating. If they have a complete obstruction, they won't be able to defecate or pass gas - not even a little. They will also have severe nausea and vomiting, sometimes so severe that they actually vomit up fecal matter.

To diagnose an SBO, your character will get an upright abdominal x-ray (they'll literally be standing to receive the x-ray) and labs to see if the electrolytes in their blood are out of whack. If they have a partial SBO (aka they're still passing gas), they can be treated with **bowel rest** and IV fluids to correct for the vomiting. They'll probably also require a nasogastric tube (NG tube)—a long tube inserted through the nose and stuffed down into the stomach—that helps promote bowel rest by

> **Bowel rest** means total abstinence from food, giving your GI tract time to heal. It's a lot like staying off a broken foot, only with a higher risk of getting hangry.

sucking fluid out of the stomach. If they have a complete obstruction, or if they've developed a fever or other signs of bowel strangulation, they'll need emergency surgery.

Having an NG tube placed is a painful and uncomfortable procedure. It can activate the gag reflex and cause pain/discomfort while being placed. However, once it's in, it usually only causes mild discomfort.

One of the most severe complications of an SBO is bowel strangulation, meaning that the bowel has twisted so much that the blood supply has been cut off. Your character will spike a fever, tank their blood pressure, experience extreme abdominal pain, and may even vomit blood. This is a surgical emergency.

Large bowel obstructions are less common and generally less severe. The most common cause is colon cancer. Most of the time, it will need to be treated with surgery, though not as emergently as in SBO.

CHOLECYSTITIS

After Clara is released from the hospital, Celine takes her children out for a celebratory dinner at her favorite French restaurant. They gorge themselves on French onion soup, brie cheese, and coq au vin. That night, after the kids have gone to bed, Celine feels that cramping pain again—the one that nearly doubled her over while she was brushing the horses. Only this time, doesn't go away. She grits her teeth, waiting, but the pain only gets worse. A wave of nausea washes over her and she runs to the toilet, vomiting up the remains of her meal. She vomits and vomits, until nothing comes up, then she dry heaves some more. Aunt Charlotte knocks on the door and asks if everything is all right. Celine tries to wave her off, but Auntie is no fool—she touches Celine's forehead, already damp with sweat, and tells her that it's time to go to the hospital.

Who gets acute cholecystitis? Just remember the 5-Fs: Fertile, Fat, Female, Fair (Caucasian), and Forty.

Acute cholecystitis is the inflammation of the gallbladder due to blockage of the bile duct leading from the gallbladder to the small intestine. Most often, this blockage is caused by gallstones—tiny crystals formed by the deposition of bile inside the gallbladder. Your character will have severe, cramping pain in their right upper quadrant (RUQ) or epigastric area, and they may feel pain in their right

A positive **Murphy Sign** is when your character can't breathe in while the RUQ of the abdomen is being pressed on. It's a strong indicator of acute cholecystitis.

shoulder as well. Other symptoms include a low-grade fever, nausea/vomiting, and anorexia.

> *In the ED—Celine is mortified to see that it's the same doctor who treated Clara—the doctor asks a bunch of questions while pressing lightly on Celine's abdomen. He presses hard just under her left ribcage and tells her to breathe in. She starts to do so, but her breath catches at the sudden pain that shoots down into her belly.*

Cholecystitis is treated with admission to the hospital for IV fluids, bowel rest, and antibiotics, but the definitive treatment is surgery. Like appendectomies, most cholecystectomies are done laparoscopically. Surgery is ideally performed within 24-48 hours of admission.

> *Much like her daughter, Celine is made nothing by mouth (NPO) and put on IV antibiotics. Twenty-four hours later, she's taken to the OR to have her gallbladder removed.*

Surgeons speak in abbreviations. A laparoscopic cholecystectomy is a "Lap chole." A laparoscopic appendectomy is a "Lap Appy."

DIVERTICULITIS

Diverticula are small bulges in the colon wall, caused by increased pressure inside the colon, usually from chronic constipation. The presence of these bulges is called *diverticulosis* and usually doesn't cause any symptoms. But if the diverticula fill with fecal matter, get blocked off, and become inflamed, your character will end up with diverticulitis.

If your character has diverticulitis, they'll have LLQ pain and fever. They may have nausea and vomiting, as well as constipation *or* diarrhea. If the doctor does a digital rectal exam, they might be able to feel a painful mass.

Diverticulitis is diagnosed with a CT scan showing the presence of inflamed diverticula. It is treated with IV antibiotics and bowel rest. If mild, it may even be able to be treated at home with oral antibiotics. However, if there are recurrent episodes or complications, such as abscess formation, bowel obstruction, or perforation, the treatment is surgery.

Digital rectal exam (DRE) is one gloved finger up the bum. It's called a digital exam because the exam is performed with a single digit, or finger. Neither patients nor doctors are particularly thrilled with this exam.

PANCREATITIS

Pancreatitis is the inflammation of the pancreas—the
organ dedicated to making digestive enzymes and proteins
like insulin. Most cases of pancreatitis are caused by
either alcohol abuse or gallstones, though viral infections,
certain drugs, and blunt trauma to the abdomen can also
cause it.

Pancreatitis is notoriously painful. The pain is usually located in the epigastric
region, but it also commonly causes chest and back pain. Nausea and loss of appetite
are also common side effects, usually due to the pain being so severe. Your character
may have a low-grade fever, a racing heart, and bruising around their belly button
or flank. The pain is worse when laying down and after eating.

Blood levels of specific pancreatic proteins (called *proteases*), along with
abdominal x-ray are usually the first step toward diagnosis. The most accurate test
is a CT scan of the abdomen.

Most people with pancreatitis only need supportive treatment, such as pain
control, IV fluids, and bowel rest. If they're vomiting up a storm, they may need
a nasogastric tube as well. However, if your character has severe pancreatitis—
including hemorrhagic pancreatitis—they'll also get a trip to the ICU and some
prophylactic antibiotics.

PEPTIC ULCER DISEASE (PUD)

If your character has ulcers, they'll have aching epigastric pain that gets worse at
night. They may also have nausea/vomiting, weight loss, and early satiety—meaning
they feel full without having eaten much.

Ulcers are usually caused by infection with
a species of bacteria called *Helicobacter pylori,*
or *H. pylori.* However, they can also be caused—
or exacerbated—by NSAID use, smoking,
alcohol, and stress. They can be located in
either the stomach or the duodenum—the
first part of the small intestines.

Ulcers are treated by suppressing acid production and eradicating *H. pylori.*
The most common treatment is called "triple therapy,"—a combination of an acid-
suppressing medication and two antibiotics. However, most ulcers will resolve with
lifestyle changes—stopping aspirin and other NSAIDs, quitting smoking, abstaining
from alcohol, and avoiding eating before bed.

ACUTE ABDOMEN

An acute abdomen is the surgical term for "sh*t is getting real." It refers to sudden, severe abdominal pain that demands urgent medical attention. If you want to see a surgeon cr*p their pants, tell them your character has had an acute abdomen for the past two hours.

If your character has an acute abdomen, they will be in terrible pain—the worst pain of their life—and they will be vomiting, or at least extremely nauseated. But, as you may have noticed, many conditions cause abdominal pain, nausea, and vomiting. What's the difference between an acute abdomen and all of the other causes of emergent abdominal pain?

The answer lies in the physical exam. First, your character will look sick. Like, really sick. Circling-the-drain sick. They may have changes to their vital signs, like increased heart rate or breathing, low blood pressure, or a fever. Second, their abdomen will be distended and rigid, and your character will exhibit "guarding"— the muscles of the abdomen tensing up with even the lightest pressure on their abdomen. Guarding is an involuntary reaction. To further prevent pain, they will lie deadly still and will cry out if someone bumps the table or tries to move them. Finally, they may exhibit rebound tenderness; increased pain when the pressure on the abdomen is released. Rebound tenderness is a sign of peritonitis— inflammation of the sack lining the abdominal cavity, or peritoneum.

> "Circling the Drain" is slang for a patient that is about to die.

If your character has an acute abdomen, it means they have a life-threatening cause of abdominal pain. The doctors won't wait for labs or imaging, they'll take them back to surgery right away. If they don't already have a good idea of what is wrong, they'll perform an exploratory laparotomy, or "Ex-Lap,"—opening up the abdomen and poking around until they find the source of your character's pain. Luckily, there's a finite number of things that can cause acute abdomen.

Life-Threatening	Organs	Symptoms	Causes
Acute mesenteric Ischemia	Blood vessels to intestines	Extreme pain, NO acute abdomen	Blood clots, plaque buildup
Intra-abdominal Bleeding	Aorta, arteries, liver, spleen	Acute abdomen, shock	Abdominal aneurysm rupture, ulcer, ectopic pregnancy
Perforation	Appendix, intestine, stomach	Acute abdomen, shock	Appendicitis, bowel obstruction, diverticulitis, inflammatory bowel disease, ulcers

Acute Mesenteric Ischemia (AMI)

At the hospital, the doctor pokes and prods Charlotte but tells her that, other than the pain, he can find nothing wrong with her. Her exam is clean and the abdominal X-ray she got on the way in was normal. He's about to send her home with some pain meds when Celine—who hasn't seen her aunt take a single pill the whole time they've lived with her—asks if she's still taking the blood thinners the doctors prescribed after she was diagnosed with a heart arrhythmia (called atrial fibrillation). Gritting her teeth against the pain, Charlotte shakes her head—she stopped those meds months ago after a friend convinced her that it was better to treat it naturally, with fish oil and magnesium.

Atrial fibrillation (See *Ch. 20: Chronic Breathlessness*) leads to clot formation in the heart. Those clots can then break off pieces that can go to the brain (causing stroke), lungs (causing pulmonary embolism), and gut (causing acute mesenteric ischemia).

Blocking off blood flow leads to tissue death (*infarction*). If that happens in the heart, it's called a heart attack, or myocardial infarction. In the brain, it's a stroke. If the blood flow to the intestines is blocked it causes **acute mesenteric ischemia**—decreased blood flow to the bowels—and it can be even more deadly than the first two.

Ischemia = not enough blood flow

Infarction = tissue death

Most cases of acute mesenteric ischemia are caused by an embolism—a blood clot formed in the heart—that traveled through the body until it got stuck in a mesenteric artery, blocking off blood flow to the intestines. The second most common cause is plaque buildup. Because of this, the same people who are at risk for heart attacks and stroke—people with cholesterol-clogged arteries and heart disease—are at high risk of acute mesenteric ischemia. If a doctor is describing this condition to your patient, they'd probably call it a "heart attack of the intestines".

The buzz phrase for diagnosis of acute mesenteric ischemia is "pain out of proportion to the exam". This phrase refers to the fact that your character is in terrible pain, but when the doctor performs the physical exam, the character looks totally normal. Your character may also have some anorexia and vomiting, but the crazy thing about this disease is how *healthy* they look—other than the blinding pain.

> Doctors don't always take patients' pain seriously, especially POC and women. If you want to kill a character through a medical mistake, a doctor missing the diagnosis of AMI because they thought the patient was exaggerating his or her pain would be, sadly, quite believable.

After this revelation, the doctor sends Charlotte for a specialized CT scan of her blood vessels. The scan shows a major artery supplying the intestine is blocked, though luckily none of the intestines have died yet. The doctor informs Charlotte, whose pain has only marginally dulled with the IV pain meds she's been given, that she's had the equivalent of a heart attack in her intestines. Charlotte then gets an echocardiogram— an ultrasound of her heart—that shows a large clot in her left atria. She's admitted to the hospital for treatment—anticoagulation and IV fluids—and pain control.

Diagnosis is through a CT scan of the blood vessels of the bowel, called mesenteric angiography, though your character will likely also get an abdominal x-ray to rule out other causes, like perforation (see below). However, if they exhibit signs of bowel infarction—low blood pressure, fast breathing, and an increase in lactic acid in their blood—they'll be taken straight back for emergency surgery.

If your character isn't circling the drain, they'll be stabilized with IV fluids and antibiotics, and given drugs to dilate the arteries or break up clots. But if any of the bowel has died, they'll need surgery to take out the dead bits.

Acute mesenteric ischemia is a deadly disease, with a mortality rate of 60-70%.[3] If bowel death occurs, it jumps to 90%.[3] Myocardial infarctions, by contrast, have a mortality rate of around 30%.[4]

Bleeding into the Abdomen

Bleeding inside the abdomen irritates the peritoneum (the sack lining the abdominal cavity). This irritation causes the symptoms of acute abdomen, including abdominal rigidity and guarding. If there is a lot of blood—and I mean a LOT—it can cause distension as the abdomen fills with blood.

Abdominal bleeding caused by trauma will be covered in *Ch. 15: Gut Wounds.*

If your character is bleeding into their abdomen, they will have severe abdominal pain and an acute abdomen. Depending on how much they're bleeding, they may also have symptoms of shock: low blood pressure, dizziness or lightheadedness, cold, clammy skin, and shallow, rapid breathing. The amount of blood they're losing—and the amount of danger they're in—depends on the cause of their bleeding.

AAA = "Triple A"

The most dramatic form of an intra-abdominal bleed is a ruptured aorta. Technically, it's a retroperitoneal bleed, as the aorta is located in the retroperitoneal space, but your character—screaming in pain and dizzy from blood loss—isn't likely to care about this technicality. And while a ruptured abdominal aorta can happen due to trauma, it is more likely to occur due to a ruptured abdominal aortic aneurysm (AAA)

An aneurysm is a bulge in the wall of an artery. AAAs are points of weakness in the muscular wall of the abdominal aorta. Most of the time, they're asymptomatic—your character will have no idea they have one unless they get a CT scan of their abdomen for something else. But if something happens—your character's blood pressure gets too high, or plaque buildup further weakens the wall, or sometimes for no clear reason at all—the bulge will break, causing a ruptured AAA.

Older individuals, particularly male smokers, are at high risk of AAA.

The classic triad of a ruptured AAA is abdominal pain, low blood pressure, and a pulsating mass within the abdomen—your character will literally be able to see the blood pumping into their abdomen. They will also quickly go into shock. The only treatment is emergency surgery.

There are other medical causes of intra-abdominal bleeding, though none are quite as spectacular as a ruptured AAA. Ulcers eroding into blood vessels lead to bleeding. Most of the time, the blood stays in the GI tract, causing an upper GI bleed but sometimes it can erode through the layers of the stomach or duodenum, leading to bleeding into the abdomen. Intra-abdominal bleeding from an ulcer is usually slow, but it can occasionally be rapid and severe, leading to shock.

Ulcers are the most common cause of upper GI bleeds.

Ectopic pregnancies occur when an embryo implants anywhere other than the uterus. If it implants inside the fallopian tube—the tiny tubes leading from the ovary to the uterus—it can grow so large that it bursts the tube, leading to dangerous bleeding. Symptoms of a burst ectopic pregnancy include one-sided, lower-abdominal pain (LLQ or RLQ), dizziness, and fainting, which may progress quickly to low blood pressure and shock.

See *Ch. 7: Childbirth* for more on ectopic pregnancies.

Perforated Organs

The most common cause of an acute abdomen is the perforation of a hollow organ—usually the intestines. It is exceedingly dangerous, as there is literal sh*t spewing into your character's abdominal cavity. It irritates the peritoneum—leading to symptoms of acute abdomen—and is a huge infection risk.

Trauma can also cause intestinal perforation (*Ch. 15: Gut Wounds*).

There are many causes of perforation, including appendicitis, bowel obstruction, diverticulitis, and peptic ulcer disease (PUD). Inflammatory bowel disease (IBD), such as Crohn's disease and ulcerative colitis, can also cause perforation. Medical procedures, such as colonoscopies and endoscopies, can also cause perforation, but the likelihood of that occurring is quite low, less than 0.2% for most routine colonoscopies.[5]

If your character has a perforation, they will have an acute abdomen—abdominal pain, rigidity, and guarding—along with high fever, nausea, and vomiting. Treatment is with emergency surgery.

BREAKING DOWN THE CLICHÉ: JUST GAS

"I think I'm dying, doc. My stomach hurts so bad, it feels like..."

Loud farting noise

"Actually, I feel better now."

This is another one of those clichés that are pretty accurate. You'd be surprised how many people show up at the ED with intense gas pain that goes away right after a foul odor fills the room.

As I said earlier, abdominal pain is the reason for about 5-10% of all visits to the ED.[1] But what do doctors find as the ultimate cause of that abdominal pain? Turns out, the most frequent cause, about 31%, is "nonspecific abdominal pain"—abdominal pain for which doctors weren't able to find a cause.[6] Now, there's no way to prove how much of that was or wasn't gas pain since there is no way to prove the diagnosis of flatulence. But the cliché of characters going to the ED (or thinking they're dying) because of gas pain probably has more than a grain of truth to it.

The fact that it won't show up on any imaging or labs, coupled with peoples' hesitance to talk about their farts, makes it very difficult to provide any real evidence that this cliché has a basis in truth. But talk to any emergency doctor or nurse, and they'll have some great anecdotal evidence. As a writer, that's probably all you need.

4. ALLERGY & ANAPHYLAXIS

Desirae is a sophomore in college. In the last few years, she's noticed that in the fall she gets a runny nose and red, itchy eyes. Sometimes when she's feeling like that, her asthma gets worse. If she goes for long walks, she brings her inhaler with her. Her tongue also tends to feel thick when she eats kiwis, so she avoids them. She grew up running around barefoot on a farm, so she's been stung by bees several times. The first few times, it hurt, but she doesn't remember much more than that. But when she was 12, a bee stung her on the thumb. Her hand swelled up like a marshmallow and she developed hives all over her body, so her mom took her in to urgent care. The doctor prescribed an EpiPen—an epinephrine autoinjector pen—and told her to always keep it with her.

> EpiPens are autoinjectors that inject epinephrine straight into the muscle.

ALLERGY

Allergies can range in severity from mild hay fever to life-threatening medical emergencies. An allergy is a specific type of immune overreaction that happens right away, called an immediate hypersensitivity. A true allergy causes a range of symptoms, from runny nose and red, itchy eyes, to hives and/or swelling of the deep subcutaneous tissue surrounding the airways and the gastrointestinal tract.

> A runny nose caused by allergies is called **allergic rhinitis**. Red, itchy eyes are called conjunctivitis.

Certain substances are more likely to result in allergic reactions. Pollen, dust mites, and animal dander are some of the most common allergies, but they tend to be mild, producing only a runny nose (*allergic rhinitis*) and itchy eyes (*conjunctivitis*). Allergies to food, such as eggs, peanuts, or shellfish, medications, and insect stings are more likely to cause more serious reactions. The most severe form of allergic reaction is called anaphylaxis.

ANAPHYLAXIS

Anaphylaxis is the most serious form of allergy: a whole-body reaction that occurs seconds to minutes after exposure. It usually starts with skin symptoms—a rash or hives—but quickly progresses to respiratory, cardiac, and sometimes abdominal symptoms. The airways swell shut, blood vessels dilate, and the lining of the GI tract swells, causing abdominal pain, nausea/vomiting, and diarrhea. Anaphylaxis can lead to asphyxiation and death.

SYMPTOMS

Desirae is studying in the quad, enjoying the warm spring day when she feels a sharp pain on the sole of her barefoot: a bee sting. Grimacing, she lifts her foot to reveal her heel already red and swollen, a raised red rash spreading up her calf. Not bothering to gather her things, she takes off running for her dorm room, trying to remember where she keeps her EpiPen. Her heart pounds as she bursts into her room, startling her roommate. She feels like she's breathing through a straw and is starting to feel lightheaded and nauseated.

If your character is experiencing anaphylaxis, they might feel:

- Lightheaded

- A sense of impending doom

- Redness, pain or itchy welts or hives all over their body

- Trouble breathing, coughing, or wheezing

- Trouble swallowing

- Abdominal pain, cramps, or nausea

- Blurry vision

- Confusion and/or trouble speaking

SIGNS

"What happened to your face?" Desirae's roommate asks. "Your eye is almost swollen shut. And you've got these red bumps all over. What's going on?"

Desirae finds the EpiPen in a back corner of a desk drawer. She wastes no time, pressing the orange end of the autoinjector into her thigh. The pain of the injection is sharp, a little like the bee sting itself.

Panting, Desirae turns to her roommate. "Call. 911." She's so out of breath, that she can barely get the words out.

If your character comes across someone experiencing anaphylaxis, they will notice a few key signs.

- **Swollen face**: particularly around the eyes, lips, and tongue

- **Trouble breathing**: the victim may sound out of breath, or they may be audibly wheezing

- **Fast heart rate:** if your character thinks to take the victim's pulse, it may be fast and thready

- **Hives**: Red, raised, itchy rash or wheals, all over the body

- **Diarrhea and/or vomiting**: especially in food allergies

- **Fainting or loss of consciousness**: fainting is usually due to plummeting blood pressure and is a sign that the victim is going into anaphylactic shock

> The medical term for hives is **urticaria**.

ANAPHYLACTIC SHOCK

Anaphylactic shock occurs when your character's immune system is so over-stimulated that their blood pressure drops precipitously. Your character will pass out, and they will be in imminent danger of death. Death by anaphylactic shock usually occurs due to either cardiovascular collapse or asphyxiation due to airway swelling or spasms.[2]

> Shock occurs when a character's blood pressure drops so low, that they can't get blood to vital organs. For more on shock, see Volume 1: Setting & Character, Ch. 14: Shock.

TREATMENT

The immediate treatment of anaphylaxis is with epinephrine. People who know they are at risk of an anaphylactic reaction are supposed to always carry an EpiPen—a bright yellow pen that auto-injects epinephrine. Realistically, that doesn't always happen. EpiPens are expensive, they can expire, and, though small and portable, are too big to fit in most wallets. It is all too easy for a character to leave their EpiPen sitting forgotten in an unused purse or drawer. But not having it could be the difference between life and death.

> The cost of EpiPens rose over 400% between 2007 and 2016, and now can cost over $500.[1] Why? Because the manufacturer had a monopoly on them, and they could.

Desirae's roommate calls 911. Desirae continues to wheeze as she leans down and pulls the stinger from her foot. After five minutes, she isn't feeling any worse, but she also isn't feeling any better, either. Her heart is still pounding. She knows she could take a second dose, but she doesn't have a second EpiPen. The paramedics arrive and administer another dose of epinephrine, and Desirae is taken by ambulance to the hospital.

Epinephrine has lots of side effects; it constricts the blood vessels and makes the heartbeat faster and stronger. It can cause a heart attack, so if your character uses their EpiPen, even accidentally, they're going to need a trip to the hospital.

After the second dose of epinephrine, Desirae still isn't feeling better. She's gasping for breath, and she's getting dizzy. Her voice sounds hoarse. The paramedic suggests they intubate her, but Desirae shakes her head in refusal, sure the second dose of epinephrine will kick in any moment. Just as they arrive at the hospital, she passes out.

A suddenly hoarse voice is a warning sign your character's airway is about to swell shut.

If your character is responding to an emergency, one of the most important rules is to address the ABCs: Airway, Breathing, Circulation. If your character's airway is occluded, the very first order of business is to get it open again; by intubating if necessary. Intubation is the process of threading a tube from the throat down into the lungs to manually keep the airway open. Intubating someone with anaphylaxis is technically challenging, which is why early intubation is preferred, if at all possible.

See <u>Volume 1: Setting & Character</u>, Ch. 13: *Approach to an Emergency* for more.

Desirae is intubated in the ambulance and rushed to the Emergency Department where she's put on a ventilator. She's given IVs in both arms and started on a myriad of drugs to calm down her hyperactive immune system, including steroids, antihistamines, and inhaled albuterol, given through the endotracheal tube. After Desirae's swelling subsides and she begins to wake up, the doctors ensure her airway swelling has gone down enough for her to breathe on her own, before pulling out the tube. She is transferred to the ICU overnight, then to the hospital floor. She goes home the next day with admonishments to always carry her EpiPen with her from now on.

BREAKING DOWN THE CLICHÉ: SICKLY SIDEKICK

*Sidekick: Are you sure this is safe? *Noisy inhaler* It looks questionable to me.*

So often, allergies and allergy-induced asthma are used to denote weakness or hypochondriac tendencies. But that simply isn't true; anyone can have allergies. Usually, those who are very careful about their allergies are doing so for good reason. I'd love to see a superhero (or supervillain) brought down by a drop of peanut oil hidden inside their morning coffee.

Many children grow out of their allergies. This is especially true of allergies to milk and eggs. Conversely, many people develop allergies to pollen and dander as adults; these allergies tend to worsen over time. If someone has one allergy, they are more likely to develop another.

It is important to note that allergies are not the same thing as intolerance or sensitivity. True allergies, especially food or drug allergies, will usually have a rash or airway component. If your character gets a stomachache from eating tomatoes, that isn't an allergy—it's heartburn. Similarly, if your character got diarrhea from a medication, it's not an allergy either—it's a side effect. Every provider has *that* patient, the one who comes into the office with a long list of "allergies" to things that make them feel tired, bloated, gassy, foggy, weak, constipated, nauseated, crampy, burpy, or give them joint pain. If you're trying to write a character who will make their doctor pull their own hair out, someone with a long list of "allergies" is a great place to start.

That said, food intolerances and sensitivities are real, and can greatly affect your character's life. A character with irritable bowel syndrome, for instance, can get bloating, constipation, gas, or diarrhea from certain foods. Many drugs have nebulous side effects like fatigue, nausea, diarrhea, or vomiting. Your character very well might have an intolerance that significantly affects their life. Just don't call it an allergy unless it is one.

5. FEVER

At first, Esteban thought it was just a cold—a runny nose and a sore throat—so he brushed it off and went to work anyway. But now that he's here, the normally comforting quiet of the library feels soporific; he keeps falling asleep at his desk. As the afternoon wears on, he begins to feel chilly, so he put on an extra sweater, then another. By the end of the day, he's shivering, a cold sweat running down the back of his neck.

> Colds very rarely cause fevers.

BACKGROUND

A FEVER IS DEFINED AS AN abnormally high body temperature—in most cases, greater than 100.4°F (38°C) when measured with an oral thermometer.[1] It can be accompanied by chills, sweating, shaking, delirium, and even seizures if your character's body temperature gets high enough.

> Normal human body temperature ranges from 97-99°F. Temperatures can be taken by mouth (oral), on the forehead, under the armpit (axillary), or up the anus (rectal). Rectal temperatures are slightly higher than oral, while axillary and forehead are slightly lower.

SIGNS & SYMPTOMS

You've undoubtedly had a fever at some point in your life, so I'm not going to spend too much time describing what it feels like. Signs and symptoms of fever include:

- **Temperature >100.4°F:** This is the only indisputable sign of a fever

- **Dehydration**

- **Hot to the touch**

- **Rigors:** Shaking and chills despite a high fever. May be accompanied by sweating, goosebumps, and teeth chattering

- **Sweating**

- **Weakness**

Instead, I'm going to spend this chapter talking about some of the causes of fever—which ones will put your character in mortal danger, and which they should be able to shrug off.

INFECTIOUS CAUSES OF FEVER

The most common causes of fever are infections. Fever is a normal—and necessary—immune response to infection with a pathogen. By increasing the body temperature, your character's immune system is making the environment less favorable towards the invader. Below is a table of some of the most common infectious causes of fever.

Pathogen = bacteria, virus, or parasite that causes infection.

Disease	Infection of…	Cause
Abscess	Trapped bacteria or foreign object	Bacteria
Cellulitis	Skin	Bacteria
COVID	Respiratory Tract	Coronavirus
Endocarditis	Heart	Bacteria or Virus
Gastroenteritis (food poisoning)	GI tract	Bacteria, Virus, or Parasite
HIV (initial infection)	White Blood Cells	Virus
Influenza	Respiratory Tract	Virus
Lyme Disease	Bloodstream	Bacteria (tick-spread)
Malaria	Red Blood Cells	Protozoa
Meningitis	Brain	Bacteria or Virus
Mononucleosis	White Blood Cells	Virus
Pneumonia	Lungs	Bacteria
Prostatitis	Prostate	Bacteria
Pyelonephritis	Kidney	Bacteria

Disease	Infection of...	Cause
Strep throat	Tonsils & Throat	Bacteria
Tuberculosis	Lungs	Bacteria

Let's go through these infections, organizing them by the primary organ that is affected.

LUNGS

COVID-19: COVID-19 is a respiratory tract illness caused by a coronavirus that can range from totally asymptomatic to complete, multi-organ failure. Like the flu, COVID-19 is spread by respiratory droplets. Our understanding of this disease is evolving so quickly that anything I write here is likely to be out-of-date before this book hits the press, so I'm just going to leave it at that.

> COVID-19 isn't the only coronavirus. Coronaviruses are all over the world and have been known to cause everything from SARS and MERS to the common cold.

That night, Esteban lies in bed, tossing and turning as he alternates between hot and cold. His muscles ache, and his head is pounding He digs around in his bedside table until he finds a thermometer—his temperature is over 101oF. He thinks about calling in sick to work but knows that he can't; there's no one to cover for him, and his boss will be livid. So, when the sun rises, he drags himself out of bed and goes to work, hoping no one will notice his cough.

Influenza: Influenza, or the flu, is responsible for the deaths of many adults and children. Responsible for nearly 50,000 adult deaths every year, pneumonia is also the #1 cause of death in children in the US.[2] Caused by an orthomyxovirus, the flu is transmitted by respiratory droplets. It causes rapid onset fever and chills, headache, sore throat, malaise, and non-productive cough. For millions of people who get sick every year, most don't need any treatment beyond rest, Tylenol, and fluids. But for those who are most susceptible—the very young, the very old, the immunocompromised, and those with significant comorbidities—the flu can be deadly.

> A **productive cough** means phlegm is brought up while coughing. A **non-productive cough** is a dry cough that doesn't bring anything up.

After a few days of gritting his teeth and trying not to look as sick as he feels, Esteban is starting to feel better. Then, suddenly, while he's eating dinner at his favorite diner on Friday night, his fever returns with a vengeance. By the time he gets home, he's coughing, and even just walking up the one flight of stairs to his flat leaves him breathless.

Pneumonia: After childbirth, pneumonia is the most common cause of hospitalizations in the US.[2] About 50,000 people die from pneumonia in the US every year.[2] Pneumonia is an infection of the lungs that causes fever, cough, chest pain, and trouble breathing. Most cases of pneumonia are caused by bacteria, but pneumonia can also be caused by viruses and even certain fungi.

Technically, there are viral pneumonias. But, with the exception of COVID, they are usually less severe than bacterial pneumonia.

Anyone, old or young, can get it. In fact, pneumonia is the most common reason for children in the US to be hospitalized.[2] However, people with compromised immune systems—the elderly, HIV-positive or cancer patients, and organ transplant recipients—are at higher risk.

After a feverish night, Esteban barely has the strength to drag himself out of bed the next morning. His cough is worse, and now he's coughing up chunks of thick green mucous. He calls his daughter, Eva to tell her not to come over with his grandkids as planned, but he can barely speak in full sentences. Eva immediately knows something is wrong and tells him he needs to see a doctor. He tries to protest—he's fine, really—but she doesn't budge. A half-hour later, she's at his door, ready to drag him to the doctor. To his horror, she drives him straight to the Emergency Department.

Pneumonia is diagnosed with a chest X-ray and blood tests. A test of their sputum—the phlegm they're coughing up—can help determine which bacteria is causing the pneumonia and will allow the doctors to tailor the antibiotic therapy.

At the ED, the doctors put a plastic clippy thing— the nurse calls it a pulse oximeter—on Esteban's finger, then a cuff around his arm that squeezes him uncomfortably. The medical assistant frowns as she takes the measurements—his blood oxygen is a little low, as is his blood pressure. She puts a clear plastic tube around Esteban's face, which blasts cool air into his nose.

A **pulse oximeter** measures the level of oxygen in your character's blood.

When the doctor arrives, she types on her computer as he talks. Esteban wishes she would look at him. She doesn't even make eye contact as she presses her stethoscope to his chest and back, telling him to breathe deeply. Afterward, she tells him that he has likely developed pneumonia secondary to the flu, but she'll need a chest x-ray to be sure. Then, she asks him to cough and spit up the resultant green goop into a test tube.

Pneumonia is divided into two main types: community-acquired pneumonia (CAP) and healthcare-acquired pneumonia (HCAP). Depending on where your character picked up their pneumonia, they will receive slightly different treatment. For example, most characters with CAP will be able to be treated at home, using oral antibiotics. However, if your character is very old, very ill, or has a bunch of risk factors, they will be admitted to the hospital. If your character has HCAP, they'll be treated in the hospital with slightly different antibiotics.

> Infections that develop during hospitalization are called **nosocomial infections**.

When the doctor returns, she tells Esteban that he has pneumonia in one lung. She's going to start Tylenol (for the fever), cough suppressants, and a course of antibiotics. Because he's over seventy, and his blood pressure and blood oxygenation are low, she's recommending he be admitted to the hospital. Esteban tries to complain, but Eva overrides him.

"He'll go," she says, shooting a glare at her father. Esteban knows better than to argue.

If your character is on a ventilator, they are at high risk of developing pneumonia; somewhere between 9-27% of all people on ventilators come down with ventilator-associated pneumonia (VAP) at some point.[3] It's one of the reasons that doctors try to wean patients off ventilators as soon as physically possible. VAP can be easy to miss, as the character can't cough or tell the doctors how they're feeling. It can also be deadly, with a mortality rate of nearly 50%.[4] If your character is put on a ventilator, be aware that they are now at high risk of this life-threatening complication.

> A character on a ventilator will be sedated but they can still feel pain and discomfort. See <u>Volume 1: Setting & Character</u>, *Ch. 20: Ventilators.*

Tuberculosis (TB): Tuberculosis—also called consumption, phthisis, or scrofula—is very popular in literature and film. From *Les Miserable* and *Moulin Rouge* to *Crime and Punishment*, writers just love killing off characters with tuberculosis. To be fair, it is an impressive disease. From the primary—usually asymptomatic—infection, to the secondary fever, night sweats, malaise, and bloody cough, tuberculosis is a dramatic way to kill off a beloved hero or heroine. And, contrary to popular belief, TB is not eradicated. It is, however, much rarer than in previous centuries.

Nowadays, your character will need particular risk factors before you can believably give them TB. People at risk of TB include recent immigrants to the United States, prisoners, HIV-positive patients, injection drug users, alcoholics, diabetics, healthcare workers, and people with certain cancers.

If your character is diagnosed with tuberculosis, they will be immediately isolated, then put on an intense, four-drug treatment regimen that lasts for six months. A PPD test—a tiny bit of TB protein injected under the skin of the forearm—is used to screen for people who have been exposed to TB. A positive PPD will necessitate a 9-month prophylactic treatment with antibiotics to prevent the reactivation of the tuberculosis.

> The medical term for coughing up blood is **hemoptysis.**

SKIN

The skin is the largest organ of the body. And it is crawling with bacteria. Depending on what layer of skin is infected, there are several different types of skin infections.

Abscess: An abscess is a swelling caused by a collection of dead white blood cells (pus) due to a localized bacterial infection. Symptoms of a skin abscess can range from mild, localized pain and redness around the swelling, to high fever, chills, nausea, and vomiting. Sometimes, the abscess leaks pus in a variety of colors ranging from white and curd-like, to brown and goopy.

> Not all abscesses form in the skin; abscesses can form around internal organs as well.

The smell of pus comes in several delightful flavors, depending on the type of bacteria involved. Most infections have only a mild smell, like cheese left too long in the back of the refrigerator. *Pseudomonas* is a particularly nasty species of bacteria that smells sickly sweet, like rotten grapes, and produces green pus. Anaerobes, a class of bacteria that can thrive in abscesses, smell the worst. Their pungent stink of sulfur and rotting meat may be enough to drive even the most veteran nurses to have a gag reflex.

Most skin abscesses can be treated at home using a warm compress. However, skin abscesses causing fever need antibiotics and drainage (cutting open the abscess to allow the pus to drain out) to prevent the infection from entering the bloodstream and causing a host of other problems.

> MRSA = **Methicillin Resistant Staphylococcus aureus.** It is a type of bacteria that is resistant to first-line antibiotics. MRSA is very hard to treat.

After a few days in the hospital, Esteban still feels awful. His sputum test showed that he was infected with MRSA, so he is on heavy-duty antibiotics. But he continues to spike fevers every night and cough up that thick, green goop that the nurse calls his 'sputum.' His doctor orders a CT scan of his abdomen and finds an abscess—a pocket of bacteria—deep in his lung. Esteban is switched to IV antibiotics.

Abscesses can also form around internal organs, such as the liver, lung, or intestines. An intra-abdominal abscess can be life-threatening. Intra-abdominal abscesses can occur after infection, surgery, or inflammatory bowel diseases such as Crohn's disease. If your character has an intraabdominal abscess, they'll have abdominal pain and fullness, a fever, lack of appetite, and nausea/vomiting. Like a skin abscess, an intraabdominal abscess is treated with antibiotics and, in some cases, drainage. If your character needs their abscess drained, it will require either percutaneous drainage or abdominal surgery. Left untreated, the infection can get into the bloodstream, causing a life-threatening infection called *sepsis*.

Percutaneous drainage uses a long a$$ needle and ultrasound of CT guidance to insert a catheter long enough to reach the abscess inside to drain it.

After several days on the IV antibiotics, Esteban begins to feel better. No longer coughing up phlegm or spiking fevers, he stops needing supplemental oxygen. He's switched to oral antibiotics, which he'll have to take for several more weeks. After one more night in the hospital, he's discharged home.

Cellulitis: Cellulitis is an infection of the skin and the surrounding tissue. Caused by bacteria, it is easily spotted by the redness, warmth, pain, and swelling of the area. Fever may or may not be present. Cellulitis is often found near breaks in the skin, such as IV sites, bites, or wounds. It's treated with antibiotics and sometimes requires hospitalization. Similar to an abscess, an untreated infection can get into the bloodstream, causing sepsis.

Cellulitis is a great potential complication if you want your character to have some serious repercussions for what initially looked like a minor wound.

INTESTINES

Gastroenteritis: Diarrhea, nausea/vomiting, and fever are the hallmarks of gastroenteritis, also known as "food poisoning." Caused by a variety of different bacteria, gastroenteritis usually gets better on its own, needing only fluids and rest as treatment. Sometimes, if the vomiting is particularly severe, your character may need to be admitted to the hospital for IV fluids and anti-nausea medications.

MOUTH & THROAT

In the weeks following her father's hospitalization, Eva makes a concerted effort

Mononucleosis: Infectious mononucleosis—popularly called "mono" or "the kissing disease"—is caused by a virus spread by saliva. It is most commonly seen in young adults and adolescents; once your character has been infected, they're immune for life.

Mono starts with a high fever (as high as 104°F) sore throat, and severe fatigue. The lymph nodes swell up, as does the spleen. The back of the throat becomes red and swollen, and the tonsils are covered in a white ooze. After a few weeks, the fever and sore throat diminish, but the fatigue and muscle pain can linger for months.

The test for mononucleosis is a throat swab called the rapid monospot test. There isn't much in the way of treatment—just rest, fluids, and Tylenol for pain and fever—but your character will need to be careful playing sports, as their swollen spleen could rupture if hit.

Eva wonders if returning to basketball will perk up her daughter, so she forces her daughter to put on the uniform and go to the next game. But when, at half-time, she mentions to the coach that Esme isn't recovering from Mono as fast as she'd like, Coach immediately calls Esme over and benches her for the rest of the season. He explains to a mortified Eva that Mono causes the spleen to swell and jostling it could result in a devastating injury.

Strep Throat, Scarlet Fever & Rheumatic Fever

All three diseases are caused by infection with a bacteria called *Streptococcus pyogenes*.

> The medical term for strep throat is **streptococcal pharyngitis**.

- **Strep throat** is a fever and sore throat caused by an infection of the throat and tonsils by the bacteria. It is diagnosed with a throat swab called a rapid strep test.

- **Scarlet fever** is an infection by the same bacteria, but with increased production of a particular toxin that leads to a red rash, skin peeling, and a red, "strawberry tongue."

While anyone can get strep throat or scarlet fever, children ages 5-15 are most susceptible. Both infections are treated with antibiotics. Untreated, these infections can lead to rheumatic fever.

- **Rheumatic fever** is characterized by fever, jerky movements of the extremities, painful joints, and heart failure. It is not contagious, but it can be life-threatening—just ask Beth from *Little Women*. If not treated properly, rheumatic fever can cause long-term heart defects, such as mitral valve prolapse and mitral regurgitation (See *Ch. 20: Chronic Breathlessness*).

ZOONOTIC (ANIMAL-BORNE) DISEASES

Lyme disease: Lyme disease is a fun one because it can cause so many different problems for your character. First, after your character was bit by a tick, they will get a rash that looks like a bullseye, called *erythema migrans*. After a few days to weeks, if they don't get treatment, the infection will spread to their bloodstream, causing fever/chills, headache, neck pain, muscle pain, fatigue, and general grossness. This is called "early localized Lyme disease."

One particularly alarming sign of early localized Lyme disease is an effect called **Bell's palsy**, where one side of the face droops due to nerve paralysis. Your character may freak out and think they're having a stroke but not to worry—symptoms of Bell's Palsy usually resolve within 2-6 months.

The symptoms of early Lyme disease usually get better after a few days. Lyme disease is rarely fatal, but if they don't get treatment, then they'll move on to a more disseminated infection. And that's where the fun begins.

Untreated Lyme disease can cause all sorts of problems. Your character could get meningitis, acute encephalitis, a nerve infection-causing paralysis, or a lack of sensation in one area of the body (called *radiculopathy*). Within a couple of months, they could get cardiac manifestations, such as arrhythmias or an irritation of the lining of their heart called pericarditis. Months after that, they

can get arthritis—especially in the knees—and even central nervous system issues, such as mild, chronic encephalitis, inflammation of the spinal cord, and nerve pain.

If it sounds like a h*ll of a lot of random, unconnected issues, you're right. That's one of the joys of giving your character Lyme disease; all of these severe, seemingly unconnected symptoms can be traced back to something as innocent as a tick bite.

But—and this is a big but—your character must get bitten by the right kind of tick: a deer tick called *Ixodidae scapularis* that is infected with the bacteria *Borrelia burgdorferi*. This tick isn't found everywhere; in fact, it is only found on deer living on the northeastern seaboard (Maine to Maryland), and in the Midwest. So, if you want your character to develop Lyme, they will need to go traipsing around in long grass in areas where deer frequent in the correct parts of the country.

If your story is set in the south, your character can't get Lyme, but they can get Rocky Mountain Spotted Fever, another tick-borne febrile disease that causes a spotted rash.

Lyme disease is diagnosed with blood tests and treated with oral antibiotics. It usually doesn't require hospitalization, unless your character gets meningitis, encephalitis, or other central nervous system symptoms. Then they'll need to be admitted for IV antibiotics.

For some people, symptoms of Lyme disease can linger for months, in a condition called *post-treatment Lyme disease*. Its symptoms are nonspecific, such as fatigue and muscle pains. To get this condition, your character must have first had Lyme disease. Unfortunately, alternative-medicine clinics and websites are popping up and misdiagnosing people who've never had Lyme disease with "chronic Lyme disease." This practice is neither helpful nor logical since there really isn't any treatment for "chronic Lyme." Furthermore, it can be downright dangerous, as symptoms of "chronic Lyme" overlap with several other concerning and very real conditions, such as fibromyalgia, multiple sclerosis, lupus, and others. If you want to use quackery to slow your character's journey to their real diagnosis (and annoy the physician in the process) "chronic Lyme" is a fantastic choice.

There is a simple blood test that can prove whether your character has been exposed to Borrelia burgdorferi. If it's negative, they can't have post-treatment Lyme disease.

Malaria

Malaria is unique in that it causes a cyclic fever—a fever that spikes every 48 to 72 hours, then goes away. It also causes chills, muscle pain, headache, nausea/vomiting, and diarrhea. Spread by mosquitos carrying protozoa that infect red blood cells, malaria is responsible for more than 600,000 deaths every year.[5]

If your character is visiting the tropics, the Middle East, or parts of Africa, their doctor will recommend Chloroquine or Mefloquine tablets as prophylaxis. However, those medications have some nasty side effects, ranging from night terrors and psychosis to heart arrhythmias. Many characters, especially those who will be staying in a malaria-endemic area for a long time, will choose not to take malaria prophylaxis. And of course, the people who live there full-time won't take medical prophylaxis. Instead, they'll do everything they can to prevent mosquito bites, including sleeping under mosquito nets and wearing (or burning) mosquito repellant.

Malaria is treated with chloroquine, but resistance to chloroquine is mounting, and chloroquine-resistant malaria can be challenging to treat.

SEPSIS

Sepsis occurs when a pathogen—usually bacteria—makes its way into the bloodstream. This causes hyperactivation of the immune system as it gears up to fight off the pathogen. The immune system does a great job of battling pathogens, such as bacteria, fungi, and viruses, but in doing so it creates the symptoms of sepsis. These include:

- Fever (>100.4°F) or low body temperature (96°F)

- Fast breathing rate (*tachypnea*)

- Fast heart rate (*tachycardia*)

- High levels of white blood cells (*neutrophilia*)

For more on septic shock, see Volume 1: Setting & Character, Ch. 14: Shock.

Diagnosis of sepsis requires at least two of the above symptoms, plus confirmation of the pathogen in the blood, usually through blood cultures. **Septic shock** occurs when your character's blood pressure drops to unsafe levels due to the immune hyperactivation.

IMMEDIATELY LIFE-THREATENING INFECTIONS

Any infection can be life-threatening. But if you want your young, otherwise healthy protagonist to get very ill, very quickly, consider these infections.

Disease	Infection of	Cause
Bacterial Meningitis	Brain covering (*meninges*)	Bacteria or Virus

Disease	Infection of	Cause
Encephalitis	Brain tissue	Bacteria or Virus
Necrotizing Fasciitis	Skin (deep)	Bacteria
Febrile Neutropenia	Any	Low white blood cells
Toxic-Shock Syndrome	Bloodstream	Bacterial toxin

BACTERIAL MENINGITIS

Meningitis is the infection of the membranes that cover the brain and spinal cord (the *meninges*). It usually starts with a fever, headache, and tiredness that is easy to mistake for a more benign illness. However, meningitis also causes sensitivity to light (*photophobia*) and a stiff, painful neck. That neck stiffness, called *nuchal rigidity*, is the hallmark of bacterial meningitis. Any doctor worth their salt will test every patient with headache and fever by asking them to bow their head forward, as if in prayer. If your character has nuchal rigidity, they won't be able to bend it, or doing so will cause pain.

> *Eva's youngest, Ernesto, is just under two years old. For the most part, he's an easy baby who loves toddling around after his older siblings. One day, she goes to pick him up for his nap—he overslept by several hours—but he doesn't wake as she lifts him into her arms. His skin is hot, and he has a speckled rash along his upper back and arms. She takes his temperature using a rectal thermometer, and it's over 104oF. She tries to wake him, but he just moans, squinting against the light.*

The characteristic triad of acute bacterial meningitis is fever, neck stiffness, and a change in mental status. This can mean that your character may feel sleepy or confused but could also be as severe as a coma. Other signs can indicate meningitis, including a rash, dilated pupils, or difficulty flexing or straightening the knees, but the definitive diagnosis comes from an examination of the spinal fluid extracted via a spinal tap (*lumbar puncture*). Your character will be asked to sit up and hunch over or curl into a fetal position in the bed while a terrifyingly large needle is inserted into the spinal canal in their lower back. The procedure shouldn't be painful—they'll receive a local anesthetic—but the size of the needle and the placement in their spinal canal is enough to terrify even the most stalwart character. Because it is so dangerous, your character will be started on IV

Aseptic meningitis, or viral meningitis, is usually mild and does not require hospitalization.

antibiotics and admitted to the hospital even before the confirmatory results of the LP come back.

Terrified, Eva drives Ernesto straight to the pediatric emergency department. As the doctor tilts Ernesto's head forward and back, the boy cries out in pain. The doctor recommends a lumbar puncture to get a sample of his cerebrospinal fluid (CSF). Fighting back tears, Eva holds Ernesto in a fetal position, while the doctor places a long, thin needle into the boy's spine. It's a testament to how sick Ernesto is that he doesn't fight them at all.

Meningitis can lead to a host of complications, including seizures, brain or spinal cord abscesses, clotting disorders, respiratory arrest, and even coma. Acute meningitis can happen very quickly, progressing from a minor headache to a life-threatening infection in as little as a few hours. Even with appropriate treatment, it is frequently fatal.

The results of the blood and CSF tests reveal Eva's greatest fear; Ernesto has bacterial meningitis and will need to be admitted to the pediatric hospital for antibiotics and monitoring.

Young people are particularly susceptible to meningitis. In fact, toddlers, teenagers, and young adults living in dorms, boarding schools, or military bases are particularly susceptible, as one type of bacteria causing meningitis is spread through the respiratory system. Lucky, there is a vaccine to prevent some of the most common causes of bacterial meningitis. Adults over 65 are given the vaccination against one type of bacteria, while all pre-teens are vaccinated against another type. However, if your character skipped their vaccinations, or is too young to be vaccinated, they would be at risk of this deadly disease.

ENCEPHALITIS

Encephalitis is the inflammation of the brain. It can occur on its own, or in conjunction with meningitis. When seen on its own, encephalitis is a rare and potentially fatal disease that is usually caused by a virus, though there are a few non-viral causes. Herpes simplex virus is one of the most common causes, causing HSV encephalitis. Other causes include West Nile virus, cytomegalovirus (CMV), varicella-zoster virus (the virus that causes chickenpox and shingles), and rabies. There are also non-infectious causes, such as autoimmune encephalitis, like Anti-NMDA-receptor encephalitis, which are caused by the immune system attacking the brain tissue.

<u>Brain on Fire</u> by Susannah Cahalan does an incredible job of describing her experience with Anti-NMDA-receptor encephalitis.

Anyone can get encephalitis, but people with autoimmune illnesses, certain types of cancer, and AIDS are at a higher risk.

The symptoms of encephalitis start with what's called a *prodrome* (an early herald of the disease) characterized by headache, tiredness, and muscle pain. But your character might start going downhill fast. Encephalitis can look like meningitis, with headache, photophobia, neck pain, and fever. However, the changes in mental status are more pronounced, with confusion, delirium, disorientation, delusions, and hallucinations. Your character might exhibit bizarre behavior, like aggression or extreme emotional swings. Your character's family may report that they are acting nothing like themselves. They may also have seizures, trouble speaking, or paralysis of half of their body.

Encephalitis is sometimes a diagnosis of exclusion, meaning it is only diagnosed when the doctors can't find any other cause for their symptoms. If your character's encephalitis is caused by a known virus, doctors might be able to detect the virus in the CSF. HSV encephalitis is associated with specific changes in the brain MRI and EEG, but this is not consistent across all causes of encephalitis. A lot of the time, there's simply no evidence for what exactly is causing your character's horrific illness. To call it frustrating is an understatement.

Worse, there isn't a cure. The treatment of encephalitis is mostly supportive, meaning that all the doctors can do is treat the complications of the disease. If your character stops breathing, they'll be put on a ventilator. If they start having seizures, the doctors will start anti-seizure meds. If your character is lucky, and the doctors find that the encephalitis is caused by HSV or CMV, they can treat it with antivirals. Mortality ranges from 2% (West Nile virus encephalitis) to 100% (rabies and acute disseminated encephalitis).[6] But even if they do survive, many will have serious neurologic sequelae, such as memory loss or seizures, that will last the rest of their lives.

Rabies causes a 100% fatal encephalitis. The only treatment is aggressive anti-rabies post-exposure vaccination prior to symptom development. Once symptoms develop, it is invariably fatal. The most common carrier of the rabies virus is bats.

If you want your character and their loved ones to go through h*ll—and *maybe* come out alive—encephalitis is the way to go.

NECROTIZING FASCIITIS

Fascia is the connective tissue deep below the skin; necrotizing means dying. Necrotizing fasciitis is a life-threatening infection of these deep soft tissues that causes massive tissue necrosis. Anyone can get it, but if your character is a diabetic, an IV drug user, or has had recent surgery or trauma, they're at a much higher risk.

The medical buzzword for necrotizing fasciitis is "pain out of proportion to exam." If your character has necrotizing fasciitis, they'll have a fever and a small lesion or discoloration of their skin. It won't look like much but when the healthcare provider touches the lesion, they will scream in pain or jump out of their chair.

Necrotizing fasciitis can progress rapidly, leading to sepsis and multi-organ failure. The treatment is emergency surgery to excise the dead tissue. Antibiotics are used as well, but the lifesaving, immediate treatment is surgery.

FEBRILE NEUTROPENIA

Febrile neutropenia is a condition that terrifies doctors. Neutropenia is a condition in which your character has very low numbers of a certain kind of white blood cell, called neutrophils, whose job it is to fight back against bacteria. However, the fever in febrile neutropenia is often indicative of a serious bacterial infection. Because the immune cells are gone, the body cannot fight off bacteria and such an infection might make your character very sick. Your character's immune system isn't fighting back because it can't and, in these instances, a fever might be the only sign that something is wrong.

Any infection can cause a fever in someone with neutropenia, though cellulitis, pneumonia, and bacteremia (a bacterial infection that has reached the bloodstream) are the most common causes. If your character has febrile neutropenia, they will be put in isolation—for their protection—and given a bunch of tests ranging from x-rays to blood cultures as their doctors scramble to try and figure out the source of the infection. They'll be put on the strongest IV antibiotics (called broad-spectrum antibiotics) immediately—even before the tests come back—and monitored closely. If they don't get better within 4-5 days (or if they don't die first), they'll also be put on IV anti-fungal medications.

TOXIC SHOCK SYNDROME (TSS)

Toxic shock syndrome is caused by a toxin produced by certain bacteria, particularly *Staphylococcus aureus* and *Streptococcus pyogenes*. The toxin works quickly and can be deadly. It starts with flu-like symptoms, such as high fever, headache, and muscle pain. Then a red, spotted rash develops, and your character will begin to have warm, flushed skin and bright red gums and tongue, known as "strawberry tongue." They may have nausea vomiting and diarrhea, confusion, and disorientation. Then, their blood pressure will start to tank. Their labs will show the beginnings of kidney failure, muscle breakdown, and dangerous drops in platelets (the blood cells responsible for clotting). Untreated, your character will die as their blood pressure plummets and their organs shut down.

> The "strawberry tongue" in scarlet fever and TSS look exactly the same—because they're caused by similar bacteria. The difference is that TSS is caused by the toxin while scarlet fever is a direct infection by the bacteria themselves.

TSS occurs when these bacteria have an ideal environment to breed and produce the toxin. The stereotypical example is in women who keep tampons in too long. However, tampons are not the only source; the bacteria can also breed in wounds or dirty bandages, burns, packed tissues or cotton balls from a nosebleed, or infected insect bites.

The first step in treatment is to remove the bacterial breeding ground, either by removing the source (tampon, bandages, etc.) or surgically draining or debriding the infected tissue. The next step is fluids and medications to stabilize their blood pressure, then IV antibiotics. As your character begins to recover, skin from their palms and soles of their feet will begin to slough off. And if your character has had TSS once, they are not immune; in fact, they are at greater risk of getting it again.

NON-INFECTIOUS CAUSES OF FEVER

Though infection is the most common cause of fever, it is not the only cause. Most of the time, non-infectious causes of fever are mild and are not accompanied by shakes, chills, night sweats, or increased heart rate. Often, these mild fevers are the first sign of blood cancer, such as leukemia or lymphoma, especially when coupled with unintentional weight loss. Below is a non-exhaustive list of some non-infectious causes of fever. It's beyond the scope of this book to detail all of them, but the general rule is that mild elevations in body temperature (99.5°F-104°F) are red flags for cancer or inflammation, while high fevers (> 104°F) are more likely to be caused by a life-threatening drug reaction.

> A low-grade fever and unintentional weight loss is a great way to introduce your character's previously undiagnosed cancer.

Cause	Condition	Fever Severity
Autoimmune	Blood transfusion	Mild
	Lupus	Mild
Cancer	Blood cancers (Lymphoma & Leukemia)	Moderate
	Neutropenic Fever	Mild but Life Threatening
	Tumor Fever	Mild, but intractable
Clots	Deep Vein Thrombosis	Mild
	Pulmonary Embolism	Mild
Drug Reactions	Antiretrovirals	Severe
	Neuroleptic Malignant Syndrome	Severe - Life Threatening
	Serotonin Syndrome	Severe - Life Threatening
	Sulfa drug allergy	Can be severe
Hormonal	Hyperthyroidism (Thyroid Storm)	Severe - Life Threatening
Inflammation	Appendicitis	Mild
	Gallstones	Mild
	Gout	Mild
	Pancreatitis	Mild
	Pneumonitis	Mild

FEVER OF UNKNOWN ORIGIN (FUO)

Fever of unknown origin is a fever that has lasted for at least three weeks (either continuously or on and off) and whose cause is still unknown despite a week of inpatient workup. If you're looking for a mysterious medical issue to foist on your character, this is a great one.

Most of the time, the fever still ends up being caused by an infection, usually something rare or hard to find, like tuberculosis or an

Often, fevers and weight loss are the first signs of blood cancers, like lymphomas and leukemias.

NATALIE DALE, MD

intrabdominal abscess. Sometimes, it's caused by a previously unknown cancer or autoimmune disease, a new drug, or one of the many non-infectious causes of fever. Often, the fever resolves without a diagnosis ever being made.

How FUO is treated depends on the severity of the fever and the frailty of the patient. If your character isn't super sick, they may not be given any treatment at all beyond inpatient observation.

BREAKING DOWN THE CLICHÉ: COUGH OF DEATH

Coughs into a handkerchief in first act

Dies of terrible disease in the third act

A cough is kind of like the medical equivalent of Chekhov's gun, especially if your character is coughing up blood. In some ways, this cliché works; there are plenty of horrific diseases that start with a chronic cough. Lung cancer, tuberculosis, heart failure, sarcoidosis, fibrotic lung disease, and chronic obstructive pulmonary disease (COPD) are a few causes of chronic cough that could legitimately kill your character.

But there are also a lot of causes of cough that aren't fatal. Colds, acid reflux, and seasonal allergies are some of the most common causes of chronic coughs, and you'd be hard-pressed to kill your character with any of those.

The other thing wrong with this cliché is that coughs are not generally the first sign of chronic or fatal disease. A mild fever—for no apparent reason—is often the first sign that your character has blood cancer, like leukemia or lymphoma. Unexplained weight loss is often the first sign of other forms of cancer, as well as many chronic diseases like inflammatory bowel disease (Crohn's disease, ulcerative colitis), Celiac disease, HIV/AIDS, dementia, diabetes, and even depression.

If you want to foreshadow that your character is going to battle an illness, go beyond the chronic cough. Once you've decided what that illness is, look up the initial presenting symptoms. Find the vaguest one (usually weight loss or fever) and sprinkle that into your story. You can still have ample foreshadowing but avoid the cliché of the bloody handkerchief.

6. SYNCOPE & SEIZURES

Francesca, a high school senior, stands at the starting line. It's her first race of the first track meet of the year; she's never been much for sports, and she only signed up for the track team to get out of the PE requirement. But now that she's here, she wants to win. Her heart pounds in her chest as she bends her knees into the set position. The starter gun booms, and she's off. Her legs pump as she forces herself to run, faster, faster, faster than she's ever run before. It's an 800m sprint—the fastest and hardest race—but it's also her best. She's giving it everything she can but as she rounds the bend to finish the first lap, the world suddenly goes black.

> Syncope is pronounced "Sing-Kuh-Pee".

FAINTING (SYNCOPE)

SYNCOPE IS THE MEDICAL TERM for fainting or passing out. It happens when, for one reason or another, the brain isn't getting enough blood flow. By definition, syncope is transient; if your character doesn't regain consciousness on their own within a minute or two, it isn't syncope. Syncope can be relatively harmless, or it can foreshadow something much worse.

CAUSES

The most common cause of syncope is fainting. Also called a *vasovagal response*, your character may faint during episodes of emotional distress, fear, pain, or fatigue. If your character has a vasovagal syncopal episode, they will know it's happening before they lose consciousness. This experience, called a *prodrome*,

> If your character faints at the sight of blood, that's **vasovagal syncope**.

may leave your character feeling lightheaded and nauseated, and they may even notice their vision darkening or hear roaring in their ears. Someone observing your character might notice that they become pale and sweaty. For the most part, vasovagal syncope is harmless in itself, though your character may hurt themselves if they fall wrong.

Another common cause of syncope is *orthostatic hypotension*, which is basically just a drop in blood pressure that occurs when your character stands up. It's very common in the elderly and in people with diabetes. Orthostatic hypotension is due to a combination of a low baseline blood pressure and a miscommunication of the part of the nervous system responsible for maintaining blood pressure. When your character stands, the appropriate reflexes don't kick in, so the blood doesn't get pumped up to the brain, and your character faints. Like vasovagal syncope, orthostatic hypotension is associated with a *prodrome*, including nausea, lightheadedness, sweating, ringing in the ears, etc.

Problems with the heart can also cause syncope. If your character has a syncopal episode due to a cardiac cause, they won't feel it coming. Instead, they'll just drop to the ground, unconscious. The exception is aortic stenosis (see below), which usually presents with dizziness and chest pain.

Cardiac causes of syncope include irregular heart rhythms (*arrhythmias*) and structural heart problems, such as narrowing of the valve leading from the heart to the aorta (*aortic stenosis)*. Common arrhythmias causing syncope include heartbeats that are too slow (*bradycardia*), too fast (*tachycardia*), or causing the heart to lose its rhythm altogether (*ventricular fibrillation,* or "v-fib"). Which cause you choose depends on your character.

If you need an older character to repeatedly faint (or fall) for no clear reason, consider *aortic stenosis*, a narrowing of the valve leading from the heart into the aorta. Aortic stenosis most often occurs in older people, usually due to plaque buildup on their valve, which becomes stiff and narrow. When their blood pressure drops, such as when they go from sitting to standing, the heart can't push enough blood through the narrowed valve, and in order to compensate, the blood flow to the brain drops, causing them to faint. Aortic stenosis is a great reason for your older character to have multiple unexplained falls and fainting episodes.

Congenital defects are ones that have been present since birth.

Acquired defects are ones that developed after birth.

On the other hand, if you want your young and healthy character to faint due to a heart problem, they will likely need a heart defect they were born with, called a congenital heart defect. **Wolff-Parkinson-White** (WPW) syndrome is a congenital heart defect that can cause deadly heart arrhythmias. Another option is a congenital problem with the heart muscle itself.

Francesca wakes up to her track team gathered around her, with worried expressions on their faces. She feels fine, other than a lump on her forehead; her teammates tell her she fell flat on her face. One of the parents—a doctor who volunteers as the medic for their team events—hurries over, stethoscope in hand. He helps Francesca sit up, then listens to her heart, frown lines deepening as he moves the stethoscope around different places on her chest. Finally, he tells her that she has a worrisome heart murmur and that she needs to go straight to the hospital.

Structural changes in the heart muscle can also lead to syncope. **Hypertrophic obstructive cardiomyopathy**, or HOCM, is the most common identifiable cause of sudden death in young athletes. It is a structural problem caused by an overgrowth of the heart muscle. Exercise, or a high heart rate, leads to manual obstruction of a heart valve, causing syncope or (if they're unlucky), sudden death. Schools and sports teams are supposed to screen for the heart murmur, but it isn't always caught in time.

A few other things can cause syncope, including low blood sugar (*hypoglycemia*), low blood pressure (*hypotension*), and strangulation or other mechanical compressions of the neck leading to decreased blood flow to the brain. Medications, especially those for high blood pressure, can cause syncope, especially if you have an elderly character whose bathroom looks like the inside of a pharmacy. But there's one cause of fainting spells that aren't syncope at all.

> **Convulsions** are uncontrolled muscle contractions. **Seizures** are electrical disturbances in the brain. Certain types of seizures cause convulsions.

> The **faceplant sign** is facial trauma (bruising, scrapes, etc.) incurred due to syncope without prodrome. Unlike in movies, people tend to fall forward when they faint without warning.

> HOCM is pronounced "hoe-kum."

SEIZURES (EPILEPSY)

Felix, Francesca's younger brother, was diagnosed with epilepsy when he was ten years old. But he takes his meds regularly and has been seizure-free for several years, so he hasn't told anyone except his best friend. Since he'd been good about taking his medications, his parents agreed to let him sit with his friends to watch his sister's track meet. Usually, they make him sit with them so that if he has a seizure, they can help him and make sure no one calls the ambulance again. He knows they mean well, but it makes him feel like a baby. So, he's excited to be sitting in the stands with his friends, sharing a bag of popcorn and talking more than watching the runners.

> Often, people with epilepsy wear bracelets explaining their condition and telling well-meaning passersby not to call an ambulance.

 NATALIE DALE, MD

Seizures are an electrical storm in the brain. There are many different types of seizures; some, but not all, cause convulsions. Lots of things can cause seizures, ranging from brain tumors and brain injury to drug overdose or withdrawal. If there is a clear reason for the seizure—alcohol withdrawal, brain tumor, brain injury, etc.—it is considered a provoked seizure. If there is no apparent cause, the seizure is considered unprovoked. Epilepsy is only diagnosed when your character has recurrent unprovoked seizures and the electrical pattern in their brain shows a particular pattern on an electroencephalogram (EEG).

SEIZURE TRIGGERS

Lots of things can trigger seizures, ranging from lack of sleep to brain infections. For people with epilepsy, the most common cause of seizures is not taking their epilepsy medications exactly as prescribed. You might think this is a stupid reason—if you have epilepsy, take your d*mn meds—but, it's more complicated than that. People with epilepsy can be extraordinarily sensitive to the levels of their medications. Taking their meds even an hour late (or an hour early) can be enough to trigger a seizure.

> An **electroencephalogram** (EEG) measures the electrical activity of the brain.

Lack of sleep and stress are also major contributors to seizures in people with epilepsy. Flashing lights can also be a trigger, as can drinking alcohol. Even things as seemingly mundane as menstrual cycles and skipping meals can be triggers.

"Hey, isn't that your sister?"

Felix turns to see Francesca collapsed on the ground, surrounded by coaches and a doctor. Fear runs up Felix's spine. He spins, searching for his parents, but they're already sprinting towards the track.

In people without epilepsy, the most common seizure trigger is alcohol withdrawal. Withdrawal from benzodiazepines and barbiturates can also cause seizures (see Volume 1: Setting & Character, Ch.17: Drugs & Addiction).[1] And while cocaine withdrawal does not result in seizures, acute cocaine intoxication can.

Other causes of provoked seizures include brain tumors, infections, stroke, fever, hyperthermia, brain bleeds or brain trauma, and extreme electrolyte imbalances.

SEIZURE TYPES

There are lots of different types of seizures. To figure out what type of seizure you want to give your character, you need to ask yourself two questions.

1. How much of the brain is involved?

2. Do I want them to be conscious throughout, or have altered consciousness?

If the whole brain is involved, it's a generalized seizure. Generalized seizures always result in altered consciousness. Your character won't remember the seizure. On the other hand, partial seizures—seizures that only affect part of the brain—can preserve consciousness during the seizure, though some cause altered consciousness as well. It's up to you to decide what kind of seizure you want your character to have.

> A **postictal state** is a state of abnormal consciousness that occurs after a seizure (see below).

If you want your character's whole brain to be involved, they will have altered consciousness and a postictal state. The most common and well-known of these full-brain seizures are tonic-clonic seizures, historically called "grand mal" seizures. Focal onset seizures occur when only part of your character's brain is involved. If your character has a focal onset seizure, you can choose whether or not they retain awareness and if they have a postictal state.

Onset	Altered Consciousness	Seizure Type	Behaviors	Postictal State
Focal onset	No	Focal onset aware (FOAS)	Retain awareness. Muscle twitching, single limb jerking, lip smacking, repeating words, picking, blank stare eye or head movements, hallucinations, numbness/tingling	No
	Yes	Focal onset impaired awareness (FOIAS)	Unaware and may be drowsy or unarousable. Behaviors otherwise similar to simple partial seizures	Yes
Generalized onset	Yes	Tonic-clonic ("Grand mal")	Sudden loss of consciousness + stiffening and jerking of all four limbs	Yes
	Yes	Atonic ("Drop")	Sudden loss of consciousness + loss of all muscle tone (drops to floor)	Yes
	Yes	Myoclonic	Sudden loss of consciousness + jerking muscles	Yes
	Yes	Absence	Sudden, brief (several seconds) loss of consciousness	No

Horrified, Felix moves to stand. He wants to run to his sister, to see if this is all a joke, to shake her until she stops lying on the ground like that. But he can't. His left big toe is twitching violently. Panic floods through him as the twitching moves up into the foot. Soon, his whole leg and arm are twitching violently. Not again….

A **Jacksonian march** is a type of focal aware seizure that spreads across the brain in a predictable pattern. Often, it will generalize into a tonic-clonic seizure.

You may have heard the stereotype that people with epilepsy smell burning tires before getting a seizure. That stereotype isn't completely wrong; people often get hallucinations of smell or taste right before a generalized tonic-clonic seizure. But that hallucination is actually another seizure, called a focal onset aware seizure (FOAS), or partial seizure.[2]

Seizures are kind of like fires in the brain—sometimes they start with a bang, other times they start in one small area and generalize to the whole brain. Auras are basically a focal onset aware seizure that is getting ready to spread to the rest of the brain. And it doesn't have to be smelling burning rubber. Auras can be experienced as:

- Hallucinations, usually smell (*olfactory hallucination*) or taste (*gustatory hallucination*)

Gustatory and olfactory hallucinations don't have to be unpleasant. I had a patient who tasted strawberries before her seizures.

- Visual disturbances (flashing lights, colors, etc.)

- Intense feelings of joy, sadness, or anxiety

- Intense déjà vu

- Stiffness, twitching, or convulsions of one extremity

- Numbness or tingling

- Rising feeling in the stomach (like the drop on a rollercoaster)

- Out-of-body experience

- Jacksonian march: numbness or twitching on one side of the body that starts small (usually in a finger or toe), then spreads, "marching" upwards to include the entire limb.

Remember, each and every one of these "auras" is actually a smaller, focal onset aware seizure that will spread and become a generalized seizure.

EXPERIENCE OF A SEIZURE

The experience of a seizure varies widely, so I'm going to focus on tonic-clonic (previously called "grand mal") seizures. If your character has a tonic-clonic seizure, they will suddenly lose consciousness and drop to the ground, their muscles become rigid as they extend outwards. This is called the *tonic* phase, and your character may stop breathing during this phase. Then, the *clonic* phase begins—a rhythmic jerking of all four extremities. During this period, they will probably lose control of their urine or feces and may bite their tongue, vomit, or even stop breathing. And while seizures only last for seconds to minutes, if your character is watching this happen, it will feel like forever.

If a seizure lasts more than five minutes, it's a medical emergency called **status epilepticus.**

If you want your character to look like they know what they're doing, have them move furniture away from the seizing character so that they can't hit anything hard or sharp while they're flailing around. They'll also check for a medical bracelet before calling 911; seizures aren't dangerous most of the time and people with epilepsy get seizures often enough that they would go bankrupt if an ambulance were called every time they seized (America!). And for the love of God, do *not* have them put anything in their mouth; biting their tongue is far preferable to choking and asphyxiating.

Finally, your character will go limp and start breathing normally again. When they wake up, they will be drowsy and confused. This is called a postictal state.

POSTICTAL STATE

The postictal state occurs after the seizure. Your character will be drowsy and confused. They may be unable to move half their body, cough, spit or salivate, or speak. They may also make repetitive motions, such as lip-smacking, face rubbing, or picking at their skin. Sometimes, they might even start doing some pretty bizarre things, like undressing, hallucinating, or speaking fluent gibberish. The seizure is over—an EEG can confirm that—but their brain isn't back to normal, either.

Your character probably won't be able to remember what happened or what they did while they were postictal. The postictal state ends when your character is back to feeling normal. While the postictal state can sometimes take hours, most of the time it only lasts 10-30 minutes. Even after the postictal state has resolved, your character may experience changes in their mood and concentration that can last for days after the event.

When Felix wakes, he's sitting on the cold metal floor between the benches. His friends are staring at him.

"Are you ok? You just…fell off your seat."

"How long?" Felix asks. He still feels a little out of it. The back of his head hurts—he probably slammed it into the metal benches at some point.

"You were down there forever."

"It was only a minute," a girl nearby says, pointing to her watch. "I timed it. I thought it might be a seizure."

"But you weren't twitching or anything," someone else cut in, "so I figured you'd just fainted. Like your sister."

Felix bites his lip; he doesn't have the energy to explain. One of the boys makes a spooky "oooooh" sound, but the girl with the watch shoots him a nasty look. Felix wonders why he doesn't recognize her.

"When you woke up, I thought you'd be ok," she continues, "but then you just kinda stared off and mumbled gibberish under your breath. Also…"

"You crapped your pants, dude," another boy cackles. Behind him, a girl snicker. The girl next to her has her cell phone out. Was she filming?

Felix flushes then reaches down. His pants are soaked in urine, and there's something warm and sticky in his underwear. He hesitates, paralyzed by the choice before him. If he gets up, he risks pieces of poop falling out of his shorts all the way to the bathroom. But he can't just stay here either. He forces himself to his feet and flees, tears streaming down his face as he hears laughter recede into the stands.

> If your POV character is the one to have the seizure, they'll need witnesses to tell them what happened. You get to decide how accurate and empathetic those witnesses are.

DIAGNOSIS & TREATMENT

Seizures can look like a lot of different things. It can look like a kid who gets lost in daydreams at school, an older woman smacking her lips, or a young, otherwise healthy man "fainting" for no reason. I even had one patient who took off her clothes and ran around a high school track.

> Atonic seizures are easy to mistake for syncope.

If your character has an unprovoked seizure for the first time, the first priority is to rule out the bad sh*t. The doctors will get blood tests to make sure they don't have low blood sugar or any crazy electrolyte balances, then a brain MRI to make sure there are no tumors or other structural anomalies. They'll also get an EEG to monitor the electrical activity of the brain, ideally within 72 hours of the seizure. If the standard EEG is negative, the workup might end there.

> For an EEG, 40 electrodes are glued to your character's scalp in a precise pattern. It takes a long time to put them on, and even longer to get the glue out of their hair.

There's a saying in neurology: "the first seizure is free." Somewhere between 8-10% of people will have an unprovoked seizure at some point in their life.[3] If your character is in that boat, they might just be in that unlucky population. Doctors will rule out the nasty causes, then shrug and write the seizure off as bad luck. If they have a second seizure, the chances they have epilepsy jump up to about 80%, and the neurologists will dig a little deeper to try and figure out the cause, usually with long-term EEG monitoring. For long-term monitoring, your character will spend 72 hours in the hospital, hooked up to the EEG monitor. They'll monitor your character while they sleep, or—if they're feeling impatient—keep your character awake to try and provoke a seizure.

> Epilepsy can only be diagnosed by seeing particular waveforms on an EEG. Not all convulsions are epileptic seizures.

The next week, Felix is brought to his doctor. She asks about the circumstances surrounding the seizure. Since he'd been taking his medications properly, but had a 'breakthrough' seizure, she decides to increase the dose of Felix's antiepileptic medicine.

If your character is diagnosed with epilepsy, they will be put on anticonvulsant medications. It can take a long time, and lots of trial and error, to find the right medication. But finding the right medication isn't the only adjustment your character will need to make.

COMPLICATIONS

Worst of all, the doctor informs Felix that, since he's no longer seizure-free, he won't be able to get his driver's license on his 16th birthday next week, as he'd planned. He'll have to keep his seizures at bay for another six months.

The aftermath of an unprovoked seizure can be far-ranging. Your character will not be allowed to drive for a while. Regulations vary by state, but it's usually around six months, with periodic medical checkups.[4] If your character is a pilot or commercial driver, they'll need to find a new career. Kids (and adults) with seizure disorders often suffer from learning disorders. But the scariest complication of a seizure disorder is status epilepticus.

STATUS EPILEPTICUS

Status epilepticus is an unrelenting seizure, a dangerous electrical storm lasting more than five minutes as it runs rampant through your character's brain. It is a life-threatening neurological emergency. Sometimes, there's an obvious cause—low blood sugar, infection, recent trauma, toxins, tumors, etc., but often, there isn't one—at least not right away. Your character doesn't have to be diagnosed with epilepsy to have status epilepticus; in fact, most cases of status epilepticus in adults are due to an underlying brain anomaly. If you were looking for a dramatic way to reveal your character's underlying brain tumor, this is it.

The medical shorthand for status epilepticus is just "status."

After it's been determined that the seizure is not due to an immediately reversible cause like low blood sugar, for instance, the first step in treatment is an injection of a benzodiazepine, such as a diazepam (given IV) or midazolam (given as in injection into the muscle). If they're still seizing ten minutes later, they're intubated and given a second-line anticonvulsant medication. If *that* fails, they're considered to be in 'refractory status epilepticus,' or RSE. RSE is treated with a barbiturate coma, one of the few indications for a true medically induced coma (see <u>Volume 1: Setting & Character</u>, *Ch. 19: Consciousness & Coma*).[5]

SEIZURES THAT AREN'T EPILEPSY (NON-EPILEPTIC SEIZURES)

Not all convulsions are caused by epilepsy. Sometimes, cardiac abnormalities can cause convulsions during syncopal events (see above). Low blood sugar, abnormal electrolyte levels, brain infections, brain tumors, and even low blood pressure can also cause non-epileptic seizures. But sometimes, doctors can't find an organic reason for the seizures, and the character is diagnosed with *psychogenic non-epileptic seizure* or PNES.

If your character has PNES, they will experience seizure-like symptoms that are not caused by electrical changes in the brain. In other words, they will have all the symptoms of a seizure—convulsions, loss of bowel or bladder control, hip-thrusting, repetitive movements— but the EEG will come back totally normal. So, if the seizures aren't caused by changes to the brain, what causes them?

PNES is a primarily female disorder that can't be diagnosed using objective tests. It's the perfect disease if you want your character to not be taken seriously by the medical community.

PNES is considered to be an extreme stress response that is often seen in people with PTSD, anxiety, mood disorders, personality disorders, and extreme life stressors. Survivors of rape and abuse frequently develop this disorder, and women are much more likely to develop PNES than men. For a long time, this condition was called "pseudo seizures," and people suffering from it were treated as attention-seeking frauds. Since PNES isn't caused by electrical changes in the brain, it can't be treated with the same medications used for epilepsy. Instead, the mainstay of treatment is therapy and treatment of the underlying psychiatric disorder. But there is still a lot of stigma surrounding PNES.

BREAKING THE CLICHÉ: ALL SEIZURES ARE GRAND MAL

"Felipe? Felipe?"

Felipe continues to stare into space, his eyes focused on something outside the window. His dad rubs at his temples. It's been a rough week. His daughter is in the hospital for a yet undiagnosed heart condition, and his middle son shat himself after another epileptic seizure. He doesn't have time to deal with his youngest son's daydreaming.

> Absence seizures are diagnosed in childhood and can often be mistaken for daydreaming or ADD.

"Damnit, Fil, don't you ever listen?"

Felipe turns, his eyes suddenly focused. "Sorry, Dad, what?"

Not all seizures are the stereotypical unconscious person writhing around like they've been possessed. Generalized tonic-clonic seizures account for only about 25% of all seizures.[6] Partial seizures (seizures in which only part of the body is affected) account for about 70% of all seizures in people older than eighteen.[7] Absence seizures, such as the one described above account for 10-17% of all epilepsies in children.[8]

7. STROKE

BACKGROUND

STROKE—THE MEDICAL TERM IS A *cerebrovascular accident*, or CVA—occurs when brain cells die, causing a sudden malfunctioning of the body. Anyone can have a stroke, though your character may be at higher risk if they have certain risk factors. There are two main types of strokes: ischemic and hemorrhagic.

ISCHEMIC STROKES

> *Giselle is watching TV with her husband, George when she notices something strange. He's eating with his right hand—clumsily since he's been left-handed his whole life.*
>
> *"George," she says, stepping forward and placing a hand on his left shoulder. But he doesn't move, just keeps watching the television.*

Ischemic stroke occurs when one of the arteries supplying the brain is blocked, depriving the brain cells of oxygen. About 85% of strokes are ischemic, and risk factors for ischemic stroke are similar to the risks for myocardial infarctions—high blood pressure, high cholesterol, diabetes, and cigarette smoking.[1] In fact, an ischemic stroke is pretty much the brain equivalent of a myocardial infarction or a heart attack.

There are two main causes of ischemic stroke: thrombosis and embolism. A thrombotic stroke occurs when a blood clot forms in the arteries of the brain. Thrombosis is usually caused by plaque buildup in the arteries. Embolic strokes, on the other hand, are blood clots that come from somewhere else in the body and get stuck in the artery. Most of the time, these embolisms come from the heart, particularly if your character has certain arrhythmias, like *atrial fibrillation*, or diseases of their heart valves (See *Ch. 2: Trouble Breathing*). Embolisms can also come from the carotid artery,

> **Atrial fibrillation** is a common heart arrhythmia that leads to the formation of blood clots in the upper chambers of the heart.

in the neck. If your character has a hole in their heart (usually a congenital malformation called a *patent foramen ovale*) the clot could come from a deep vein thrombosis or DVT (See *Ch. 1: Chest Pain*).

Ischemic strokes cause sudden and dramatic symptoms called *neurological deficits* (see below). These deficits—such as facial droop, arm weakness, or trouble speaking—occur suddenly and are not usually accompanied by pain.

HEMORRHAGIC STROKE

A *hemorrhagic stroke*, on the other hand, occurs when there is bleeding on the brain. These bleeds are usually caused by weakened blood vessels, such as aneurysms—outpouching of the wall of the blood vessel. While these types of strokes are rare, hemorrhagic strokes are more common in younger people. One study found that 50% of all hemorrhagic strokes occurred in people under the age of 45.[2] So if you're looking to give your young character a stroke, hemorrhagic is probably your best bet.

Hemorrhagic strokes look different than ischemic strokes. First, they usually start with a sudden, intense headache. Often described as "thunderclap headaches," these headaches come on suddenly and are often associated with signs of increased pressure in the brain, like vomiting and loss of consciousness. There are two main types of hemorrhagic stroke: intracerebral and subarachnoid.

Intracerebral hemorrhage (ICH) is bleeding directly into the brain tissue. It's the second most common type of stroke and is usually caused by high blood pressure.4. Blood thinners, brain tumors, alcohol, and illicit drugs like cocaine and amphetamines, also increase the risk.4 While large hemorrhages tend to present with sudden and severe headaches along with nausea/vomiting, and loss of consciousness, smaller hemorrhages may not cause a headache at all. Instead, a small hemorrhage might only cause a focal neurologic deficit, mimicking an ischemic stroke.

Subarachnoid hemorrhage (SAH) is a brain bleed that occurs just outside the brain tissue. The buzz-phrase for a subarachnoid headache is the "worst headache of their life." Other symptoms include a stiff neck (due to the irritation of the lining around the brain), nausea/vomiting, sensitivity to light (photophobia), confusion, double vision, and even seizures. Focal neurologic deficits, such as trouble speaking, facial droop, or one-sided paralysis are also common.

The most common cause of a subarachnoid hemorrhage is trauma (See *Ch. 12: Traumatic Brain Injuries*). However, the next most common cause is a burst berry aneurysm—a bulging or outpouching of a blood vessel within the brain. Most aneurysms don't cause any symptoms until they burst, so if you're looking for a

 NATALIE DALE, MD

sudden way to suddenly kill off a character, a subarachnoid hemorrhage caused by a burst aneurysm might just be your ticket.

Most brain aneurysms cause no symptoms. However, if you're looking to foreshadow your character's soon-to-burst aneurysm, there are a few symptoms you can leave as clues for your reader. Most berry aneurysms occur towards the front of the brain. Symptoms may include a headache that always occurs in the same spot (usually right behind one eye), one eyelid that droops, or blurry/double vision.

<u>**Signs & Symptoms**</u>

Giselle steps in front of the television.

"George, you're dropping crumbs…" she trails off as she sees George's face, the left side of his lips pulled down.

"Give me your hand—no, the other one," she snaps as he lifts his right hand towards her.

"I did," he replies, clearly annoyed that she's standing between him and his program. Giselle, remembering her father's stroke when she was a child, knows it is time to call 911.

FAST

The easy, CDC-approved way to look for the common signs of stroke is to use the mnemonic FAST.

F = Facial droop
A = Arm weakness
S = Speech difficulty
T = Time to call 911

This acronym is often printed on signs at clinics and hospitals; having a character read this sign might be a good way to foreshadow things to come.

Facial droop occurs when the muscles in the face are no longer innervated by the brain. The lower edge of the lips drops, and your character will be unable to smile or bare their teeth on that side. To test for facial droop, have your character ask the victim to smile.

Arm weakness is another common sign of stroke. They may be able to move it a bit (weakness), or they may be completely paralyzed. The arm may also feel numb. Leg weakness is also common in stroke. To test for arm weakness, your character should ask the victim to raise both arms with their eyes closed, then see if one drifts downward.

Speech difficulty may mean that your character is stuttering, slurring their words, or having difficulty making words. They may even speak in gibberish. For the test for speech difficulty, have your character ask the victim to repeat a simple phrase; something easy, like "I went to the store today"—no tongue twisters!

If you want to quickly signal to your reader that your character is having a stroke, you can use the FAST mnemonic and most people will understand what is happening. However, if you want to dive deeper into the world of stroke, you'll need to understand neurologic deficits and which deficits tend to occur together.

NEUROLOGICAL DEFICITS

The ambulance takes George and Giselle to the hospital, despite George's assertations that nothing is wrong. Once they're in a room, a neurologist who introduces herself as Dr. Gao performs a thorough neurologic exam over George's objections. She asks him to smile, but he can only smile on the right side of his face. He follows her fingers with his eyes, but only to the right. When she snaps her fingers in the left side of his face, he doesn't even blink. She asks him to lift his arms, then his legs—both times he only moves the left. When she picks up his left arm, it drifts slowly down. He's able to name and remember several objects, but when the doctor asks him to draw a clock, he draws all the numbers on the right side. When she asks if that's what a clock looks like, he insists that the drawing is correct.

Contralateral means symptoms occur on the opposite side of the body as the brain injury. **Ipsilateral** means symptoms occur on the same side as the injury.

A stroke produces *neurological deficits*—abnormal bodily functions due to injury of a specific part of the brain. For the most part, neurologic deficits occur on the opposite side of the body from where the brain injury happened. So, if your character's stroke occurred on the left side of their brain, they'll have symptoms on the right side of their body. The exception is the eyes, which are stupidly complicated (more on that later).

It is also important to note that the brain has slightly different functions on the left vs. right side, called hemispheres. It also experiences "handedness," meaning that the brain tends to have a dominant hemisphere. For the most part, the dominant hemisphere is the one where language is processed. For instance, if your character is right-handed, their language center will be on the left side of the brain. If they're left-handed, it's a little more complicated; about 70% of left-handed people process language on the left hemisphere, but 30% process language in the right hemisphere.[3] As a writer, this means you can use left-handed characters to throw off the doctors when they come into the ED with signs of a stroke, especially if they forget to ask the all-important question: is your character left or right-handed?

Common neurologic deficits include:

Facial droop is the weakness of the muscles in the face. In stroke, this weakness usually affects the lower half of the face—the forehead is often spared, meaning your character will be able to lift their eyebrows. If you want to make your relatively young character develop stroke-like symptoms (without actually giving them a stroke), you can give them **Bell's Palsy**, a nerve palsy that causes drooping of the upper and lower face. Bell's palsy is self-limiting, meaning that it almost always improves on its own, though some medications can hasten recovery.

Limb weakness, or *paresis*, occurs on the opposite side of the body (contralateral) to the location of the injury. Severity can range from mild weakness to complete paralysis.

Neglect means that your character will completely ignore half of their body. It is a crazy phenomenon to observe. Your character might completely ignore everything, even large objects, or other people, on their neglected side. If your character is asked to draw a clock, they'll cram all the numbers into the one side they can acknowledge. They may even refuse to use that half of their body, despite having no weakness or paralysis. Crazier yet, they often have no idea that they have a deficit. This is called *anosognosia*. Spatial neglect can be a subtle sign of stroke if you're looking to delay a character's diagnosis.

> Having a deficit but not realizing it is a neurologic condition called **anosognosia**.

Sensory deficits, like hand numbness, occur contralateral to the location of the injury. Sensory deficits include the inability to feel soft touch, pressure, pain, and temperature.

Speech difficulty, called *aphasia*, comes in two different forms. *Broca's aphasia*, also called expressive aphasia, causes difficulty speaking. Your character will stutter and struggle to find the appropriate words, but they will be able to understand what is said to them. *Wernicke's Aphasia*, on the other hand, causes difficulty understanding language. They'll be able to speak fluently and easily, but their words will make little sense and they won't be able to comprehend speech.

Dysarthria is another type of speech difficulty, but it is not a problem with language processing. Instead, it is caused

> **Broca's aphasia** is incredibly frustrating for the person suffering from it. They understand what is going on and just can't find the words they need. People with **Wernicke's aphasia**, on the other hand, don't tend to notice their deficit.

by weakness or paralysis of the muscles of the tongue and voice box. Dysarthria causes slurred and slowed speech. Your character won't have any difficulty finding or understanding words, they'll just have trouble physically forming the words.

Vision changes are extremely complicated. The neurologic pathways leading from the retina to the brain tend to cross and uncross at crazy intervals. I don't recommend going into heavy detail on vision changes, since it is elaborate. Instead, here are a few high-yield facts to keep in mind.

- Loss of vision in one eye (unilateral vision loss) is an eye or nerve problem, not a brain problem.

- The brain splits the visual field (i.e., the area your character sees) into four quadrants. Most types of strokes will cause *hemianopia*, meaning loss of half of a visual field. This means your character won't be able to see anything on one side of their nose, and their eyes will deviate to the opposite side. To test for hemianopia, have your character leave both eyes open, and place a divider (a hand works) on the nose. Despite having both eyes open, they won't be able to see anything on the opposite side of that divider.

> **Visual field =** the left/right, top/bottom of your character's vision.

RARE NEUROLOGICAL DEFICITS

There are also some rare neurological deficits that, as a writer, you might find will fit well into your story. These deficits are a bit more unusual but common enough that no one will bat an eyebrow if you throw them into your story:

- **Abulia** = loss of motivation, willpower, or ability to make decisions

  o Can also be seen in people with mental illness

- **Acalculia** = loss of previous ability to perform simple calculations

- **Achromatopsia** = inability to perceive colors

- **Agraphia** = loss of previous ability to write

- **Alexia** = loss of ability to read (but can still write)

- **Anosognosia** = inability to comprehend their illness or deficit

  o Can also be seen in patients with mental illness

- **Apraxia** = inability to perform movements on command

- **Ataxia** = loss of control of muscles

- **Disinhibition** = loss of filter, inability to control reactions, increased impulsivity

- **Prosopagnosia** = inability to recognize faces, even of familiar people

LOCALIZING THE LESION

Unfortunately, you can't just throw a bunch of neurologic deficits together to give your character their symptoms. This is because the types of neurologic deficits that occur are determined by where in the brain the problem lies. Because of this, certain deficits tend to occur together, allowing doctors to figure out where the stroke occurred based on the symptoms your character is exhibiting; this is called *localization* or *localizing the lesion*. It's the bread and butter of neurology, and one of the most incredible and fun things about the specialty. But it is also way too complicated to get into too much detail here. Instead, I'll go over the three most common areas where strokes occur and describe how your character would look and feel if they had a stroke at that location. Finally, I'll talk about the dreaded basilar artery stroke, more commonly known as "locked-in-syndrome."

> Neurologic deficits usually occur on the **opposite** side of the body from where the injury occurred. So, if your character's stroke is on the right side of the brain, they'll experience left-sided symptoms.

Side of the brain: The side of the brain—fed by the middle cerebral artery (MCA)—is the most common location of a stroke. In fact, almost 90% of strokes occur in this area.1 A stroke in this region can cause a lot of problems. These include:

- Weakness, paralysis, and/or loss of sensation on the opposite side of the body from the lesion.

    o Arm and face weaknesses most common

- Loss of half their visual field (*homonymous hemianopsia*)

- Difficulty speaking (*aphasia*) if the stroke occurred on the left hemisphere (more common)

    o Left MCA strokes may also cause acalculia, agraphia, alexia, apraxia, and dysarthria

- Neglect of the left half of the body if a stroke occurred in the right hemisphere

    o Right MCA strokes may also cause anosognosia

Front of the brain: The front of the brain, fed by the *anterior cerebral artery* (ACA), is where executive functioning and personality reside. For this reason, strokes here tend to cause personality and cognitive changes, including abulia, executive dysfunction, and disinhibition. Leg weakness and urinary incontinence also occur with ACA stroke.

> **Executive functioning** is your character's ability to plan, organize , and control their behavior.

Back of the brain: The back of the brain, fed by the *posterior cerebral artery* (PCA), is where visual processing occurs. Strokes here mainly cause vision changes, such as double vision (*diplopia*), visual changes, and even cortical blindness—a condition wherein the eyes work, but the brain can't process the input. Your character will be unable to see, though they may vehemently deny being blind. They may also exhibit *blindsight*—the ability to navigate a maze or catch an object thrown at them, despite being unable to see. Other visual dysfunctions stemming from PCA stroke include:

> There are many different types of visual field defects that can occur in a **PCA stroke**, depending on the exact location.

- Alexia without agraphia: Inability to read without losing the ability to write.

- Achromatopsia: Inability to perceive colors.

- Prosopagnosia: Inability to recognize faces.

Strokes in this area can also cause sensory loss and difficulty controlling the limbs (*limb ataxia*).

Base of the brain: Along the base of the brain runs a single large artery, called the basilar artery. A stroke here results in a terrifying condition called locked-in-syndrome, in which your character loses all control of every muscle in their body except for a few tiny muscles in their eyes. Their consciousness is preserved, meaning that they are awake and cogent, but unable to move, literally, locked inside their body. The only muscles they can move are those of their upper eyelid and (sometimes) the upper eye, meaning that they can blink and move their eyeball upward: that's it.

Since they can't control their diaphragm—the muscle that controls breathing—they need to have a ventilator breathe for them. They also can't swallow, so they'll need to be fed through a tube in their stomach. They'll be fully conscious and able to think and feel everything going on around them, but unable to move or communicate complex ideas. I'm a pretty creative person, but I have trouble thinking of a worse fate.

DIAGNOSIS

After the exam, Dr. Gao orders a CT of George's brain. When it comes back, the doctor says that George has had an ischemic stroke—he needs to be given clot-busting medications and admitted to the hospital.

When your character arrives at the ED with symptoms of stroke, they'll get a quick neurologic exam from the doctor before being whisked back for a head CT to look for blood and rule out a hemorrhagic stroke. After that, if they're stable, they'll be given a brain MRI, along with several blood tests. They may also be given an echocardiogram to look for possible sources of a clot.

TREATMENT

Treatment of stroke is time-dependent; the faster your character gets treatment, the more likely they are to recover. If your character has an ischemic stroke, and it's been less than 3 hours since their symptoms started, they'll probably be given clot-busting medications called thrombolytics. If your character is at a large teaching hospital—a large, tertiary hospital usually associated with a university—they will instead thread a wire through an artery in their groin and into the vessels of the brain to manually pull out the clot, a procedure called *percutaneous vascular intervention* (PCI). However, if it's been more than 24 hours since symptoms set in, the treatment is just to give aspirin and hope for the best.

If your character has a hemorrhagic stroke, their options are even worse. The blood is already on the brain, so all the doctors can really do is control the blood pressure, stop any medications that might worsen the bleeding (such as aspirin and blood thinners), and control the pressure in the brain itself. Sometimes, neurosurgery can be performed to try and stop the bleeding and minimize the pressures in the brain.

Small intracerebral hemorrhages generally have a good prognosis. Large subarachnoid hemorrhages have the worst prognosis.

Brain bleeds, such as hemorrhagic strokes, are one of the few legitimate reasons your character might be put into a therapeutic coma—the medical term for a "medically-induced coma." Blood on the brain irritates the brain tissue, causing brain swelling. Since the brain is encased in the skull, if the brain swells too much, it will squelch out of the hole leading into the spinal cord, compressing the brainstem and killing your character. In order to prevent this, doctors may give your character sedating medications to quiet their brain and minimize swelling (called a therapeutic, or medically induced coma). But remember: this procedure is only done if your character is already in very, very bad shape. Do not expect them to wake up from a therapeutic coma without some serious brain damage.

RECOVERY & PROGNOSIS

After a few days in the hospital, George is beginning to improve. He still won't look to the left, but he at least acknowledges there might be a problem. He is discharged to a rehabilitation hospital.

Time is tissue; the faster your character receives care, the better their chances are for recovery. However, it can be difficult for doctors to predict who will recover and who will not. As a writer, you can use this uncertainty to your advantage.

Recovering from a stroke is a long process. On average, your character will need to stay in the hospital for about five days for an ischemic stroke; eight if the stroke was hemorrhagic.[5] But your character probably won't get to go home straight from the hospital. Instead, they'll be sent to a rehabilitation hospital.

Rehabilitation hospitals are inpatient facilities that specialize in getting patients back to their previous level of functioning. To do this, they provide physical therapy, occupational therapy, and speech therapy, along with nursing and medical care. Along with stroke patients, rehab hospitals also treat victims of traumatic brain injury, recent amputees, people with major fractures, and heart attack victims, among other things. If your character has had a stroke, they should expect to stay at the rehab hospital for about two weeks—longer if their deficits are more severe.

For more on the setting of a rehabilitation hospital, see Volume 1: Setting & Character, Ch. 7: Other Settings.

STROKE LOOK-ALIKES

If you want your character to have symptoms of a stroke, but you don't want them to have residual brain damage and a long-term path to recovery, there are a few conditions you can use to mimic a stroke.

TRANSIENT ISCHEMIC ATTACK (TIA)

A TIA is basically a reversible stroke. Blood flow to an artery in the brain gets blocked and your character has all the symptoms of a stroke. But then the blockage is spontaneously cleared without any medical intervention, and the symptoms go away. TIA is often considered a precursor to a bigger ischemic stroke. So, if you're looking to foreshadow a bigger stroke coming down the pipeline, TIA is a great option.

A TIA will not show up on imaging like a CT or MRI of the brain. For this reason, TIA's can be easily dismissed or overlooked by medical professionals. If you're looking to widen a schism between your character and the medical community, having their TIA symptoms dismissed is, unfortunately, a realistic situation.

MIGRAINE

You'd think that it would be pretty easy to tell the difference between a migraine and a stroke, but there is some crazy overlap. First, migraine auras can simulate a stroke. Auras are sensations that precede the actual headache portion of the migraine. Typical auras include flashing lights or blurry vision, but they can also mimic a stroke. Some of the stroke-mimicking auras include:

- Numbness or tingling on half the body

- Difficulty speaking or inability to speak

- Loss of vision in one eye

- Vertigo (feeling like the world is spinning)

There are also migraines called *hemiplegic migraines* that are characterized by numbness, weakness, or even complete paralysis on one-half of the body. These symptoms can last for hours or even days, only for the headache to set in later.

Like with TIA, migraines do not cause any changes to the brain imaging. Migraines can easily be confused with a TIA. But unlike stroke and TIA, migraines usually start slowly and ramp-up. And while people with migraines have an increased lifetime risk of having a stroke, it's not the blaring warning signal that a TIA is.

BREAKING DOWN THE CLICHÉ: THE MEDICALLY INDUCED COMA

> *"We had to put your wife into a medically induced coma after her car accident. We'll give her body some time to heal, and in a few months, she'll wake up and you'll be able to talk with her."*

In Volume 1, I devoted an entire chapter to comas, and I spent a lot of that chapter talking about the mythical "medically induced coma." But this is an important concept (and one that writers seem to get wrong a lot), so I'm going to cover it again here, just not quite as in-depth. If you want a full description, please see <u>Volume 1: Setting & Character</u>, Ch.19: Consciousness and Coma.

A coma is a description of a state of consciousness—it is not a diagnosis in and of itself. If your character is in a coma, it means that they are unresponsive to external stimuli. Your character's level of consciousness will be graded on the **Glasgow Coma Scale** (see *Ch. 12: Traumatic Brain Injuries*); a score of < 8 is considered a severe injury.

Comas don't just happen; your character needs an underlying reason to be in a coma. There are lots of reasons your character could be in a coma, including:

- Lack of oxygen to the brain (*Anoxic brain injury)*

- Strangulation, asphyxiation, or drowning

- Ischemic stroke

- Carbon monoxide poisoning

- Hemorrhagic stroke

- Traumatic brain injury

- Electrolyte imbalance

- Diabetes (blood sugar that is too high or too low)

- Drugs and alcohol

Ischemia = lack of blood supply to cells, tissues, or organs.

If your character is in a coma, their prognosis is generally determined by the cause of the coma AND the duration of time spent in the coma. Comas due to drugs, alcohol, and diabetes usually have a better prognosis if they are reversed quickly. Comas due to lack of oxygen (*anoxic injury*) have the worst prognosis. Most comas last for no more than 2-3 weeks, but the ones with the best chance of a full recovery usually last for minutes to hours. The longer your character is comatose, the less believable their recovery will become.

A therapeutic coma—the medical term for a "medically induced coma"—occurs when doctors give medications to induce a coma. It is a last-ditch treatment option, used only when doctors need to dampen brain function as much as physically possible. There are only two scenarios (technically three) where doctors use a therapeutic coma: **refractory status epilepticus** and **increased intracranial pressures**.

Refractory status epilepticus (RSE) is a condition of continuous seizures that are not responding to anti-seizure medications. These unrelenting seizures are caused by an electrical storm in the brain; the purpose of a therapeutic coma is to use medications to dampen as much of that electrical activity as possible to quell the storm. It's a little bit like dousing a grease fire by smothering it with a blanket.

For more on seizures, see *Ch. 6: Syncope & Seizures.*

Increased intracranial pressures (increased ICP) - high pressure inside the skull—is caused by brain swelling. The normal response of tissue to injury is swelling (think about a sprained ankle or jammed finger)—and the same is true of brain tissue. But the brain is encased in the hard, immoveable casing of the skull. So, when the brain tissue starts to swell, it has nowhere to go—except for the hole in the base of the skull leading down into the spinal cord. If the brain squishes out into this hole, it cuts off the brainstem and kills your character. This is called *brain herniation*, and it is inevitably fatal. Increased ICP is most often caused by brain bleeds (the blood irritates the brain tissue, causing more swelling), but can be caused by other types of brain injury as well. A therapeutic coma decreases swelling by decreasing brain activity and is used alongside a whole host of other therapies (including neurosurgery) to lower the pressures in the brain.

The third reason for a therapeutic coma isn't a coma at all—it's general anesthesia. Anesthesiologists use medications to make your character fall unconscious and unresponsive to all external stimuli. After the procedure, they reverse the effects of the anesthesia, and your character wakes up. The only real difference is that, for general anesthesia, your chara cter doesn't have any underlying condition that will keep them in the comatose state after the medications are reversed.

A therapeutic coma is a last-ditch effort to quiet down the brain and prevent your character from dying. It is not used to give them time to heal injuries anywhere else in their body. It also is not a long-term strategy; people are in a therapeutic coma for a few days, not weeks or months.

Finally, if your character needs to be placed in a therapeutic coma, they are very, very ill. So ill that they will probably die; mortality for RSE is around 40-60%, while mortality for brain injury with a GCS <8 is nearly 80%.[1,2] Furthermore, if your character survives, they will almost undoubtedly have a residual brain injury and will live out the rest of their life with severe disability. Even with a "good recovery" (a designation applied to less than 10% of coma patients) most will still have disabilities severe enough that they can no longer work.[3]

While recovery from comas certainly happen, the chances of your character recovering from a severe anoxic brain injury leading to a long-term coma are abysmal. They're more likely to win the lottery and be bitten by a shark the same day.

I'm fixating on these recovery statistics because coma recovery is an overused trope that has real consequences. It broke my heart to see how many families clung to the thought of their loved ones "waking up" from their coma. They'd seen it happen so often—in books, tv, and movies—that they truly believed it would happen to them. They spent hundreds of thousands of dollars, went into incredible debt, and spent weeks/months/years holding out hope, only for their loved one to die of complications of the coma, which is by far the most likely outcome. So, before you put your main character into a coma, please consider the real-life ramifications of treating a miraculous recovery like it's an everyday expectation.

8. PREGNANCY & CHILDBIRTH

Himari hasn't slept in nearly 72 hours. She's 37 weeks pregnant and has been having contractions every 6-10 minutes for the last three days. She called her midwife when the contractions started, but she told Himari not to go into the hospital until her contractions were less than five minutes apart and lasting for at least an hour. Since then, Himari has done everything in her power to get comfortable—warm baths, aromatherapy, even a Tylenol PM to help her sleep, but nothing helps. How the #$% is she supposed to sleep when it feels like her uterus is trying to turn itself inside out every six minutes?

> The 5-1-1 rule states that women should go to the hospital when their contractions are 5 minutes apart, and last 1 minute each, for at least 1 hour.

ANATOMY 101

FOR THOSE OF YOU WHO failed sex ed, here's a quick overview of the human reproductive system. *Ovaries* produce and ripen eggs (*ova*). Every month, one spits out an egg, which travels down the *Fallopian tube.* If met by a man's *sperm*, it becomes fertilized and implants in the *uterus,* which has prepared all month with a bloody lining that will ultimately become the *placenta*. The *cervix*—the tight, muscular entrance to the uterus—keeps the fetus safe inside while it gestates. If the egg isn't fertilized, it gets washed out, along with the remains of the lining in a bloody rush called *menstruation.*

When it's time to be born, the uterus contracts, forcing the fetus's head downward onto the cervix to soften and open it (this process is called *cervical ripening*). The fetus is pushed down the vaginal canal, squeezing between the pubic bone (*pubic symphysis)* and the tailbone (*coccyx),* to emerge from the vagina as a baby.

PREGNANCY

Pregnancy is one of those weird things that is at once totally natural and completely terrifying. Most writers probably have a good idea of what a normal pregnancy should look and feel like (many of you have probably experienced it yourselves), so I'm going to keep this section brief.

PREGNANCY TIMELINES

A normal pregnancy lasts about 40 weeks; the first trimester is defined as weeks 1-12, the second trimester is weeks 13-26, and the third trimester lasts from week 27 to delivery. Babies born before 37 weeks are considered premature; less than 28 weeks are extremely premature. Babies born at 24 weeks or less have a 0-10% chance of survival.[1] Babies delivered after 42 weeks are post-term.

About one in ten infants are born preterm.[1] Many go on to live healthy lives but the earlier a baby is born, the harder it will have to fight to survive.

Definition	Timeline
Preterm Delivery	20-37 weeks
Full Term Delivery	37-42 weeks
Post term Delivery	>42 weeks

When Himari was 26 weeks pregnant, she thought she was having contractions, irregular mildly painful cramping that came and went with no apparent pattern. Himari had panicked, scared she was going into preterm labor and called her midwife. They turned out to be nothing more than Braxton Hicks contractions. Now, Himari can only laugh at herself for imagining that those contraction were real labor.

Braxton Hicks contractions are mild, irregular, and do not cause cervical change.

Pregnancy is dated from the first day of the woman's last period. Weirdly, this means that the woman won't conceive until two weeks after the start of pregnancy. Most women won't find out they're pregnant until they're about five to six weeks pregnant; even the earliest home pregnancy tests can't detect pregnancy until around the first day of her missed period, or the fourth week of pregnancy. This period of uncertainty is a great source of tension for your characters. There's the old "pregnancy scare" trope (a woman having unprotected sex, then having to wait two whole weeks to

A woman's due date is just an estimate—only about 5% of women deliver on their due date. If the baby is born anywhere from 37-42 weeks, they are considered on time **(full term)**.[2]

find out if she's gotten knocked up), but there's also a lot of room for more original storylines. Your character may find out she's pregnant, only to realize that the seemingly innocuous blood pressure medication she's on causes horrible birth defects when taken in the first trimester. Conversely, your character may be trying for pregnancy and takes the test too early, thus receiving a heartbreaking (but false!) negative. The world's your oyster on this one.

GRAVIDITY & PARITY

Doctors refer to a woman's obstetrical history in terms of gravidity (# of pregnancies) and parity (# of children); a woman who is G3P2 has been pregnant three times and has two living children. The third pregnancy may have ended in abortion, miscarriage, stillbirth, or even death after birth. Doctors generally don't use this terminology when talking to their patients, but it will generally be the first thing out of their mouths when talking to other healthcare providers.

> The medical term for a woman who has never given birth is **nulliparous**.

PRENATAL & OBSTETRICAL CARE

There are four types of practitioners who care for pregnant women and deliver babies. Whomever they chose as their healthcare provider, your character will visit them at least eight times for routine prenatal visits during their pregnancy—more if she has preexisting conditions or develops worrisome symptoms.

Midwives are healthcare professionals specializing in pregnancy, childbirth, and preventative women's health. They care for women at low risk of complications from pregnancy/childbirth and can facilitate either home or hospital births.[2] They cannot perform cesareans, though they can assist the physician who does.

Family Practice Physicians are doctors specialized in providing primary care and provide pregnancy care to low-risk women. Historically, family physicians delivered babies as well, but with the rise in litigation in the US, this practice is becoming less and less common.[3] Most can't perform caesarian deliveries (c-sections), as they are not trained as surgeons.

> A **c-section** is a surgical procedure used to deliver a baby.

Obstetricians-Gynecologists (Ob/Gyn) are doctors who specialize in women's health. They care for all sorts of women, ranging from low risk to relatively high risk, and almost always have their patients deliver their babies in a hospital setting. They can perform c-sections and are the most common choice for pregnant women.

Maternal-Fetal Medicine Physicians (MFM), also called perinatologists, are Ob/Gyn doctors specializing in high-risk pregnancies. They can perform specialized procedures, such as *amniocentesis* (testing the amniotic fluid for genetic conditions in the body) as well as c-sections. If your character needs an MFM doctor, they will have to deliver in the hospital with close monitoring.

> If your character has preeclampsia, she should be seen by an MFM doc.

The first ultrasound, called the dating ultrasound, usually occurs around 8 weeks of pregnancy and gives your character a clear idea of her due date. At 18-20 weeks, during the anatomy ultrasound, your character will be able to find out the biological sex of their baby. But this ultrasound (or the blood test called a 'quad screen' that occurs around the same time) can also reveal a horrible truth; genetic or anatomic anomalies that indicate the fetus will not survive out of the womb. In real life, this is one of the most heartbreaking situations a woman can find herself in. But in writing, it presents an excellent opportunity for a no-win situation: carry the baby to term, knowing that it will die shortly after birth, or choose the despised "late-term abortion."

> Medically, there's no such thing as a "late-term abortion." Most medical and surgical abortions occur before 13 weeks, but when they occur later, they are referred to by the method and week in which they occurred (i.e., surgical abortion at 18 weeks).

PREGNANCY EMERGENCIES

PREECLAMPSIA & ECLAMPSIA

If you've ever watched a period drama, someone probably died of eclampsia; it's a time-honored way of killing off beloved female secondary characters. But what *causes* preeclampsia? The short answer: no one really knows.

Preeclampsia is defined as high blood pressure coupled with protein in the urine, indicating that the kidneys are shutting down. Your character will get severe headaches, nausea and vomiting, abdominal pain, and trouble breathing. Preeclampsia usually starts after 20 weeks. If it is mild, your character will be watched carefully, then induced—given medications to begin labor—at 37 weeks. If it is severe (super high blood pressures, lots of protein in the urine, or evidence of liver damage) they'll be induced as early as 34 weeks and given magnesium to prevent seizures.

Eclampsia happens when your character's blood pressures get so high, that they start having seizures. This is a life-threatening emergency, and requires immediate delivery of the baby, along with IV magnesium. If she survives, the mother may continue having seizures for up to six weeks after giving birth.

HYPEREMESIS GRAVIDARUM

Hyperemesis gravidarum is severe, refractory nausea/vomiting that can cause significant weight loss, dehydration, and electrolyte disturbances. Unlike its milder cousin, *morning sickness*, hyperemesis gravidarum can be severe enough to require hospitalization. Both morning sickness and hyperemesis gravidarum are caused by the rising hormone levels, including the fetal hormone β-hCG; nausea can begin as early as 4-8 weeks into pregnancy, peaks around week 12, and (usually) goes away by week 20.

> **Morning sickness** is a misnomer; the nausea can strike at any time of day!

ECTOPIC PREGNANCY

An ectopic pregnancy occurs when the embryo implants somewhere other than the uterus, usually the fallopian tube. This embryo cannot survive to become a baby. If things go well, it will die, and your character will miscarry the pregnancy without ever being the wiser. But if the embryo doesn't die, it can continue to grow, and cause symptoms, such as abdominal pain and vaginal bleeding. If this happens, your character should go to the doctor, where she will have an ultrasound that will show the pregnancy outside the uterus. Then, she'll be given a medication called methotrexate to end the nonviable pregnancy. If she doesn't go to the doctor, or if she doesn't realize she's pregnant, the embryo will continue to grow and eventually will burst the delicate fallopian tube, causing a ruptured ectopic pregnancy.

> In young women, ectopic pregnancies may be mistaken for appendicitis.

A ruptured ectopic pregnancy is a life-threatening emergency. Your character will feel sudden, sharp abdominal pain, or pain in her low back or shoulders. She may feel dizzy or may even faint. If this happens, get your character to the hospital for emergency surgery.

NORMAL LABOR & DELIVERY

After a few hours, Himari's contractions are closer together and lasting long enough that her husband grabs the pre-packed baby bag and drives them to the hospital, where they're immediately shown to their room. They're met by Himari's midwife, who performs a quick exam and informs Himari that she is already 6 cm dilated and is now in active labor.

Labor is divided into three distinct stages. The first stage starts at labor onset and ends once the cervix is 10 cm dilated. The second stage goes from complete dilation to delivery of the baby, and the third stage ends at the delivery of the placenta.

FIRST STAGE (ONSET OF LABOR TO 10CM DILATED)

A. Rupture of membranes

Rupture of membranes (the medical term for water breaking) is often the first sign that labor is about to begin. Your character may experience a dramatic rush of clear or yellowish fluid like you've seen in the movies, but most of the time, it'll feel more like they're wetting their pants. Sometimes, the trickle of fluid is so subtle women aren't even sure if their water broke or not.

B. Early labor

The first stage of labor is the longest, and it is split into two parts. Early labor can last for days. For nulliparous women, it lasts for an average of 20 hours, though that time (thankfully!) tends to decrease with subsequent children.

During early labor, contractions are less strong and further apart. Unlike what you see on TV, early contractions are generally uncomfortable, but not scream-through-your-teeth painful (that comes later). Since women in early labor will be there for a while, they're encouraged to go for walks, take baths, listen to music—pretty much do anything to distract them from what's coming.

C. Active labor

Active labor starts when the cervix is 6 cm dilated. Your character's contractions will get stronger, longer, and closer together. She may have leg cramps or feel nauseated (or like she needs to poop). This is when she goes to the hospital. There, she'll be monitored throughout her active labor, which usually lasts for four to eight hours; the rule of thumb is that the cervix dilates at a rate of about 1 cm per hour, though this can vary widely.

Three hours later, Himari's contractions are now so strong and close together that she can barely grit her teeth and breathe through them. Her husband holds her hand as she squeezes his. She wants to push, but the midwife says she isn't dilated enough; pushing now may increase the swelling of her cervix

> The **cervix** is the muscular opening of the uterus. It's spent the last 9 months keeping the baby from falling out. Now, the baby's head presses against the muscle with every contraction, forcing it to soften and open, or dilate, until it's big enough for the baby's head to fit through—approximately 10 cm.

> Doctors measure the cervical opening with their fingers. It is a remarkably low-tech procedure.

---

and increase the chance of tearing. Himari is close to tears when she finds out her cervix is now only 8 cm dilated. She is so tired she doesn't know if she will be able to push when the time comes. Finally, she asks the midwife if she can still get an epidural. She hadn't wanted one—her plan was for an "all-natural birth"—but right now, she would do anything to sleep.

If your character is going to get an epidural, it will happen during active labor. An epidural is an anesthetic medication injected into the spinal canal that numbs your character from the waist down. An epidural lasts for about eight hours and can significantly slow the progression of labor.

A few minutes after deciding to get the epidural, Himari is introduced to the anesthesiologist, who explains the procedure. She sits on her bed, hunching forward as the doctor injects numbing medicine into her lower spinal column. She tries not to look at the ginormous needle on the tray beside her, but when she hunches forward to let the doctor insert the needle, she feels nothing more than a slight pressure. Within a few minutes, her contractions are less painful. After ten minutes, she can't feel a thing. She lies down and immediately falls fast asleep.

SECOND STAGE (10CM TO DELIVERY OF BABY)

The second stage of labor begins when your character's cervix is dilated to 10 cm. That's when she starts pushing. The second stage of labor can last anywhere from minutes to hours and finishes with the delivery of the baby.

Himari is woken by the midwife less than an hour later. Her cervix is 10 cm dilated; it's time to push. She does so, though it's a weird sensation—more pressure than pain—as her uterus contracts. Part of her wishes she could walk around, bearing down as she'd been taught, but her legs are too numb. Holding her husband's hand and breathing deeply, she pushes down every time she feels that odd pressure.

THIRD STAGE (DELIVERY OF BABY TO DELIVERY OF PLACENTA)

The third stage of labor ranges from delivery of the baby to delivery of the placenta, or afterbirth. This is the fastest stage of labor, usually lasting only five to thirty minutes, though it can take up to an hour.

POSTDELIVERY CARE

As soon as the baby is delivered, there is a flurry of activity. The umbilical cord is cut, then the baby is handed over to the waiting pediatrician, who will suction the nose and mouth, calculate the APGAR score, and give the baby antibiotic eye drops and a shot of Vitamin K.

While this is happening, the doctor/midwife will evaluate the placenta, making sure no chunks are missing. If there are any chunks missing, your character may have retained placenta, which could bleed and/or cause infection. Then the infant is placed in mom's arms, often still covered in blood and *vernix caseosa*, a curd-like white film that protects the newborn's skin as it transitions out of the womb.

> **APGAR score**—given at 1 & 5 minutes of life—is calculated based on baby's breathing, muscle tone, and heart rate.

OBSTETRICAL EMERGENCIES

PRETERM LABOR & PREMATURE RUPTURE OF MEMBRANES

Preterm labor occurs if your character goes into labor between 20 and 37 weeks. The goal of treatment is to prevent labor by giving medications and fluids to slow contractions. Mom will also get a shot of steroids (which helps the baby's lungs develop) and another round of antibiotics, so a baby that comes early has a better chance at survival.

Premature rupture of membranes (PROM) means mom's water broke before 37 weeks even though there are no signs of premature labor. PROM is dangerous to both mom and baby because it means the cervix (the protective muscular neck of the uterus keeping baby inside), is now open and able to conduct all those delightful vaginal bacteria up into the uterus. The only hope at this point is to try to prevent infection while keeping the baby inside for as long as possible. If no infection occurs, the baby is delivered at 34 weeks. But if mom shows signs of amnionitis (fever and foul-smelling vaginal discharge indicating an infection of the amniotic sack), it is treated with IV antibiotics and immediate delivery of the baby, no matter how premature.

> Amnionitis is fatal if left untreated!

POOR POSITIONING

Babies are meant to come out headfirst and face down, called a *cephalic presentation*. If it's in any other position (sideways, bum-first, sticking a limb out where it shouldn't be), it's called **fetal malpresentation**, and it can make vaginal birth

> Bum-first births are called **breech** and account for 3% of all pregnancies.[6]

almost impossible. The doctor or midwife will perform a set of maneuvers to turn the infant, but even if they're successful in doing so, the fetus must be carefully monitored in case the umbilical cord becomes trapped during the maneuver. In that case, an emergent c-section might still be necessary.

Shoulder dystocia occurs when the baby's shoulder gets trapped at the pubic bone. It causes prolongation of the second stage of labor and the unique "turtle sign": the fetal head retracting back into the vaginal canal after pushing. Most cases of shoulder dystocia can be fixed with special maneuvers, but if the baby won't budge, it's time for a c-section.

FETAL DISTRESS

After three hours of pushing, Himari feels as if she's gotten nowhere. The midwife, concerned by the baby's lack of progress, fetches the obstetrician on call. After examining Himari, he places a small disc onto her belly, held on by a belt and connected to a machine that spits out a jagged line that looks kind of like an EKG. The doctor informs her that the device is monitoring her baby's heart rate, along with the strength of her contractions. As she grits her teeth through another contraction, the doctor's pleasant expression dips into a frown. Three contractions later and the doctor has seen enough; her baby's heart rate is "not reassuring"—whatever that means. He tells her she needs a c-section.

During hospital births, the fetal heart rate is continuously monitored using Doppler scanning on the mom's belly. The fetal heart rate slows during contractions; these are called *decelerations*. Some types of decelerations are normal, but late decelerations (meaning the heart rate slows *after* a contraction) are a sign that the fetus isn't getting enough blood to its brain and is an indication for immediate delivery.

> Doctors call these decelerations "decels."

UTERINE RUPTURE

Bleeding is normal during labor, but excessive bleeding is a sign that something is going wrong. A uterine rupture (a complete tear in the wall of the uterus) is one of the most dramatic and life-threatening reasons for hemorrhage during labor.

If your character has a uterine hemorrhage, they've probably had a prior c-section, or have given birth several times. She'll be laboring normally when suddenly severe pain will lance across her lower abdomen (at the site of her c-section scar if she's had one). The shape of her pregnancy belly will change, as her uterus is suddenly no longer able to exert any force and the baby that was being pushed down into her vaginal canal shoots back upwards. The doctor or midwife monitoring down below will notice the head of the baby disappear from the vaginal canal and there will be signs of fetal distress.

Uterine rupture is a surgical emergency requiring an immediate c-section.

CESAREAN DELIVERY (C-SECTION)

Himari, wearing only a hospital gown and a blue scrub cap, is wheeled into the OR, the hairs on her arms pricking at the sudden cold. The anesthesiologist gives her another dose of the epidural after he's helped her onto the cold table. The doctor places a tall, vertical curtain over her chest so she can't see the bottom half of her body. Her husband, dressed in pale blue scrubs and a disposable scrub cap of his own, enters the OR and hurries over to hold her hand. She squeezes it gratefully, as another contraction racks her body. She's so terrified—for her baby, for her surgery—that she barely feels her gown being drawn up and the antiseptic wiped over her abdomen. The doctor steps up, already dressed in a blue paper gown, and quickly explains the surgery, but she can't hear his words over the frantic buzzing in her mind. She nods, she already signed all the paperwork, after all, then the surgeon steps behind the curtain. Minutes later, she hears a wailing cry, and the doctor steps around the curtain and places her daughter in her arms. She's so entranced she barely notices as her husband cuts the umbilical cord.

Only obstetricians—doctors who completed an Ob/Gyn residency—can perform cesareans.

A cesarean, or c-section, is one of the most incredible surgeries I've ever seen. The obstetrician steps up, makes a precise horizontal slice just above the pelvic bone, makes a few more cuts, then pulls out a baby! The whole thing is over in minutes; the rest of the surgery is just stitching the uterus and skin back together. I watched my fair share of surgeries in medical school and residency, but I have yet to see anything quite match the miracle of the cesarean.

INDICATIONS

Contrary to popular opinion (which seems to view cesarean delivery as mostly stemming from comfort or convenience), there are lots of reasons your character might need a c-section, even if it isn't necessarily a medical emergency.

1. **Prior c-section**: If your character has had a previous c-section, every subsequent birth will also need to be a cesarean, or else she'll risk uterine rupture. That being said, this trend has seen some change in recent years, with some obstetricians being more open to "VBAC," or vaginal delivery after c-section.

2. **Failure to progress**: If your character has been in active labor for 20 hours or more but the baby isn't moving, she probably needs a c-section. This is the most common reason for unplanned c-sections.

3. **Fetal distress**: If there are signs that the baby is not doing well—particularly if there are signs that the umbilical cord is getting squished (*cord prolapse*)—it's time for a c-section.

4. **Big baby + small pelvis**: (*Cephalopelvic Disproportion*): Sometimes, the head is just too big for the hole. The pelvic joints relax during labor to help the baby fit. Baby's skull isn't yet fused; this allows its skull to squeeze through (have you ever noticed how babies' heads look kind of pointy when they first come out?). But at some point, bone meets bone, and there's just no getting through.

> Historically, **forceps** were used for fetal malposition and difficult births. If the doctor is properly trained on them, they work better than other vaginal-assist methods. However, if misused, they have a high rate of complications. In the age of c-sections, doctors are not getting the training, and forceps-assisted deliveries are falling out of favor.

5. **Poor positioning of baby** (*Fetal malposition*): There are maneuvers doctors can perform to try and reposition the baby, but if those fail, it may be time for a c-section.

6. **Poor positioning of the placenta** (*Placenta previa*): Sometimes the placenta attaches itself to the uterus so that it blocks the exit. Usually, this condition shows up as painless bleeding during the third trimester, so mom will have time to schedule her c-section in advance.

7. **Maternal illness**: If mom has an active STD (such as genital herpes), cervical cancer, or other trauma to the vagina, abdomen, or pelvis, she will need a c-section. If the mother dies, a c-section will be performed to try and save the baby.

POSTPARTUM EMERGENCIES

After the baby (and placenta) are delivered, there are still risks and conditions your character can develop related to childbirth.

POSTPARTUM HEMORRHAGE

While it's normal for your character to bleed during and after childbirth, too much blood (around 0.5L for a vaginal delivery) is called postpartum hemorrhage. Depending on the cause, postpartum hemorrhage can range from a minor annoyance to life-threatening. Worldwide, postpartum hemorrhage is the leading cause of maternal death.[7]

Many conditions can cause postpartum hemorrhage—the placenta was in the wrong place (*placenta accrete*) or didn't fully come out (*retained placenta*), vaginal tearing, prolonged labor, etc. But the most common cause is *uterine atony*, the uterus's failure to contract down into a hard ball of muscle to close off all those blood vessels that used to be attached to the placenta.

Treatment of postpartum hemorrhage depends on the cause. Treatments range from uterine massage (literally massaging the uterus through the abdominal wall to promote contraction) to suturing tears. If the bleeding absolutely cannot be stopped and the mother's life is in danger, she may require an emergency hysterectomy (removal of her uterus).

FEVER

Two days later, as Himari is recuperating in the hospital, her husband notices that she feels hot to the touch. A nurse comes in and takes her temperature, it's 100.7°F. The doctor from yesterday - Himari can't remember his name— returns and examines her. When he touches her lower abdomen, it feels sore and painful to the touch. He then orders some blood and urine tests and tells her it's probably endometritis (an infection of the uterus). He starts her on an antibiotic that is safe for breastfeeding and informs her she won't be going home until the fever resolves.

Low fever in a woman who has just given birth is always something that should be checked out; most of the time, it will just go away, but a fever can be a sign of something seriously wrong.

Often, the fever is due to infection. Common infection sites include the uterus (*endometritis*), urinary tract, or the surgical incision site after a c-section. If she's breastfeeding, she may develop an infection of her nipples (*mastitis*). But postpartum fever could also be due to a blood clot in her legs (a deep vein thrombosis) which can break off and cause a potentially life-threatening pulmonary embolism (see *Ch. 1: Chest Pain*).

DEPRESSION

After three days in the hospital, Himari and her daughter are sent home. But less than a week after returning home, Himari finds herself tearful, crying for no reason, and feeling like she's a terrible mother. Her husband does what he can to comfort her, but he is gone most of the day at his job, which does not provide any paternity leave. After two months of insomnia, poor appetite, and near-constant feelings of hopelessness and guilt, Himari begins to wonder if her baby would be better off if she were dead.

Postpartum blues is a mild depression characterized by mood swings, crying, irritability, sleep changes, loneliness, and feelings of vulnerability. It starts within a few days of delivery and resolves within two weeks. It is also extremely common; somewhere between 60-80% of women experience some form of the "baby blues."[8]

Postpartum depression is, by definition, more severe. Postpartum depression is a major depressive episode that occurs within 1 year of giving birth. If your character has postpartum depression, she will feel sad, down, and hopeless. She may have trouble sleeping, have lost interest in activities she previously enjoyed, and have thoughts of suicide (see *Ch. 9: Suicide*).

> Minor trauma occurring in the 2nd and 3rd trimester can adversely impact pregnancy.

When Himari tearfully reveals her feelings to her husband, he encourages her to talk with her doctor. She's started on an antidepressant—one that's safe for breastfeeding mothers—and connected with a therapist who will text with her, so she doesn't have to find time to go to appointments. She doesn't feel better right away, but after six weeks on the medication, she's beginning to feel like herself.

Postpartum psychosis is the most severe postpartum psychiatric manifestation. If your character has postpartum psychosis, she will develop psychotic symptoms (hallucinations and delusions) within two weeks of giving birth. She may also experience other symptoms of postpartum depression, particularly guilt and hopelessness.

Postpartum depression and postpartum psychosis are serious, life-threatening illnesses that require emergent treatment.

BREAKING DOWN THE CLICHÉ: MISCARRIAGE FROM FALLING DOWN THE STAIRS

"You can't be pregnant."

"I am. The condom broke, I told you."

"Absolutely not. I won't allow some gold-digger tramp to trap me like this."

pushes her* *she falls down the stairs* *he stares in horror

cuts to the hospital

"I'm sorry, ma'am. You appear to have miscarried."

A few things wrong with this one. First, only major trauma (catastrophic injuries such as hemorrhagic shock or splenic rupture) can cause miscarriage in the first trimester. Minor trauma, falling down the stairs for example, is not associated with miscarriage.

Second, and more importantly, the vast majority of miscarriages are due to genetic anomalies in the embryo, meaning that nothing the mother did could have changed the outcome. Not all pregnancies result in live births. In fact, 10-20% of known pregnancies end in miscarriage.[3] Since most miscarriages occur before the 8th week of pregnancy (before many women even know they're pregnant) the true prevalence is likely to be closer to 25 or 30%.[4]

Third, miscarriages don't "happen." They aren't a one-and-done event; they take days, weeks, sometimes months for the physical symptoms to abate. Even in the best situation, such as an early spontaneous loss, the miscarriage will last about as long as a heavy period (5-7 days, for those of you without a uterus). Under less ideal circumstances, such as a later miscarriage, or an incomplete or missed miscarriage (see below) your character could cramp and bleed for several weeks.

Fourth and finally, miscarriage isn't a medical term. Loss of pregnancy prior to twenty weeks gestation is called an abortion. After twenty weeks, a miscarriage is called a stillbirth. There are many different types of abortions. A **spontaneous abortion** occurs when the fetus dies unexpectedly in the womb, then passes out through the vagina. Medical and surgical abortions are triggered by a pill or surgical procedure, respectively. But sometimes, the fetus doesn't pass on its own.

> A dilation and curettage (D&C) is the procedure used in a surgical abortion.

A **missed abortion** occurs when the fetus dies in the uterus but does not pass. Missed abortions are often diagnosed by a lack of heartbeat on ultrasound. An **incomplete abortion** occurs when part of the fetus passed, but other parts remain inside. An incomplete abortion is a high risk for infection. If your character is in this situation, she not only has to go through a miscarriage, but also has to go through the trauma of taking an "abortion pill" and/or getting a surgical procedure to clean out her uterus, called a *dilation and curettage* (D&C).

A missed or incomplete abortion is a heartbreaking situation for anyone; make it tougher by forcing your character to receive her healthcare through Planned Parenthood. In order to get the care she needs, she'll typically have to walk through the gauntlet of protesters screaming at her not to kill her baby—the baby she wanted but is now dead and decomposing inside her.

SYMPTOMS OF MISCARRIAGE

Symptoms of a miscarriage include abdominal pain, vaginal bleeding, and discharge that last anywhere from a few hours to several weeks. Your character's experience of a miscarriage will vary depending on how far along in the pregnancy they were. Many women miscarry without even knowing it, and simply experience a longer or heavier period than usual. Women who miscarry later in pregnancy will experience more cramping, heavier bleeding, and may even be able to identify fetal parts amongst the discharge.

No matter how far along the pregnancy was when it happened, miscarriages are painful and heartbreaking. Above, I've only listed the physical symptoms of miscarriage; the emotional and psychological toll it takes is equally, if not more, impactful.

When I say heavy bleeding, I mean heavy bleeding. Bleeding through multiple pads an hour, bathroom looks like a crime scene kind of bleeding.

9. SUICIDE

Isaac has a wonderful life. He gets good grades, has two loving parents, and a super-hot boyfriend who shares his passion for campy horror films and '80s power ballads. He attends an art school where, instead of being bullied for being a dancer, he's popular because of it. Isaac knows that he's lucky. Maybe too lucky. He can't help but feel like he doesn't deserve this life. That there's something wrong inside him, and when everyone finds out, they'll hate him.

FROM *ANNA KARENINA* TO *JAVERT*, literature is full of famous suicides. Sensationalism and oversimplification of suicide have led to a misunderstanding of the act and may even be responsible for copycat suicides (see "Real Talk" below).[1] So how can you—the author—write about suicide without glorifying or minimizing it? The first step is understanding it.

BACKGROUND

Suicide is the intentional act of killing yourself; a suicide attempt is the act of trying to kill yourself. The term "successful" suicide is considered outdated, as many people who attempt suicide later regret it. Instead, the terms *completed suicide* or *incomplete suicide attempt* are used.

Suicide is, unfortunately, very common. It is the 10th leading cause of death in the US; in 2019, there were nearly 1.4 million suicide attempts and more than 47,000 deaths from suicide.[2] While white, middle-aged men are the most likely to commit suicide, certain other populations are at high risk.[2] The leading cause of maternal mortality is suicide, and women who are pregnant or recently gave birth are at very high risk of attempting suicide.[3] Teenagers are also a high risk; in 2019, suicide was the second leading cause of death among 13—19-year-olds, with LGBTQ youth 2-6 times more likely to attempt suicide than their heterosexual peers.[4]

SUICIDAL IDEATION

Ever since he got his driver's license last year, Isaac drives himself and his little sister to school, rather than take the bus. On their route is a sharp curve with a sturdy oak tree just a few feet off the road with a white cross draped in fake flowers planted just in front of it. Every time Isaac drives by that corner, he wonders what it would be like to slam on the gas and drive straight into the tree. The thought frightens him, but also feels...right, somehow. Sometimes, he even presses down on the gas, accelerating towards the curve. Then he looks over at his sister, inevitably engrossed in her phone, and eases on the brake, taking the curve slowly.

Suicidal ideation (SI) means your character is thinking about wanting to die, or not wanting to be alive anymore. It comes in two forms: passive and active. Passive SI indicates that your character is thinking about dying, even wishing they were dead, but are not planning on killing themselves. If your character has active SI, it means they intend to kill themselves, and may even have a plan for how to go about it.

SI is a key component of depression and several other mental illnesses, but your character doesn't need to have a mental illness to have SI. About 9% of people worldwide have experienced SI at some point in their lives.[5] And SI doesn't look the same for everyone; in fact, SI can vary significantly in intensity and type even in the same person. The presence of SI does not necessarily mean that your character will commit suicide, and its absence does not mean they are safe.

> **Myth:** Asking about suicide will make people more likely to attempt suicide.
>
> **Fact:** Open and honest communication about suicidal ideation actually decreases the risk.

CAUSES OF SUICIDE

Isaac was diagnosed with depression and anxiety when he was twelve, back when he was still in a normal school and getting bullied for being a "ballerino." He took pills for a while, but they made him feel dizzy and gain a bunch of weight, so he stopped. Then he transferred to the Art School, and everything got better. Well, almost everything.

Overwhelmingly, the cause of suicide is mental illness; one study estimated that 60% of all suicide attempts were due to depression.[6] Substance use disorders (such as alcohol use disorder or opioid use disorder), and psychosis are the next most common causes, though other mental illnesses, such as bipolar disorder, post-traumatic stress disorder (PTSD), eating disorders, borderline personality disorder, schizophrenia, and anxiety can all contribute. One study that looked at the brains of those who had completed suicide estimated that more than 90% had a mental illness.[7]

But there are factors other than mental illness that influence suicidality. Chronic pain and chronic illnesses can lead to suicide, as can hopelessness. Recent life events, such as flunking out of school or getting fired, can also contribute. Often, someone driven to attempt suicide will have several of these risk factors.

The biggest risk factor for suicide is previous suicide attempts.[4] Other risk factors include male gender, being unmarried, single, or living alone, and feelings of hopelessness.[4]

> People who have completed suicide are more likely to have a diagnosis of major depressive disorder AND a recent major life stressor[7].

WARNING SIGNS

One day, while taking a break from Fortnite, Isaac leans back against his boyfriend, Idris's shoulder. "I'm so tired," he whispers.

Idris wraps an arm around his shoulder, kissing the top of his head. "Me too. I was up all night studying for that chem final. Mr. O is a killer."

Isaac shakes his head. He'd been up all night too, though he wasn't studying. He'd just stared at the ceiling, wishing he could fall asleep and never wake up. He's been doing that a lot lately. He'd even spent a few hours googling the least painful way to kill yourself, though he'd made sure to delete his browsing history afterward.

"It's not that. Don't you ever get tired of living?"

"What do you mean?"

Isaac's chest tightens at the horrified look on Idris's face. "I mean, dancing, classes, applying to colleges," he improvises. "It's exhausting."

Idris looks relieved. "I mean, yeah, it's hard. But what else are you going to do, not dance?" He chuckles at his joke. "I know you've been down lately, which is why I'm cool with us not hanging out with the gang as much. But the day you stop dancing is the day I'll be really worried."

Isaac swallows against the sudden lump in his throat. "Round two?" He leans down to grab the controller, making sure Idris can't see the tears brimming in his eyes. He hasn't wanted to dance in a very long time.

> **Myth:** You can't know if someone is suicidal.
>
> **Fact:** Like any disease, there are signs of suicidality, though people may do their best to hide it.

Like any disease, suicide is characterized by a constellation of signs and behaviors that are observable to others. These are warning signs that will indicate to your other characters that your main character is contemplating suicide. Not everyone will show all of these signs—people with mental illness are often masters of disguising their true feelings—but there will usually be at least a few signs for your characters to pick up on. These signs are split into two broad categories: things your character says, and the things they do.

A few days later, Isaac's sister stays home from school due to a cold. As he's passing the tree, Isaac slows to a crawl. He takes the next right, driving around the block until he's back at the tree. He does this over and over—he's not exactly sure why—until he gets a text from Idris.

Where ru? 1ˢᵗ period's almost over!

Horrified, Isaac snaps out of it and drives straight to school, hurrying inside.

- Things they say:

    o Feel hopeless, trapped, misunderstood, or alone

    o Feel tired of being alive, or that they have no reason to continue living

    o Look for a way out

    o Express interest in suicide (even joking)

    o Threaten to kill themselves

> If someone jokes about suicide, your characters should take them seriously until proven otherwise.

- Things they do:

    o Make a will or give away treasured possessions

    o Withdraw from their friends and family

    o Sleep or eat too much or too little

    o Have dramatic mood swings

    o Seem restless, anxious, or agitated

    o Research methods of killing themselves

    o Act impulsively

    o Reckless behaviors

> Impulsivity increases the risk of suicide attempts, as up to 50% of suicide attempts are not premeditated.[6]

    – Erratic driving

    – Excessive drug/alcohol use

o Collect materials for suicide attempts (hoard pills, buy a gun, etc.)

o Revisit site/materials for planned attempt (the bridge where they intend to jump, the safe where the gun is stored)

o Write letters or notes to be opened by loved ones after their death

METHODS

By the time school is over, the road is covered in a thin blanket of snow. Isaac kisses Idris goodbye, then sits in his car, waiting for the engine to warm up. It was a terrible day. He failed his chemistry test, got detention for skipping first period, and was passed over for the role of Snow King in the upcoming Nutcracker performance. But he isn't sad. He isn't sure he can feel sad anymore. The world just feels gray, gray as the clouds stretching to the horizon in every direction. He's been feeling like this for so long, that he doesn't think it can ever end. When he rounds the bend and sees the tree, he doesn't stop to think. He just presses on the gas.

Methods for suicide are generally split into two categories: violent and non-violent. Violent methods of suicide include the use of guns, jumping from a height or under a train, cutting, car crash, drowning, and self-immolation. The main nonviolent method is poisoning, either through medications, illicit drugs, drinking poisonous fluids, or inhaling poisonous gas. Men are more likely to utilize violent, high lethality methods, and thus are more likely to die from suicide.[4]

DRUGS USED IN SUICIDE

Substances used in suicide attempts range from illicit drugs to over-the-counter medications. Drugs commonly used in suicide attempts include:

- Alcohol

- Anti-anxiety medications

- Antidepressants

- Illicit drugs

- Opioids

Fatal overdoses are often due to a combination of medications.

Kids are more likely to use over-the-counter medications in overdose attempts.

- Over the Counter Medications

- Sleeping pills

GUNS IN SUICIDE

Violent methods—especially firearms—have a higher lethality, meaning your character is more likely to die if they use a gun. Firearms alone account for more than 50% of deaths from suicide in the US.[4] Men are more likely to use guns than women, but that's just averages—there are plenty of women who have used guns in suicide attempts.

OTHER METHODS

As the tree zooms closer, fear rears up inside him, and he slams on the brakes. The car skids and the rear crashes into the tree. The airbags shoot outward, pummeling him with the force of its eruption. When everything is still, Isaac sits in his seat, breathing hard. He feels battered and bruised, and can barely take a breath in, but he's alive. He knows he should feel relieved, but the grayness is back. He struggles to get out of the car—the passenger side is crumpled, but he can still get his door open—then dials home.

"Mom," he says, his voice croaking, "I got in a car accident. Can you come to get me?

Other methods used to commit suicide include jumping from heights or in front of cars or trains, drowning, hanging, suffocation, and even self-immolation.

I'm deliberately not going to go into the specific methods; I don't want this to become a how-to guide. If you are writing a suicide scene, I hope you will do the same and leave the details vague.

TREATMENT

SUICIDAL IDEATION

The treatment for suicidal ideation is to treat the underlying cause. If your character has depression presenting with SI, the treatment is therapy, close monitoring, and medications. Sometimes, *electroconvulsive therapy* (ECT) is used for extreme depression, or if the depression is not responding to medications.

Most of the time, if your character has SI, they will be treated on an outpatient basis. However, if their symptoms become severe enough that they—or someone close to them—are concerned that they are a danger to themselves, they'll be taken to the emergency department for evaluation.

For more on ECT, see *Ch. 16: Mental illness.*

At the ED, the doctor will evaluate your character based on the presence/severity of their mental illness, the intensity of the SI, and their access to lethal means of killing themselves. Not everyone with active SI needs to be admitted to the inpatient psychiatric hospital. In fact, the goal is to keep people out of inpatient hospitalization as much as possible; psychiatric treatment takes time, and inpatient hospitalization doesn't do much except prevent your character from hurting themselves while they're waiting for the meds to kick in. For that reason, only those who exhibit an intent to kill themselves *and* have a plan or means to do so will be admitted. Evidence of poor judgment, poor social support, or increased impulsivity also increases the case for admission.

SUICIDE ATTEMPT

At the hospital, the doctors poke and prod Isaac, shining a light into his eyes and asking if he hit his head. Isaac just shakes his head, unable to form words. Finally, the doctor asks Isaac's mom to leave the room.

"Can you tell me what caused the accident?" the doctor asked, her voice kind but firm.

Isaac just shrugs.

"Did you lose control?"

He shakes his head.

"Was it intentional?"

Isaac can't bring himself to shake his head. The doctor sighs, then leans forward, trying to meet his eyes.

"Isaac, did you try to kill yourself today?"

Isaac's head dips into the smallest nod. The doctor reaches out and touches him on the shoulder. "I'm sorry you're having such a rough time, Isaac. But I'm glad you're here. You're in the right place. Have you been having thoughts of suicide, or feelings of hopelessness?"

Isaac nods.

"Have you lost interest in things you normally love?"

Isaac nods again. She asks a long series of questions, to which Isaac either replies with a nod or a shrug. Finally, she leans forward to catch his eye again.

"Do you still feel like you want to kill yourself?"

A lump rises in Isaac's throat but he nods anyway.

If your character attempts suicide, they'll be brought to the ED, even if they didn't manage to do much damage to themselves. They'll be seen first by an ED physician. If your character doesn't need medical hospitalization, your character will be admitted directly to the inpatient psychiatric ward. But if their injuries are severe enough to require medical hospitalization, they'll be admitted to a medical floor and placed on suicide watch.

If your character attempts suicide without causing much damage they still need to be brought to the ED, as subsequent attempts may be more lethal.

In the hospital, they'll be treated for their injuries. For example, if they tried to shoot themselves, they may be taken for immediate surgery. If they took pills, their stomach will be pumped or they'll be given activated charcoal to bind up the poison, and given a reversal medication, like Narcan or Flumazenil, if appropriate. Only once they are medically stable will they be transferred to the inpatient psychiatric ward.

Narcan is a drug that reverses opioid overdose. **Flumazenil** reverses benzodiazepine overdose.

VOLUNTARY AND INVOLUNTARY ADMISSION

After their conversation, the doctor asks Isaac if he wants to tell his mother. He nods his agreement the doctor calls Isaac's mom back in and informs her of their discussion. Since Isaac remains actively suicidal and has shown a high level of impulsivity, the doctor recommends admission to a pediatric psychiatric ward. Isaac balks at this, but the doctor tells him it will likely only be for a few days, a week, max. Then she leaves the room, giving Isaac and his mother time to talk. By the time she returns with the paperwork, Isaac is ready.

Mental health is given higher levels of protection under HIPAA. Though exact rules vary by state, most teenagers have the right to pursue mental healthcare without parental permission.

The first step to inpatient psychiatric admission is voluntary admission; your character will sign a bunch of paperwork saying that they agree to be admitted. Rules vary by state, but most of the time, if your character is voluntarily admitted, they are also able to leave at any time. They also will have the right to refuse treatment at any time, as long as they are not an imminent danger to themselves or others. The vast majority of people in psychiatric wards are voluntary admits.

If your character refuses to be admitted to a psychiatric hospital but is found to be an imminent danger to themselves or others, they can be detained involuntarily. Involuntary admission varies state by state, but for the most part, your character will be held against their will in the inpatient facility for a few days. Then there will be a trial to determine if they need to continue to be held and for how long. But remember—even if your character is admitted involuntarily, they still have the right to refuse treatment. If your character has legal capacity then they get to make all of their own decisions about their medical care, even if they were admitted involuntarily.

However, the courts can determine that your character lacks the capacity to make such decisions. Judges have the authority to force people to adhere to a treatment plan, including taking medications, but only if the doctors can prove that they are unable to understand their psychiatric and medical conditions, and therefore cannot make informed decisions. It's a high bar. Real-life isn't like *One Flew Over the Cuckoo's Nest;* forcing someone to take medication without the approval of the courts can get medical providers in serious legal trouble.

> **Myth:** If your character is admitted to a psychiatric hospital, they lose all control over their treatment.
>
> **Fact:** People admitted to psychiatric hospitals still have the right to refuse treatment, even if they were admitted involuntarily.

> Not all involuntary admits are due to suicide. Often, involuntary admits are for people with complex medical and psychiatric needs who are simply unable to care for themselves due to their mental illness.

PSYCHIATRIC WARD

The psych ward is nothing like what Isaac has seen on tv. It looks more like the pictures of college dorm rooms, with their double rooms, fluorescent lights, and a communal bathroom. The only difference is that there are no windows, and the door handles slope downwards to prevent hanging attempts, he's told.

> Psychiatric hospitals can be private or public. Some are attached to general medical hospitals, while others are freestanding.

On the psychiatric ward, your character will be started on medications (or ECT) and closely monitored for improvement and side effects. They will spend most of their day in group therapy, learning skills for coping with mental illness. Specialists visit the ward to instruct the patients in art therapy, pet therapy, music therapy, etc. Your character will also be assigned both a counselor and a psychiatrist.

Isaac sees a psychiatrist for his intake appointment. She starts him on antidepressants and an antipsychotic, but after that first day, he only sees her for about ten minutes each morning. Instead, he spends hours in group therapy, learning coping strategies and practicing meditation. But there are still too many hours in the day. Isaac spends most of his extra time reading or doing Sudoku puzzles from the book his mom brought for him.

Though your character will meet with both their psychiatrist and therapist every day, their roles on the inpatient ward are different than you might imagine. Psychiatrists (medical doctors specializing in diseases of the mind) are primarily interested in your character's response to medications and will probably spend less than 20 minutes each day with your character. Therapists spend more time, usually an hour a day, providing one-on-one counseling and behavioral therapy. But most of your character's time will be spent in group activities, and they'll even have free time in the evenings.

The inpatient psychiatric ward is a unique setting. It is a locked ward, meaning patients can't leave, with specific personnel and multiple modifications made to prevent people from hurting themselves. If you're going to set any part of your story in a psych ward, make sure to visit one first.

Doorknobs in inpatient psychiatric wards are sloped to prevent patients from trying to hang themselves.

PARTIAL HOSPITALIZATION & INTENSIVE OUTPATIENT PROGRAMS (IOP)

After a few days in the psych ward, Isaac is discharged to an intensive outpatient program. Since he isn't allowed to drive anymore, his mom drives him every morning to a building across the road from the hospital, dropping him off before she leaves for work. There, he spends all day in more classes. At 5:30, his dad picks him up and brings him home. When he's home, he can feel them watching him all the time. He isn't allowed to take his own meds, and his parents locked the alcohol cabinet, though Isaac has never been a drinker. It's infantilizing, but his parents keep reminding him that it's for his own safety.

If your character isn't an immediate danger to themselves, but still has active SI, they will be placed in partial hospitalization or an intensive outpatient program. Your character will get to sleep in their own bed, but they'll spend their days at an outpatient facility. Like on the inpatient ward, they'll have group therapy classes scheduled from 9-5 and meet every day with a counselor. A psychiatrist will oversee their treatment and will check in at least every few days.

Being a part of a partial hospitalization or IOP is a big commitment for the people taking care of your character. Because your character is still a suicide risk, they won't be allowed to do anything that could result in their death. They can't drive, can't cook (all the knives should be hidden or removed from the house), and can't even be responsible for taking their meds. All the alcohol, medications, and potentially dangerous substances (like bleach or lye) have to be locked away. Your character is never allowed to be alone, except when they're sleeping. This means that they need constant supervision during the hours they aren't at the hospital. Needless to say, it's a lot of work, and not everyone has social support. If your character doesn't have the support for partial hospitalization or IOP, they'll be admitted to the inpatient ward, just to be safe.

> *Nearly two months after the car crash, Isaac is feeling more like himself. His parents are no longer watching him so carefully, and he's once more in charge of his own medications. When his parents finally allow him to drive, he drives straight past the tree without giving it a second thought.*

BREAKING DOWN THE CLICHÉS

There are a lot of tropes, stereotypes, myths, clichés, and misunderstandings that surround suicide. Falling into these tired habits is not only bad writing but can contribute to the stigmatization (or glorification) of suicide.

CRY FOR ATTENTION

If your character attempts suicide through a less-than-lethal means, or attempts, then calls 911 right after, they will undoubtedly be met with skepticism from friends, family, and even medical professionals, as to whether or not they really "meant it." Some may even go so far as to say that the attempt was simply a "cry for attention," that they were never in any danger of actually hurting themselves.

> Medical professionals (especially in the ED) are notorious for rolling their eyes behind the backs of "frequent flyers" who make trivial suicide attempts on a regular basis. Your character may need to fight for the care they need.

There are several reasons a suicide attempt may not be fatal. First, many people immediately regret their actions and realize that they want to live. The lucky ones get the chance to call 911 and get help. Second, people don't always know what methods will be most lethal or how to carry out their plan, such as not knowing how to tie a sturdy knot or having no idea what dose of a drug or poison they need to take. Third, suicide is often an impulsive act; while stockpiling, writing suicide notes, and revisiting a plan are all signs of suicidal ideation, not everyone makes plans. One study found that 87% of suicide attempts were impulsive, while only 13% were planned.[8]

Some suicide attempts really don't look like

> These tenuous suicide attempts are more frequent in people with **borderline personality disorder**.

they are "trying" at all, or like they want to be stopped. I had one patient take six Tylenol, then call 911 to say she'd overdosed. Another tied a pair of (stretchy) nylons to the doorknob, wrapped them around her neck, and immediately yelled to her boyfriend that she was hanging herself. A third posted pictures of himself with a gun to social media, saying that he was ready to end his life. When the police showed up ten minutes later, he was waiting for them. Turns out, he didn't even know where his parents kept the ammo.

While some people call these sorts of attempts a "cry for attention," mental illness specialists call it a "cry for help." People who intentionally make less-than-lethal suicide attempts usually do so because they are experiencing extreme emotions that they don't know how to handle. They are in a psychiatric emergency and need help. Anyone who has made a suicide attempt—even a half-a\$\$ed one—is more likely to attempt again. And subsequent attempts may very well be more lethal. For this reason, all suicide attempts should be taken seriously, no matter how trivial.

> Self-harm, such as cutting or burning, is another example of a "cry for help" that deserves immediate medical attention.

DRIVEN TO SUICIDE

One of the first rules I learned as a writer is that, if your character is content, you're probably doing something wrong. The "driven to suicide" trope takes this to an extreme, making the character so miserable, guilty, horrified, or heartsick that they chose to end their life.

It's understandable why writers fall into this trope; it's dramatic, it's heartbreaking, and it's at least partially true. People who commit suicide often do so after a major life stressor.[7] There might even be situations where it is logical for your character to end their life, such as concentration camps, or a painful, terminal diseases for which there is no cure. But ending your own life is hard; most people cannot take that step without an underlying brain pathology. If your character doesn't have an underlying mental illness, you have to think long and hard about why and how they're jumping to such an extreme.

> Spoiler alert!

Overwhelmingly, most people who attempt suicide have an underlying medical illness. For me, this absence of the mental illness component is the missing piece in the "driven to suicide" trope.

Some books have done a great job showing the interconnected nature of mental illness and suicide. *The Bell Jar* is the obvious example, but modern writers such as Brandon Sanderson (*The Way of Kings*) and Gail Honeyman (*Elinor Oliphant is Completely Fine*) are great examples that intertwine mental illness into the story *before* the suicide attempt is brought up.

Too many books, movies, and TV shows start with suicide attempts. The protagonist is talked off the ledge, someone important to the protagonist commits suicide, etc. It may set off a murder investigation, bring, people together, or cause the main character to rethink their life. Either way, suicide acts as the inciting event.

The problem with this trope isn't just unoriginality; it can be actively harmful. Starting with a suicide doesn't give context to the complexities of suicide. Often, it is blatant sensationalism, intended only to draw in the audience. At its worst, portraying suicide in this way risks glorifying the act of suicide. When that happens, it can lead to a dangerous phenomenon: copycat suicides.

REAL TALK: COPYCAT SUICIDE

Sadly, copycat suicide is a real phenomenon. Suicide methods used by celebrities are five times more likely to be used by the general public in the months following their death.[9] In 2016, two five-year-olds died by hanging themselves, mimicking a suicide that they'd recently watched on TV.[9] In 2017, two teenagers in California committed suicide shortly after watching a particular episode of *13 Reasons Why*; their parents believe their deaths were directly triggered by the show and sued.[10]

Copycat suicides are so common that the phenomenon has a name—the Werther effect. In 1774, Goethe published *The Sorrows of Young Werther*, in which the eponymous character shot himself in the head, then died slowly and with great suffering. The publication of this book was followed by so many suicides of people dressed as Werther, and using the exact same method, that the book was banned all across Europe.

As a writer, you need to be aware of this phenomenon. Please note that I'm not saying you shouldn't write about suicide. I'm just asking that you do your research and treat the act with as much complexity and dignity as you would any other life-threatening illness. Ensure your book does not glorify suicide or treat suicide as the only way out. By the same token, do not turn your book into a how-to manual for someone looking to kill themselves; keep the details vague, or make them up altogether. You could save someone's life.

After the publication of Final Exit, a book which promoted asphyxia as a suicide method, deaths by asphyxiation rose 313%.[11] The book was found on the scene of 27% of those deaths.[11]

10. POISONING

Jerry is a jack-of-all-trades. Jerry is not very bright. Jerry is not going to survive this chapter.

THERE ARE A LOT OF potential poisons in the world; there's no way I can cover them all. Luckily, I don't have to. Some excellent books have already been published—including one written by my former medical school physiology professor—that cover the typical poisons in great detail. Instead of reinventing the wheel, I'm going to use this chapter to discuss some unusual poisons that your clever antagonist might be able to get their hands on.

Please remember, I'm not writing a how-to guide for poisons. For that reason, I'm not going to spend a whole lot of time on actually acquiring these potential poisons, or how you'd get an unsuspecting character to ingest/touch/inhale the substance. I'll leave those logistical concerns up to your clever characters.

ARGON

Today, Jerry is helping out at a manufacturing plant. He wiggles into the crawlspace beneath a machine and is in the process of inspecting the welding when he loses consciousness.

Argon is a noble gas that is heavier than air. It is odorless, colorless, and tasteless. When your character breathes the argon in, the gas will settle in the lungs, and they won't be able to breathe it out. As they breathe in more and more of the gas, it will displace the regular, oxygen-containing air. Eventually, your character's lungs won't have enough oxygen to pull into the bloodstream and your character will die. This is called inert gas asphyxiation.

SYMPTOMS

There are no symptoms of argon poisoning*.

Yup, you read that right. After breathing in the argon, your character will walk around, feeling totally normal; until they pass out and

*Some people may get a mild headache or feel vaguely dizzy, nauseated, or fatigued right before passing out.

die. This lack of symptoms occurs because of the way your body feels asphyxiation. Turns out, all the symptoms you feel when you're struggling to breathe—anxiety, fear, chest tightness, etc.—are due to the buildup of carbon dioxide in the blood. Normally, you breathe in oxygen and breathe out carbon dioxide, so if the carbon dioxide is building up, it usually means there isn't enough oxygen in your blood. Your body only notices the low blood oxygen levels until the levels are dangerously low.

With argon poisoning, your character is still exhaling normally. They're getting rid of the carbon dioxide—and thus have no symptoms of asphyxiation—without getting the oxygen that the brain desperately needs. It's a beautiful illustration of human physiology at work.

> Nitrogen gas asphyxiation, a proposed method for state executions, is another form of inert gas asphyxiation.

DETECTION

Since argon isn't absorbed into the blood, it isn't detectable on blood or urine tests. But, if your character is very clever, they might think to test gas samples from the lungs for argon levels. They might also be able to find increased argon in the lung tissue.[2] But these are not routinely performed tests—your medical examiner character would have to be looking for them.

> *Jerry wakes up in the ambulance with an oxygen mask blowing full force into his face. Apparently, there was an argon leak, and the crawlspace wasn't properly ventilated. His coworkers had performed CPR and had even held him upside-down to try and get the argon out. When Jerry asks the paramedic if holding him upside down really worked, she just shrugged and said, "Doesn't look like it hurt."*

> Turning the victim upside-down is one way to get the argon out. CPR, forced ventilation, and 100% oxygen work better.

ARSENIC

A byproduct of iron and lead mining during the industrial revolution, arsenic was widely used to kill all sorts of vermin throughout the 20th century, though it has since been replaced by anticoagulant rodenticides.[1] Arsenic is tasteless, colorless, flammable and soluble in water. When heated, it smells of garlic. If your character has been poisoned with arsenic, their breath may smell garlicky.[3]

Symptoms of arsenic toxicity vary by dose. At high doses, symptoms of arsenic poisoning include nausea, copious vomiting, and bloody diarrhea, leading to severe dehydration. Death is usually due to cardiovascular collapse secondary to hypovolemic shock. However, at lower doses, the symptoms of gastrointestinal distress are present but less severe. Other symptoms of low dose poisoning include headaches, muscle cramps, irregular heart rhythms, nerve damage, seizures, and coma.[1,3] Your character might survive for weeks with these symptoms, only to die of organ failure within a few months.

Changes to the victim's skin, hair, and nails may help your astute character determine that they are a victim of arsenic poisoning. Hair loss and pale white lines in the fingernails, called *Mees' lines*, may appear after acute poisoning. Dark patches on the skin (*hyperpigmentation*) and raised, scaly skin patches (*keratoses)* that look like "dewdrops on a dusty road" are signs of chronic arsenic poisoning.[3] Blackfoot disease—similar in appearance to gangrene of the foot—is another potential sequela of chronic arsenic poisoning.[3]

Since chronic arsenic poisoning was so easy to mistake for other conditions, it was a favorite poison throughout the 20th century. Now urine tests can be used to test for suspected arsenic toxicity. Acute arsenic poisoning is treated with airway/blood pressure support, IV fluid, blood infusions, and medications called chelating agents that bind up the free arsenic in the blood. If your character had a large, acute ingestion, they might need to have their stomach pumped (*gastric lavage*) and be given large doses of polyethylene glycol (also known as the colonoscopy prep) to flush the arsenic out of their system.[3]

DIMETHYL MERCURY

Dimethyl mercury is a colorless liquid that smells slightly sweet but if your character can smell it, they're as good as dead. This molecule is highly toxic and invariably fatal even at minuscule doses. But what makes it a really fun poison for writers is that symptoms don't start for weeks to months after exposure. Let me start by telling you a true story.

Karen Wetterhahn was a professor of chemistry at Dartmouth college when, in August of 1996, she spilled two drops of dimethyl mercury onto her gloved hand.[4] Five months later, she began to have some mild neurologic changes—numbness and tingling in her feet—that quickly escalated to trouble walking (*ataxia*), loss of vision, slurred speech, and a whooshing sound, as if she had water in her ears.[4] She was diagnosed with mercury poisoning—the mercury level in her blood was almost 100 times greater than the threshold for toxicity—and only then did she remember the two drops of dimethyl mercury spilled on her glove.[4] Despite aggressive treatment, she slipped into a coma less than three weeks after the start of her symptoms and died a few months later.[4]

To recap, this molecule can be administered through contact with skin, symptoms don't show up for months after exposure, and once symptoms show up, it is inevitably fatal. Mystery, crime, and thriller writers—you're welcome.

NICOTINE

Jerry uses e-cigarettes. For business, he has to fly across the country, so he packs his e-cig and the liquid cartridge in his carry-on. Halfway through the six-hour flight, his cravings are so intense that he feels like he might jump out of his skin. He can't smoke on the plane—but there's nicotine in the cartridge, right? He dumps half the contents into his ginger ale and chugs the whole thing. It tastes bitter.

Nicotine, the addictive molecule in tobacco, is a highly toxic molecule that is heat stable. It can be ingested or absorbed through the skin (nicotine patches) and oral mucosa (chewing tobacco). The most common administration of nicotine, however, nicotine is inhalation (cigarettes, cigars, e-cigarettes, etc.).

When inhaling tobacco, it is very difficult to absorb enough nicotine for a fatal dose. A lethal dose of nicotine for a 150 lb. adult is about 50-60mg; the dose from inhaling a cigarette is usually only 1-2mg.[5] However, with the advent of liquid nicotine from e-cigarettes, a lethal dose is much easier to come by. One e-cigarette container has around 24 mg of nicotine, in 20 mL of fluid. That means it only takes 50 mL—less than ¼ cup—of e-cigarette fluid ingestion to kill a grown man. Remember, this is a heat-stable substance; it can survive burning, baking, and boiling.

SYMPTOMS

A half-hour later, Jerry starts feeling sick. He runs to the bathroom, where he empties his stomach. He's sweating, his head hurts, and the muscles of his hands keep cramping. He returns to his seat, only to have to race back to the restroom again. This time, it's coming out the other end.

Symptoms of nicotine poisoning are split into the early phase (15 minutes-1 hour) and late phase (30 minutes—4 hours). These symptoms are due to overstimulation of the parasympathetic response—the "rest and digest" system that acts as a counterpoint to the sympathetic "fight or flight." Symptoms of nicotine poisoning include:

- Gastrointestinal symptoms

    o Nausea and vomiting

    o Diarrhea

- o Abdominal pain

- o Increased salivation

- Increased sweating (*diaphoresis*)

- Poor coordination and trouble walking (*ataxia*)

- Headache

- Involuntary muscle twitching (*fasciculations*)

- Fast heart rate

- High blood pressure

As he's walking back to his seat, an angry-looking flight attendant asks if he's had anything to drink. Jerry shakes his head, but he's having trouble standing. He's breathing fast and heavy, and his hands keep shaking. When they land, the flight attendant calls an ambulance.

Symptoms of severe poisoning include:

- Convulsions (See *Ch. 6: Syncope and Seizures*)

- Low blood pressure

- Paralysis

- Slow breathing rate and trouble breathing

- Slow heart rate

- Death

Death is due to either paralysis of the diaphragm, leading to asphyxiation, or the combination of a slow heart rate and low blood pressure leading to the collapse of the cardiovascular system.

> The half-life of nicotine is about two hours.

DETECTION

At the emergency department, the doctors tell Jerry that the nicotine levels in his blood were very high; he consumed the equivalent of an entire pack of cigarettes all at once.

Levels of nicotine (and its metabolite cotinine) will be detectable in the blood and will be extremely high for up to 3 days after the ingestion.[5] It will also be detectable in the urine for up to 3 weeks. If your character is a nicotine user, they will have elevated nicotine levels at baseline. But the nicotine levels after poisoning will be much higher than expected for normal nicotine use.

POISONOUS MUSHROOMS

After his e-cig debacle, Jerry decides to take it easy. He retires to a cabin in the woods and learns to forage mushrooms. One day, he finds a beautiful white mushroom growing between the roots of a tree. He pops it in his mouth.

Mushrooms of the *Aminata* family contain a deadly poison called an amatoxin. The toxin is stable under both heat and drying. It is also highly lethal, with a mortality of around 80%.[5] While there are several different species that contain the toxin, two species—*Amanita phalloides* and *Amanita bisporigera*—are two of the most toxic.

Amanita phalloides, also called "death cap mushrooms," are nondescript, white-brown mushrooms, commonly found in wet environments all over the world. *Amanita bisporigera,* called "The destroying angel," are pristinely white and grow beneath mixed forests in the grass. These mushrooms have no distinctive smell or taste and are easily misidentified for other forms of edible mushrooms. In fact, many who have ingested these mushrooms claim that they tasted quite delicious.[6]

SYMPTOMS

The next morning, Jerry starts vomiting. It's the nicotine poisoning all over again—but worse. Severe belly pain, copious vomiting, and so much diarrhea it feels like he's peeing out of his bum. Jerry can't drink enough water. He wonders if this is how he's going to die.

At first, amatoxin poisoning is asymptomatic, a period called the "silent phase." The first stage of amatoxin poisoning begins around 6-12 hours after ingestion and is characterized by severe gastrointestinal distress: nausea, vomiting, abdominal pain, and extreme watery diarrhea.[6] The diarrhea can be so severe that your poisoned character could die of dehydration. Treatment at this stage of poisoning is to give large volumes of IV fluids.

Jerry doesn't die. It was the worst 24-hours of his life, but he isn't dead. He's starting to get better. Maybe he's not so bad at this foraging thing after all.

By days 2-4 after ingestion, your character will start to look better. They may even think that they're through the worst of it. But they'd be wrong. Because while your character is looking better, the amatoxin is wreaking havoc on their liver.

The next day, Jerry's daughter, Joni, comes to visit. She thinks his skin looks yellow, so she tells him to go to the doctor. He refuses. She returns the next day

Around day 3, your character will start to become jaundiced, starting with a yellowing of the whites of their eyes. Then their liver will fail, causing their kidneys to fail. Symptoms include delirium, jaundice, mood/personality changes, drowsiness, muscle twitching (*myoclonus*), hand flapping (*asterixis*), decreased urination/dark urine, swollen abdomen (*ascites*), and problems with coordination and memory. Finally, your character will die of fulminant liver failure. The only treatment is a liver transplant.

DETECTION

Amatoxin is difficult to detect in the blood, as the toxin moves quickly out of the blood and into the cells. It can be detected in urine using special tests, but they are not widely used in forensic laboratories.[7]

RODENTICIDES

Rodenticides (rat poison) are a unique form of pesticide because they are intended to kill mammals. For that reason, they can also be highly toxic to other mammals, including dogs, cats, and humans. And your character can buy them at their local home and garden store. There are several different classes of rodenticide.

ANTICOAGULANTS

The most commonly used types of rat poison work as potent blood thinners, causing the rodent to bleed to death. Depending on the active ingredient, these rat poisons are highly toxic when ingested, inhaled, or even absorbed through the skin.[8] Two of the most potent active ingredients include brodifacoum, sometimes called "super warfarin," and bromadiolone. Other anticoagulant active ingredients include chlorophacinone, diphacinone, and difenacoum.

These rodenticides work by chewing up Vitamin K, which the body needs in order to clot. It's the same mechanism used by Warfarin, the famous medical anticoagulation drug. In fact, Warfarin was the first anticoagulant used to kill rodents, starting in the 1950s.[1] Because the poison has to use up the Vitamin K, it takes several days of poisoning (anywhere from 1-9 days) before symptoms show up. Even large doses can be asymptomatic for as much as 72 hours after ingestion.

The primary symptom of anticoagulant poisoning is, unsurprisingly, bleeding. If your character is exposed to one of these drugs, they will notice that they bruise easily and may bleed excessively from minor wounds. They might have recurrent

---

nosebleeds, heavy menstrual bleeding, and blood in their urine. Even a small injury—hitting their head on a doorframe or getting punched in the abdomen—could cause severe bleeding and even death.

Because doctors put their patients on warfarin all the time, it is very easy to test for this type of poisoning: just check a Vitamin K level as well as coagulation labs, such as PT/PTT and INR. It's also pretty easy to treat; give Vitamin K along with a type of pro-clotting blood product called fresh frozen plasma. IV fluids and blood transfusions may also be required. However, it is plausible that your poisoned character might not notice the early signs of poisoning—easy bruising, heavy periods, etc.—until the minor injury causes them to bleed out.

NON-ANTICOAGULANT RODENTICIDES

Bromethalin is a neurotoxin that causes swelling in the brain (*cerebral edema*). It is used as a single-dose rodenticide and is rarely fatal in humans. However, it is highly toxic to animals, including cats and dogs.[8]

Cholecalciferol (also known as Vitamin D) causes death in rodents by increasing the levels of calcium and phosphorous levels in their blood to dangerous levels.[8] Signs of cholecalciferol poisoning include nausea/vomiting, weakness, frequent urination, kidney stones, and kidney failure. It is rarely fatal in people, as it is difficult to ingest enough to cause serious toxicity.[8]

Strychnine is a widely popular poison in fiction, but not a very popular rat poison. In fact, only certified applicators are allowed to use it.[1] Despite its extremely bitter taste (or perhaps because of it), strychnine was used as a "health tonic" for centuries. That being said, strychnine poisoning is a horrible way to die. Strychnine is a colorless neurotoxin that causes uncontrollable muscle contractions throughout the body, resulting in exceedingly painful convulsions.

Sometimes called "awake seizures," your character will be awake and able to feel pain for several minutes, as the muscles of their face contract into a horrific smile (*rictus sardonicus*), their back arches (opisthotonos), and their hands clench to fists. They might die from asphyxiation, due to spasms of the muscles of the airway blocking off their ability to breathe. Or they could die from organ failure due to proteins and electrolytes spilling into the bloodstream as the intensity of the contractions leads to a breakdown of the muscles. Death usually comes within a few hours.

In the presence of water and acid, such as in the stomach, zinc phosphide transforms into phosphine gas, an organophosphate like sarin gas. It is particularly toxic for animals like rats

See *Ch. 2: Trouble Breathing* for more on organophosphate poisoning.

and mice who cannot vomit. In humans, ingestion causes headache, restlessness, dizziness, trouble breathing, and copious vomiting that smells of garlic. Severe ingestions result in fluid filling the lungs (*pulmonary edema*), low blood pressure, irregular heart rate, trouble walking, sweating, fatigue, vision changes, seizures, coma, or death.[8]

TETRODOTOXIN

Tetrodotoxin (TTX) is a neurotoxin that causes muscle paralysis. It is heat stable, meaning the toxin will not lose potency when cooked or boiled. Famously derived from the pufferfish in the form of Fugu, a Japanese delicacy, TTX is also found in high concentrations in other species, including the blue-ringed octopus, certain sea slugs, snails, crabs, and starfish. But TTX production isn't limited to the sea. Several species of frogs and newts, including the pacific northwest's rough-skinned newt, produce TTX in their skin as a defensive mechanism.

SYMPTOMS

TTX intoxication can begin anywhere from 15 minutes to 6 hours after ingestion.[9] Symptoms of TTX poisoning begin with numbness and tingling (paresthesia) around the mouth. It is for this symptom that Fugu has become popularized. These effects may or may not be accompanied by nausea, vomiting, or diarrhea. As the intoxication spreads, the numbness will spread to the face, tongue, and hands/feet, causing slurred speech and poor coordination. Other early symptoms include excess salivation, abdominal pain, headache, and sweating.

Aphonia = inability to speak due to problems with the voice box (larynx) or mouth.

Aphasia = inability to speak due to problems with the brain.

As the toxin progresses, your character will experience ascending paralysis and an inability to speak (*aphonia*). They may also experience cardiovascular problems, such as low blood pressure, slow heart rate, or heart arrhythmias, and their skin may blister and rub off. They will still be conscious.

Eventually, the paralysis will reach the diaphragm, the muscle required to breathe. Their blood pressure will tank, their heart rate will drop, and they make experience heart arrhythmias. Death is usually due to respiratory failure due to the paralysis of the diaphragm. They may or may not be completely conscious as they suffocate to death.

TREATMENT

There is no antidote for TTX. The mainstay of treatment is to perform gastric lavage (pump the stomach) immediately after known ingestion. Once symptoms begin, treatment is to intubate and mechanically ventilate the victim until the toxin can leave their system. Even with treatment, mortality hovers around 50%.[9] Death usually occurs in the first 24 hours; if the victim survives beyond that, their prognosis is good.[9]

DETECTION

The easiest way to detect tetrodotoxin is by sampling the food (usually seafood) that was ingested. If that isn't possible, it is possible to detect TTX in the blood and urine. However, it is technically challenging to do so and is not a routinely ordered test.[9]

POISON ACCOMPLICE: DMSO

Dimethyl sulfoxide is a chemical compound, beloved by chemists because it will dissolve almost anything. It's absorbed through the skin—and will take anything dissolved in it with it. This means that your character could take a substance that would usually need to be ingested orally, dissolve it in DMSO, then apply it surreptitiously to the victim's skin. It isn't toxic on its own, but it does increase the effects of certain medications, such as blood thinners and sedatives. And it's available over the counter.

BREAKING DOWN THE CLICHÉ: FAMOUS POISONS THAT AREN'T THAT LETHAL

DIGOXIN POISONING

The fox wore gloves, lest he touches the beautiful flower and be slain by its poison.

I grew up on a farm, and the gorgeous foxglove flowers were *persona non grata*. I was taught that the towering flowers were poisonous, not only to me but to our animals. Like the fox in the story, my dad always wore gloves when dealing with the plants. Turns out, foxglove plants are definitely poisonous. They're just not that deadly.

Leaves, flowers, and stems of the foxglove plant are toxic.

The foxglove plant famously produces a class of toxins called *cardiac glycosides*. Of these, digoxin is the most famous and is commonly used in modern medicine. The cardiac glycosides work at a cellular level to both increase the contractile strength of the heart and slow the electrical signaling, resulting in slower, stronger contractions of the heart. For that reason, digoxin is commonly prescribed to patients with heart failure and heart arrhythmias, such as atrial fibrillation.

Digoxin is famous for its narrow therapeutic window, meaning that the dose at which people get the benefit of the medication is very close to the dose where they get side effects. Side effects of digoxin include nausea/vomiting, drowsiness, slow heart rate, and visual changes resulting in a yellow halo around lights. It's been hypothesized that Van Gogh, famous for the yellow halos in his famous *Starry Night* and other paintings, was experiencing low-grade digoxin toxicity.[1]

While it doesn't take a very high dose to experience side effects from digoxin, it takes a remarkably high dose to be fatal when ingested orally—somewhere between 20-50 doses taken all at once. Since the foxglove plant has an even lower concentration of toxins, your character would have to eat a veritable foxglove salad to develop toxicity, as did this husband-and-wife, who mistook foxglove plants in their yard for kale, and lived to tell the teale.[10] If your character is a child, a small animal, or if they receive the dose intravenously, much smaller doses may be fatal.

OLEANDER HONEY

The old woman gathered honey
made by bees
fed exclusively
from her oleander trees.

She sold her honey
to a man down the way.
No one looked twice
when he passed away.

You've probably heard some version of the oleander honey story. And while oleander plants are poisonous, there are a few things wrong with this myth. First, oleander flowers do not produce nectar, so bees won't make honey from it. Second, it takes a lot of oleander flowers to kill.

Oleander produces several different toxins, but they're all cardiac glycosides and so have similar effects to digoxin. Symptoms of ingestion are similar to digitalis poisoning, including gastrointestinal upset, visual changes, slow heart rate, and heart arrhythmias. These symptoms appear around 2-4 hours after ingestion.[11]

The lethal dose of oleander varies depending on the part of the plant ingested, the exact species, the time of year, and the size of the person who has ingested it. Adults are unlikely to die from oleander ingestion, but a lethal dose is much easier to achieve in a child. One study found that it would take about 4 grams (2 tablespoons) worth of packed leaves to achieve a fatal dose in an adult.[11] While this large of a dose is sometimes seen in intentional ingestions (suicide attempts) it would be difficult for someone to accidentally ingest this amount.

PART II: TRAUMA

11. HEAD, NECK & THROAT INJURIES

Kunal is walking home from his favorite bar when he realizes he forgot his wallet. He's only a few blocks away, so he turns straight around. As he's passing the alley leading to the bar, he sees something move in the shadows. He turns just in time to see a knife glinting in the streetlight, then pain shoots up the left side of his scalp.

BACKGROUND

THE HEAD AND NECK ARE incredible structures. The head houses, not only the brain, but the eyes, the tongue, and all the tiny nerves that allow for taste and smell and facial movement.

The neck is a thin stalk that not only holds up our heavy head but is also the conduit that connects our brain (not to mention our nose and mouth) to the rest of the body. The delicate **spinal cord** runs through the neck, protected only by a bony casing of **cervical vertebrae**. Hollow tubes, such as the **esophagus** and **trachea**—the windpipe—connect the mouth and nose to the stomach and lungs, respectively. Huge blood vessels (the carotid artery and the jugular vein) run superficial and close to the skin. There's even an entire organ encased in the neck—the butterfly-shaped **thyroid**—that sits just in front of the trachea and regulates the body's metabolism.

No wonder the neck is such a good target.

SKULL AND SCALP INJURIES

SCALP INJURIES

Kunal spins away, reaching automatically to touch the side of his head. His fingers come away bloody.

Cuts to the scalp (*scalp lacerations*) bleed like h*ll, but they aren't usually life-threatening. The exception is if a large portion of the scalp is ripped from the skull. Medically, it's called an *avulsion*

> Scalp wounds are almost always stapled, rather than sutured, closed..

injury, but you've probably heard of it by the outdated (and slightly racist) term "scalping." Scalp injuries are treated by washing the wound, clamping off major blood vessels, and stapling the laceration closed. Your character will also receive imaging to rule out underlying skull fractures.

SKULL FRACTURES

The skull is very thick, so it takes a lot of force to crack it. If your character has a skull fracture, they'll have pain and swelling at the affected area and may be bleeding or leaking a serous (thin) pink fluid from their nostrils or ears. Skull fractures come in four basic flavors: simple, depressed, open, and basilar.

Simple fractures are like cracks in the pavement—a line that does not distort the overall integrity of the skull. The main treatment is to clean the area and assess for underlying brain damage.

Depressed fractures occur when part of the skull is crushed inwards, towards the brain. From the outside, it will look like a dent in your character's head. If your character has a depressed skull fracture, they made need neurosurgery to relieve the pressure on the brain.

Open fractures are characterized by bone fragments breaking through the skin. These require immediate surgery to protect the brain from infection.

Basilar skull fractures occur when the base of the skull is fractured. While basilar skull fractures are often missed on x-rays, there are important signs your character might exhibit. The first is "Battle's sign," or bruising behind the ear. The second— "raccoon eyes,"—is bruising around the eyes. Both signs are indicative of major blunt facial trauma that can cause basilar skull fractures. The third, and most worrisome sign is a pale pink fluid (cerebrospinal fluid) leaking from your character's ears or nose.

Cerebrospinal fluid (CSF) is the clear fluid that surrounds and cushions the brain.

While basilar skull fractures are a sign that your character experienced significant trauma, there isn't much doctors can do to treat it. Your character will be admitted and, assuming there's no sign of acute brain bleeding, managed expectantly.

Expectant management is the medical term for "watch and wait."

While there aren't a lot of treatments for basilar skull fractures, there are things medical professionals should absolutely avoid if your character is suspected of having a basilar skull fracture. The most important of these is the placement of nasogastric tubes (NG tubes) and nasogastric intubation. Anything going into the nose should be avoided like the plague. This is because a basilar skull fracture could provide an opening for the tube to snake into the brain, rather than your character's throat, giving them all sorts of brain damage. If you're looking for a classic, tragic medical mishap, look no further.

FACIAL INJURIES

Though the face may look solid, it's made up of a collection of rather fragile bones. Sports injuries, motor vehicle crashes (MVCs), falls, or even just a punch to the face can be enough to fracture some of these structures.

LOWER JAW INJURIES

With the right amount of force, the lower jaw (the *mandible*) can be broken or dislocated. A broken jaw is painful, especially at the site of the break. There will be swelling around the jaw and the surrounding face, which leads to stiffness, trouble chewing, and, a few hours later, bruising. Your character may also bleed from the mouth and feel as if their teeth have come loose. If they touch the site of the break, it will feel tender, and they may be able to feel bone crunching against bone.

If your character dislocates their jaw, it will also be painful, but the pain will be more related to movement. They may feel as if their teeth don't line up, or they can't shut their mouth, causing difficulty speaking and excessive drooling.

Lower jaw injuries are diagnosed with an x-ray and will be wired shut during recovery, meaning your character gets to spend the next several weeks eating through a straw.

MID-FACE FRACTURES

Major blunt force trauma to the face results in a distinctive pattern of fractures that occur along lines of weakness in the bone structure. There are three main types of facial fractures:

1. A horizontal fracture along the upper jaw (*maxilla*), just above the front teeth

2. Twin vertical fractures along either side of the nose

3. A horizontal fracture extending behind the eyes and across the bridge of the nose.

This pattern of facial fractures, called *Le Fort fractures* by those in the know, are a sign of significant trauma. They are associated with major complications, including difficult intubation and CSF leaks.

OTHER FACIAL FRACTURES

A fist swings out of the darkness, slamming into his nose. Kunal feels it crunch, then a metallic tang fills the back of his mouth.

Broken Nose (Nasal Fracture): Noses are easy to break because the nasal bones are thin and weak. Signs of a nasal fracture include bleeding, swelling, and bruising. Pain is usually sharp and intense at the moment of the break, but the pain quickly fades to a dull throb. If the bones are displaced (i.e., the nose looks crooked), and your character goes into the ED in time, the doctor can carefully, and with anesthesia, realign the bones and place a splint. Severe breaks (or those that have gone too long without getting fixed) require surgery.

Your character snapping their own nose back into place (or having someone else do it for them) is a great way cause permanent damage. The exception is martial artists and boxing coaches, who have had hands-on experience.

Broken Eye Socket (Orbital Fracture): The eye sockets are relatively fragile, while the orbit (the bony ring around the eyes) is strong. A fractured orbit indicates severe trauma and requires immediate repair by a plastic surgeon. A crack in the thin bones behind the eye, called the orbital floor, requires less force but can sometimes result in entrapment of the muscles and nerves of the eye, preventing its normal movement.

EYE INJURIES

Injuries to the eye are not for the faint of heart. Even the most minor injury can be enough to turn a reader's stomach.

Bloody Eye: There are two types of bloody eyes. The first, a ***subconjunctival hemorrhage,*** is a bloody pool on the white of the eye. It looks worse than it is. Caused by bleeding from the small blood vessels in the space between the white of the eye (sclera) and the eye's clear coating (conjunctiva), a subconjunctival hemorrhage is painless and will go away on its own.

The second, ***hyphema,*** looks like blood filling the iris and pupil. It is caused by blunt trauma to the eye; if your character gets a black eye from getting punched in the face, they might also develop hyphema. Unlike subconjunctival hemorrhage, hyphemas often require treatment; most of the time, that's just bed rest and steroid drops, but if the hyphema is causing increased pressure in the eye, your character may need it drained—a giant needle straight to the eye.

 NATALIE DALE, MD

Foreign Bodies: You've had dust in your eye at some point in your life; you know that gritty feeling as your eye tears up and you can't stop blinking. Most foreign objects are relatively harmless (dust, eyelashes, mascara, etc.) and can be removed with careful washing at home. If your character has shards of glass, wood, or metal embedded in their eye, they'll need to go to the ED to get them removed.

Ruptured Orbit: Also known as a punctured eyeball, a ruptured orbit occurs when something penetrates the outer layer of the eyeball, causing the fluid to drain away and the eyeball itself to collapse. Unsurprisingly, this is an ophthalmologic emergency that often results in blindness in that eye.

PENETRATING NECK INJURIES

Penetrating injuries are anything that cuts, stabs, or blasts through your character's skin and tissue, causing an open wound. Penetrating injuries cause lacerations (cuts), perforations (when an object passes cleanly through tissue), and punctures. High-energy projectiles, such as bullets, can also cause *cavitation* injuries and shockwaves.

When discussing penetrating injuries to the neck, the first step is to describe the mechanism of injury, such as stabbing vs. gunshot wound. The second step is to describe *where* the injury occurred. And no, 'the neck' is not specific enough. When talking about trauma, the neck is divided into three zones: the root, mid, and upper neck.

> **Cavitation injuries** are due to a large cavity formation around the path of the bullet. **Shock waves** cause injury via energy transfer. Both can cause severe injury.

The root of the neck extends from the collarbone to the Adam's apple. It's the most dangerous zone for penetrating injuries because the great vessels (the aorta and vena cava) run just beneath the collarbone. The mid-neck extends from the Adam's apple to the base of the jaw; most neck injuries occur here. The upper neck goes from the base of the skull and poses a challenge should your character need surgery since there are a lot of important structures packed into a very small area.

No matter the zone, your character will develop symptoms based on the organ that was involved. But remember, the neck is small, and the organs, nerves, and blood vessels are packed tightly together. If your character has an injury to one, others are likely injured.

BLOOD VESSELS

Thinking fast, Kunal presses the palm of his hand hard against the gash in his neck, trying to hold pressure on the wound. He doesn't have much time; he needs to get to the hospital. But first, he needs to escape.

In the root of the neck, the big concern is laceration of the great vessels: the *aorta* and *vena cava*. The aorta is the muscular artery that conducts blood from the heart to the rest of the body; the vena cava is the giant vein that brings the blood from the body back to the heart. Perforation of either will cause your character to bleed out in seconds.

In the mid and upper neck, the main concerns are the *carotid artery* and the *jugular vein*. The carotid artery and jugular vein run vertically and parallel to each other, on the sides of the neck. Laceration of the artery can cause high velocity spurting of blood, and your character will bleed out in anywhere from 5-15 seconds.[1] Laceration of the jugular vein will cause slower (but still high volume) bleeding; your character will still bleed out within minutes. Since the artery runs below the vein, it's possible to nick the vein without hitting the artery, but the reverse is rarely true.

> More about spinal cord injuries in *Ch. 12: Spine & Spinal Cord Injuries.*

The carotid artery and jugular vein are the biggest vessels in the neck, but they are not the only ones. Smaller vessels that run along the front of the neck will bleed if cut, but not enough to make your character bleed out quickly. A fun artery no one ever talks about is the *vertebral artery*, which runs along the side of the spine, providing blood to the spinal cord. Cut that vessel in the neck, and you've got some crazy neurologic symptoms, like *Brown-Sequard Syndrome* (see *Ch. 13: Spine & Spinal Cord Injuries*), which causes paralysis on one half of the body and loss of sensation on the other.

ESOPHAGUS

The esophagus connects the mouth to the stomach. As part of the gastrointestinal system, it is the conduit for all sorts of nasty bacteria. Perforation of the esophagus causes those bacteria to spill out into the neck or chest cavity, causing all sorts of infections if your character doesn't get antibiotics right away.

If your character has a perforated or damaged esophagus, they will feel significant pain and will resist moving their neck. Swallowing will be painful, and they may bleed from the mouth, or have blood-tinged saliva. They may also feel a crunching or popping under the skin of their neck, called *crepitus*.

Crepitus is caused by air bubbles forming under the skin. It's a sign that a hollow organ has been perforated.

WINDPIPE

The windpipe extends from the mouth down to the lungs and is made of the larynx, or voice box, and trachea. Externally, you can see the larynx; it's the Adam's apple.

Signs of damage to the larynx and trachea include changes in voice or a hoarse voice, drooling, difficulty breathing, stridor, and neck swelling. Coughing, swallowing, breathing, and even moving their tongue will be painful. If there's an obvious wound, there might be a sucking sound or pink froth that appears to bubble with every breath. The skin around the wound could exhibit crepitus.

Stridor is a high-pitched wheezing sound caused by blockage of the windpipe.

If there's any concern that the trachea might have been cut, doctors will need special equipment to intubate without causing serious damage.

NERVES

Several different nerves run through the neck; cutting one can result in a whole host of weird symptoms, including a drooping smile, trouble swallowing, a hoarse voice, or even tongue deviation! Most major nerve damage occurs due to injuries in the upper neck.

SPINAL CORD

We'll talk in detail about injuries to the spinal cord in Chapter 12, but it is very possible for a penetrating object (bullet, knife, etc.) to nick or sever the spinal cord, causing a whole host of problems.

TREATMENT

Treatment of penetrating neck injury is somewhat controversial. Some surgeons want to operate on every victim since neck wound victims can go downhill quickly,

Intubation is dangerous if your character has a penetrating injury to the neck. Providers may need to use guided techniques, such as bronchoscopy, to intubate safely.

while others support conservative management: watching and waiting. It can be a source of tension between providers; the surgeon who doesn't want to perform unnecessary procedures vs. the ICU physician who doesn't want the victim dying on their watch. How would your character feel, if their loved one was caught between the two?

BLUNT FORCE INJURIES

As Kunal focuses his energy on his assailant, he feels something cold slip around his throat. He's yanked backward as someone—a second assailant—tightens a belt around his throat.

Blunt force injuries cause damage through force of impact. It can cause broken vertebrae, strokes, and swollen soft tissue that has the potential to block off your hero's airway. Potential mechanisms for blunt force injuries to the neck include falls, car crashes, hangings, strangulation, and assault.

STRANGULATION

Kunal kicks and fights, but his assailant holds firm. His lungs scream for air, and he feels like his eyes might pop out of his head. As the world starts to go black, the first assailant steps forward, patting Kunal's empty pockets. Just as he's slipping out of consciousness, Kunal feels a warm wetness drip down his legs.

Strangulation is defined as the use of external pressure around a victim's neck to cut off air and blood supply.2 It takes less than 11 lbs. of weight to completely occlude the blood vessels.3 Strangulation can be accidental or intentional; the mechanism of strangulation can be manual (hands gripping throat) or utilizing a ligature, such as a rope, scarf, or belt. Accidental strangulation happens most often in children, while most adult strangulations are due to assault, homicide, or suicide. Women are particularly at risk of being strangled, due to intimate partner violence.[3]

> While choking and strangling are often used interchangeably, **choking** refers to an internal airway blockage, while **strangulation** refers to an external one.

As suddenly as the pressure came, it's gone. Kunal crumples to the ground, the world coming back into focus. He clutches his neck, gasping for air, barely registering his assailants' hasty retreat. Moments later, someone kneels beside Kunal. It's the bartender, holding a gun in one hand and Kunal's wallet in the other. He presses a towel to Kunal's neck and calls 911. The ambulance arrives, and Kunal is brought to the nearest trauma center, where is quickly whisked back to surgery for repair of the laceration.

Getting strangled is a terrifying and painful experience. As it's happening, your character will feel not only the pain of whatever is around their neck, but also the panicked feeling of needing to breathe and the fear of dying. After 30 seconds of strangulation, your character will lose control of their bowels and bladder. They may lose consciousness, though they will quickly regain it after the strangulation has ceased (providing they aren't dead or seriously brain damaged).

When your character wakes up, their voice will be hoarse and raspy. They may have pinpoint bruises (*petechiae*) on their face, broken blood vessels in their eyes (*subconjunctival hemorrhage*), pain and tenderness along their neck and throat, and trouble swallowing. They'll develop bruising (finger or ligature marks) along their neck, though in darker skinned characters, the bruising may be hard to see.

> Doctors aren't often taught how to look for skin changes in dark skinned individuals, contributing to the under-treatment of people of color. In your writing, it can be a source of conflict between your character and the medical establishment.

When Kunal wakes from surgery, he feels battered and bruised. It hurts to swallow, to move his neck, to breathe—but he's alive. His neck is bandaged where the knife cut him, and he can feel bruises along the line where the belt nearly strangled him. He spends a few nights in the hospital before going home to the care of his sister.

Near-strangulation has both immediate and long-term consequences for your character. Immediately, the symptoms all have to do with there not being enough oxygen getting to their brain. They might have seizures, strokes, and brain swelling that can lead to permanent brain damage. This is particularly true if your character was strangled to the point of passing out.[2]

A month later, Kunal is playing basketball with friends when he collapses to the ground, suddenly unable to speak or move the right side of his body. He's taken to the hospital, where he's diagnosed with a stroke and given a clot-busting medication. No one knows for sure, but Kunal's doctors think it was probably caused by his assault a month prior.

Long-term consequences of strangulation are mainly due to bruising and tissue swelling. If your character survived near strangulation, they could still die of suffocation, as their

> Long-term consequences of strangulation are a great opportunity to play with reader expectations.

airway swells up in response to the strangulation forces on their neck. Similarly, near strangulation could cause a clot to break off of the carotid artery and travel up to the brain, giving your character a stroke hours, or even days, after survival of the initial strangulation attempt.

HANGING

There are three ways to die from hanging: suffocation due to a crushed windpipe, lack of blood flow to the brain due to compression of the arteries and veins in the neck, and a fractured cervical vertebra that severs the spinal cord.

This last mechanism is considered the most humane, as it causes instantaneous death. It does so by creating a specific fracture of the second cervical vertebra (C2) called the "hangman's fracture." To guarantee that this is how the victim will die, the knot of the noose is placed under their neck, and they are dropped from a calculated height.[4] This method (called the long drop) is supposed to be a more humanitarian method of execution. It is still used for capital punishment in some countries today, including India.[4]

> Historically, the short drop was the most common method of hanging. It is also the most common method for suicides via hanging.

The short drop—kicking away a stool or dropping the floor out from under the victim with the noose around their neck—is less pleasant. Death can take anywhere from 5 to 45 minutes, and it is horrible to watch as the victim kicks, spasms, and seizes. However, it is also survivable. Particularly if your character was somewhat responsive at the time of the incident, it is very possible that they could walk out of the hospital without any long-term brain damage.

BROKEN NECK (FRACTURED CERVICAL VERTEBRAE)

In Volume 1, I talked about the ABCs of the medical response to an emergency: **A**irway with c-spine protection, **B**reathing, and **C**irculation. The first step—Airway—require the addition of "with c-spine protection" because of the dangers inherent to a broken neck.

Neck fractures are some of the most dangerous injuries your character can incur. A bone shard in the neck can sever the spinal cord, and BAM, your character is paralyzed for life. That's why it's so important to protect the neck if there's any chance at all that the cervical vertebrae (aka the seven bones that hold up the head and protect the spinal cord) could be

> For more on the medical response to emergencies, see <u>Volume 1: Setting & Character</u>, *Ch. 13: Approach to an Emergency.*

injured. For this reason, anyone with significant trauma, MVCs, falls, etc., will be placed in a c-collar until their c-spine can be cleared.

Fractured cervical vertebrae can be unstable. They can slip and sever the spinal cord at any moment, particularly if the neck is moved, resulting in paralysis. This can happen at any point during care, including:

> **Whiplash** is a legal term (not a medical one) for strained neck ligaments caused by acceleration/ deceleration injuries.

- Moment of impact

- Moving the victim (out of harm's way, in order to be ventilated, onto the stretcher, etc.)

- Placing the victim on a stretcher

- Transport in the ambulance

- Transferring the victim from the gurney to the bed

- Transferring the victim onto the surgery table

> Done incorrectly, any one of these transfers could shift an unstable vertebra and cause paralysis for your character.

If your character has a fractured cervical vertebra, they'll have a stiff, painful neck with a limited ability to move their head. If someone touches the bone itself, it will be exceedingly painful. If there's no tenderness over the bone, chances are good that there's no fracture, and the doctors will take off the c-collar.

BREAKING DOWN THE CLICHÉS

PULLING OUT THE KNIFE

> *Tara Sunder is in the fight for her life against her evil nemesis. She thinks she's finally got him, when he leans down and pulls a knife from his boot, stabbing her in the neck. She manages to throw him off her—and off the cliff behind them—but the knife stays embedded in her flesh. She checks over the cliffside to make sure her nemesis is dead, then pulls out his knife, spits on it, and throws it after him.*

Don't. Pull. Out. That. Knife. Or the shard of glass, or the sword, or the metal rod. If something is penetrating your character's flesh, do not—I repeat, DO NOT—pull it out. Unless you wish your character to suffer even more catastrophic injury, of course.

When something is embedded in your character's body, it puts pressure on the blood vessels, keeping them (relatively) shut. When you pull the penetrating object out, it not only reinjures the surrounding flesh, but it also relieves the pressure on those blood vessels, allowing them to bleed to their heart's delight. For this reason, your character should always wait until they have access to prompt medical attention. For injuries where it's unlikely to cause significant bleeding—such as the hand or foot—that may just mean a place with bandages, pain meds, sutures, and antiseptic. However, if there's any chance the penetrating object has nicked a major artery, the object shouldn't be moved until your character is actually in the OR. This includes any injuries to the neck, groin, armpit, abdomen, chest, or skull.

INJECT IN THE NECK

"He's getting stronger! I'm not going to be able to hold him."

Doctor walks up, injects medication into patient's neck

Patient drops immediately

Movies love injecting characters—particularly ones who are agitated or violent—straight into the neck. And every time, the injected medication starts working in seconds. In truth, medical professionals rarely administer medications into the neck. There are several reasons for this.

> For more on methods of medication administration, see FAQ #2.

First, super-fast-acting medication needs to be given intravenously (IV), and injecting medication into a vein is quite difficult. To inject a medication intravenously, your character will first have to find the vein, then carefully insert the needle, then inject the meds. This isn't something you can do in the middle of a fight. The easiest way to inject medications intravenously is if the character already has a catheter inserted—usually in the hand or the crook of the elbow. All the provider needs to do is inject the medications through the IV.

Second, injecting into a vein *in* the neck is even more difficult because the veins there are located relatively deep. Sometimes doctors do, in fact, need to administer medications into the big vein in the neck, called the *internal jugular vein*. To do so, doctors need to perform a small surgical procedure, called *intrajugular vein cannulation*, to gain IV access. There is no way your character could do *that* during a fight.

Third, injecting straight into the neck can have disastrous consequences. The internal jugular vein carries a lot of blood; puncturing it could cause massive bleeding into the neck, called a *hematoma*. Worse, the carotid artery runs right beneath it. If the doctor tries to jab the neck and they miss by even a few centimeters, they've punctured the carotid artery and your character will bleed out. And don't even get me started on all the important nerves your character could hit with that needle.

Third, injecting into the neck vein, rather than any other vein, won't make the medications take effect any faster. Veins drain blood from the body into the heart, the internal jugular vein drains blood from the head. That means that, if your character actually managed to inject into the jugular vein, the medications wouldn't go straight to the brain; the meds would first be carried down to the heart and would then traverse the same path as if they had been injected into a vein in the arm or hand.

12. TRAUMATIC BRAIN INJURIES

Layne is riding their bike to work. They're riding fast; they're late for a big presentation, and since they're only going a few blocks away, they didn't bother putting on a helmet. They're almost there when a car door opens right in front of them. They don't have time to stop—their bike slams into the door, and they are thrown forward, tumbling head over heels. The last thing they see is the pavement rising up to meet them.

BACKGROUND

Traumatic brain injuries (TBI) are both common and devastating. Almost three million TBIs are diagnosed in the US every year; nearly one-third are children.[1] And TBIs can cause nasty sequelae; nearly half of those hospitalized for a TBI will have a long-term disability.[1] So, if you're giving your character a TBI, make sure to think about what long-term effects it might have.

Regardless of the underlying cause, symptoms of TBIs include headache, nausea/vomiting, confusion and drowsiness, slurred speech, memory loss, disorientation, personality, and cognitive changes, and dizziness. TBIs that cause damage in one particular part of the brain, such as brain bleeds (*hematomas)*, will have focal neurologic deficits specific to both the area of the brain and the side of the body that was injured.

Focal neurologic deficits are problems with a specific part of the brain that affect a particular area of the body, See *Ch. 7: Stroke* for more.

When Layne wakes up, they're lying on the road, surrounded by strangers. Their head is pounding, and when they reach up to touch the back of their head, their fingers come away bloody. As lights and sirens barrel down the narrow street, Layne realizes someone must have called 911.

If your character was hit in the head, especially if they've lost consciousness, they'll need to be evaluated by a medical provider. This will include asking questions regarding the mechanism of injury, assessing their score on the Glasgow

Coma Scale (see below), and performing a neurologic exam. Depending on the severity of the injury and your character's symptoms, your character may also need brain imaging.

IMAGING

Brains are imaged using two modalities: the CT scan and the MRI. A CT scan is basically a 3D x-ray. CTs are great for showing blood on the brain, as well as bony fractures, so they are usually the first step in imaging after TBI. Brain MRIs use electromagnetic waves to provide a detailed view of the structures of the brain and are used for imaging that needs a higher level of detail, such as tumors or autoimmune lesions.

CLASSIFICATION OF TBI

The severity of a traumatic brain injury can be measured by three factors: the Glasgow Coma Scale score (see below), the duration of the loss of consciousness, and the duration of posttraumatic amnesia. And while a positive finding on head CT places your character in a moderate-to-severe category, they could still have a severe TBI even if the imaging looks normal.

Measure	Mild	Moderate	Severe
Glasgow Coma Score	13-15	9--12	3-8
Duration LOC	< 30 min	30 min - 6 hrs.	> 6 hrs.
Duration PTA	0-1 day	1-7 days	> 7 days
Head CT	Normal	Normal or Abnormal	Normal or Abnormal

GLASGOW COMA SCALE (GCS)

When the paramedics arrive, one goes to talk to the bystanders while another—a tall man with a thick black beard—sits Layne down on the curb and asks them a barrage of questions. Layne answers to the best of their ability, telling him how they flipped their bike over the car door and lost consciousness for a few minutes. They're able to answer all his questions easily, until he asks what day it is. Suddenly unsure, Layne looks around for clues. They're wearing nice slacks and their favorite blouse—work clothes, though they're now covered in blood—and the morning sun is already hot. They make a guess—Tuesday?— and see the paramedic's thick eyebrows furrow in concern.

The Glasgow Coma Scale is used to evaluate the level of consciousness after a head trauma. It has three components: eye-opening, motor response, and verbal response. Each behavior category ranges in score from least responsive to most. In all three categories, least responsive means no response.

Behavior	Response	Score
Eye Opening	Does Not Open Eyes	1
	Opens to Painful Stimulus	2
	Opens to Voice	3
	Opens Spontaneously	4
Motor Response	No Movement	1
	Arms/Legs straight, back arched (*"decerebrate posturing"*)	2
	Arms flexed; legs turned inward (*"decorticate posturing"*)	3
	General movement to pain	4
	Specific movement to pain	5
	Obeys commands	6
Verbal Response	No vocalizations	1
	Incomprehensible sounds	2
	Inappropriate words	3
	Appropriate words but confused	4
	Appropriate words and oriented	5
	Total	**3-15**

The severity of a head injury is classified by the GCS score. A GCS of 14-15 is mild, a score of 9-13 is moderate, and 3-8 is severe. Remember, a GCS of 3 is the lowest possible score.

POSTTRAUMATIC AMNESIA (PTA)

Posttraumatic amnesia, which occurs after a brain injury, impairs your character's ability to make new memories. Your character will be confused, asking the same questions over and over as they try to figure out what is going on. And while they'll remember who they are, they might have trouble recognizing their friends and family. They may also act out of character, becoming aggressive or rude. PTA is self-limited, meaning that it will stop on its own without treatment, and usually only lasts for minutes to hours. Rarely, it can last weeks or even months. The more severe the head injury, the longer the PTA will last.

> If your character emerges from a coma, they will likely have PTA.

CONCUSSION

The paramedic informs Layne that he thinks they need to be taken to the hospital. Layne disagrees; they feel fine. And anyway, what could the doctors possibly do for them at the hospital? They had a concussion a few years back, and the doctors hadn't been able to do anything about it. They found nothing on the CT scan and hadn't given them any medications to help the blinding headache. Layne had spent months feeling like their brain was inhabited by an angry alien: daily headaches, trouble concentrating, trouble controlling their temper, even trouble remembering what led to the concussion in the first place. But they'd gotten better eventually, no thanks to the doctors. What was the point in taking an expensive ambulance ride if nothing could help?

> **A&Ox4** is medical shorthand for alert and oriented to time (the date), person (who they are), place (where they are), and why (what brought them to the doctor).

A concussion is a diffuse brain injury that occurs when your character's brain sloshes around inside the skull after getting hit or shaken. Lots of things can cause concussions, ranging from car accidents and physical attacks to sports injuries. Most of the time, your character won't lose consciousness at the time of injury or will be unconscious for only a few seconds.

SYMPTOMS

After the injury, they'll have a headache, nausea/vomiting, confusion, and may feel tired or lethargic. Other symptoms include sensitivity to sound and light, ringing ears,

> **Post-concussive syndrome** happens when the symptoms of the concussion last for more than three months.

dizziness, blurred vision, mood changes, cognitive changes, and trouble sleeping. Your character may even have some memory loss, but don't go overboard, it isn't the global amnesia you may have seen on daytime television. Most of the time, it just means they won't be able to remember the events leading up to the concussion, (retrograde amnesia), or will have difficulty forming memories after the injury (posttraumatic anterograde amnesia).

SEVERITY

Concussions are graded by severity. Severity is determined by the duration of symptoms and whether your character lost consciousness. The higher the grade of the concussion, the longer your character's recovery will take.

Grade	Mental Status	Duration of Symptoms	Loss of Consciousness
Mild (Grade 1)	Confused/Posttraumatic amnesia	< 15 min	No
Moderate (Grade 2)	Confused/Posttraumatic amnesia	> 15 min	No
Severe (Grade 3)	Confused/Posttraumatic amnesia	> 15 min	Yes

DIAGNOSIS

Concussions don't show up on CT or MRI scans; there are no visible physical changes. Similarly, they won't show any focal neurologic changes on the physical exam. Instead, concussions are diagnosed clinically. Treatment is focused on managing symptoms, such as headache, ringing in the ears, vertigo, and memory problems.

Vertigo = the sensation that the world is spinning.

PROGNOSIS

Concussions can take a long time to heal (weeks to months), but in general, people do recover. Most of the symptoms are worst in the first 7-10 days, and they usually clear up within three months. If symptoms persevere beyond three months, your character has persistent post-concussive syndrome, in which symptoms can last up to a year.

Chronic traumatic encephalopathy (CTE) is brain damage caused by many repeated hits to the head.

One of the most dangerous things your character can do after a concussion is to get

NATALIE DALE, MD

right back in the action. If your character gets hit on the head, then gets back up and keeps on doing whatever they were doing, watch out! A second hit can aggravate the first injury, causing *second impact syndrome*—severe brain swelling that can lead to death.

Repeated concussions, even mild ones, can lead to *chronic traumatic encephalopathy*—a progressive brain disorder characterized by anterograde amnesia, mood swings, confusion, disorientation, and trouble making decisions. As the disease progresses, the memory problems worsen, as does the personality changes, and they develop the typical symptoms of Parkinson's disease: tremor, muscle stiffness, poor balance, and slowed movements. CTE is strongly associated with contact sports, primarily football. Phillip Adams, an NFL player, was found to have severe CTE on autopsy after he'd shot and killed six people and then himself.[9]

SHEARING INJURY (DIFFUSE AXONAL INJURY)

Diffuse axonal injury (DAI) is an acceleration/deceleration injury. It occurs when the brain is thrown so violently against the skull that the long axons of the neurons are sheared off. It requires a high-force mechanism of acceleration and deceleration, such as motor vehicle collisions, long falls, and high-velocity sports injuries.[2] It is both one of the most common, and most devasting, types of traumatic brain injury.

> **Shaken baby syndrome** is at type of diffuse axonal injury.

DAI presents as a loss of consciousness, usually for at least six hours. Those few who regain consciousness usually exhibit signs of permanent brain damage. However, most people who survive DAI are left in a permanent coma.

> A concussion is the mildest form of diffuse axonal injury.

Like concussions, DAI doesn't show up very well on imaging. Instead, the diagnosis is made based on the mechanism of injury and your character's presenting symptoms. If your character survives DAI, they will have long-term brain damage and will need significant rehabilitation.

BRAIN BRUISE (CEREBRAL CONTUSION)

A cerebral contusion is bruised brain tissue, caused by the brain slamming against the skull. It causes focal bleeding and, 24-72 hours later, swelling. Cerebral contusions are serious injuries that cause both direct and indirect damage to a focal point of the brain. They're diagnosed with a CT scan and neurologic exam, including a GCS score. The lower the GCS score, the less likely they are to survive, but even those with the best prognosis tend to have residual deficits.

Sequelae of cerebral contusions include seizures, cognitive and personality changes, lack of smell, impaired concentration and memory, coma, and death. The exact symptoms your character will experience will be based on the specific location of the bleed itself; a bleed at the front of the brain may be more likely to have changes in personality and smell, while a bleed located near the left temple is more likely to have changes in language. It's beyond the scope of this chapter to delve into the regions of the brain, but I covered it briefly in *Ch. 7: Stroke*. If you know where your character is going to get hit, look up what that part of the brain does. It can guide you when you're writing your character's symptoms.

BRAIN BLEEDS

The brain is a highly vascularized organ and there are lots of blood vessels, both within the brain and along with the protective coverings of the brain. There are several different layers of protective coverings around the brain. From the outside-in, the layers are the scalp, the skull, the thick *dura mater*, the spidery *arachnoid mater*, the delicate *pia mater*, and the brain tissue itself. Depending on the layer in which the bleed is located, your character will have different symptoms.

> If your character gets an "epidural" during labor, it means she had numbing medications injected into the epidural space in her spinal cord.

EPIDURAL HEMATOMA

Epidural hematomas are caused by arterial bleeding that collects between the skull and the protective dura, called the *epidural space*. Because the dura is thick, somewhat rigid, and attached to the skull in specific places, an epidural bleed results in a pool of blood between the skull and this thick outer layer. Epidural hematomas are most commonly caused by a strike to the side of the head, near the temple.

Epidural hematomas present in a very specific way. Your character, usually young and healthy, gets hit on the head and falls unconscious. Then they wake up, insisting that they're fine, though they have a bit of a headache. As the headache worsens, they get progressively more and more drowsy until, just a few hours later, they fall unconscious again, and this time, they won't wake up.

> The period time after your character wakes up until she passes out again is called the **lucid interval**.

As Layne is signing the refusal of transport paperwork, the pounding in their head intensifies. They feel tired, all they want is to go home and curl up in bed. Hiding a yawn, they hand the paperwork back to the bearded paramedic.

He reminds them to go to the hospital if they start feeling worse, then asks how they're going to get there. Layne lies, making up a story about calling a friend, but the paramedic's exchange worried looks. A bystander steps up and says something to the paramedic about how Layne wasn't slurring their words like that earlier. The paramedic returns and pleads with Layne to let them take them to the hospital. They finally agree, it seems like less work than trying to convince the paramedic they're fine.

Mechanically, as the artery continues to bleed, the collection of blood grows, pushing on the brain. But the brain is encased in a hard skull—what happens when there's too much crammed into too little space? The brain begins to herniate, squishing down through the only hole it can find, the one at the base of the skull where the brain connects to the spinal cord. Once the brain herniates, it squishes the brainstem, which controls your character's most basic life functions, and then your character dies.

By the time they arrive at the hospital, all Layne wants is to go to sleep. As they're rolled into the ED, they're surrounded by a flurry of people in white coats and scrubs, poking needles into their arms and shining lights into their eyes. Someone stays with them as they're rolled down the CT scanner, a machine that looks like a white donut whose nonstop whirring makes them want to tear out their eardrums.

Epidural hematomas are diagnosed by a head CT showing a lens-shaped collection of blood on the brain. The treatment is emergency neurosurgery. About 20% of people with an epidural hematoma will die because of it.[3]

After returning from the CT scan, a doctor enters Layne's room and tells them that they have a brain bleed called an epidural hematoma. They're going to need emergency surgery. Begrudgingly, Layne agrees, and they're quickly whisked back to the OR.

If I had to pick a favorite medical condition for writers, it would be the epidural hematoma. The stakes are high (life-threatening brain bleed in an otherwise healthy and young character), there's a ticking clock, and there's serious potential for a missed diagnosis. So much tension!

SUBDURAL HEMORRHAGE

A subdural hemorrhage is a collection of blood in the space between the *dura mater* and the *arachnoid mater*. The bleeding is venous, rather than arterial,

> The **dura mater** is the thick lining closest to the skull. The **arachnoid mater** is a transparent, spidery membrane that fits between the dura and the **pia mater**—the thin lining closest to the brain.

so it happens over a longer timescale than the epidural hematoma. Subdural hematomas can be acute—meaning the blood pools and begins causing symptoms in a matter of hours—or chronic. Subdural hemorrhages can occur after minor trauma, particularly if your character is older or on blood-thinning meds.

Like other types of TBIs, subdural hematomas present with headache, nausea/vomiting, and disorientation. Acute subdural hemorrhages are particularly dangerous. Symptoms, particularly the headache, appear suddenly and are quite severe. Without prompt neurosurgical treatment, your character will herniate and die.

Chronic subdural, on the other hand, can take months to show up. They are more insidious and cause chronic changes, say in personality or memory that your other characters might chalk up to dementia or old age. If you're looking for a reversible cause of dementia or want your elderly character to have long-term sequelae of a fall that was "no big deal," a chronic subdural hematoma is a great option.

SUBARACHNOID HEMORRHAGE (SAH)

Subarachnoid hemorrhage is a brain bleed that occurs between the delicate *pia mater* and the soft layer called the *arachnoid mater*. SAH causes a sudden, intense headache—the worst headache of your character's life—along with weakness, dizziness, and a decreased level of consciousness. They may even have seizures. Doctors sometimes call this a "sudden drop" headache.

The most common cause of SAH is trauma, but it can also be caused by a burst aneurysm.

See *Ch. 7: Stroke* for more on SAH & ICH.

INTRACEREBRAL HEMORRHAGE (ICH)

Intracerebral hemorrhage, bleeding inside the brain tissue itself, is the fourth and final type of brain bleed. ICH doesn't have to be caused by trauma; in fact, ICH is often caused by high blood pressure. However, if ICH is present after a traumatic injury, it's probably a bad sign; traumatic ICH is associated with a mortality rate of up to 50%.[3]

PENETRATING BRAIN INJURIES

This probably goes without saying, but anything stabbing, poking, or blasting through brain tissue is not good news. That said, there are certainly survivable penetrating cerebral traumas. The most famous case is Phineas Gage, who had a railroad iron blown into his left eye, through his brain, and out top. He lived to tell the tale, but his personality was forever altered; a quiet, reliable young man turned into an aggressive alcoholic bully who couldn't keep a job.[4]

I wouldn't recommend doing anything quite so spectacular to any of your characters, sometimes the truth is stranger than fiction. But the brain is super unpredictable, so you can get away with some pretty insane injuries, so long as there are real consequences. If your character is going to get stabbed or shot in the head, here are a few rules of thumb.

> The moral of Phineas Gage's story is **not** that you can give your character whatever horrific injuries you want, and they might still survive. The moral is that if you mess with the brain, there had better be consequences.

1. The most important brain function (for survival) is the brainstem, located at the base of the skull. A gunshot to the back of the throat ("swallowing the gun") is more likely to be fatal than a shot to the temple.

2. Bullets move fast, causing *cavitation injuries* (See Ch 11: Head, Neck, & Throat Injuries). Even a straight shot through the brain is going to cause an impressive amount of damage.

3. Do *not* pull out the ax! If your character has something sticking out of their skull or brain, for the love of G-d, leave it in there until they get to an experienced neurosurgeon.

4. Check for entry and exit wounds; the exit wound will likely be much bigger (and messier) than the entrance wound.

5. Unlike gunshot wounds to other parts of the body, bullet fragments in the brain should be removed to prevent infection and abscess formation.[5]

BREAKING DOWN THE CLICHÉS: BLOWS TO THE HEAD

BLOWS TO THE HEAD THAT CAN...KNOCK SOMEONE OUT

He was on top of her, pinning her to the floor. She could smell his fetid breath and feel his saliva pooling on her neck as he growled.

"Wolf," she whispered, praying that saying his name would bring him back to her, "it's me!"

But it was a futile hope. He raised his head and howled, his pointed fangs glistening in the moonlight. Then something moved in the shadows, almost too fast to see. Something black and heavy collided with the side of Wolf's temple and he crumpled to the floor. A woman appeared behind him, holding the bloodied tire iron in one hand.

"Don't worry," she said, kneeling beside Wolf's crumpled body, "He'll wake up in a few hours. He'll have a headache when he does, but he'll be ok."

He probably won't be ok. A hit to the head hard enough to cause someone to lose consciousness, even for just a few seconds, is going to cause some damage. At best, he'll have a concussion and all the headaches, nausea/vomiting, confusion, blurry vision, and ringing ears that go along with it. At worst, he'll have a skull fracture and a life-threatening brain bleed. Without medical attention, he may never wake up at all.

> See FAQ #3 for more on the repercussions of knocking someone unconscious.

The longer your character is out cold, the more likely they are to have severe damage. Unconsciousness lasting seconds to minutes may be mild enough to only cause a concussion; unconsciousness lasting more than 20 minutes is a sign of moderate to severe brain injury. If it lasts more than six hours after head trauma is a sign of severe injury, usually diffuse axonal injury, which has a very poor prognosis.

That said, it *is* technically possible to knock someone out with a single punch. Boxers can do it, as an experienced martial artist. But that's usually when they're fighting someone less experienced and/or drunk, AND they get the perfect punch in. Even for professionals, a knockout punch is a very rare occurrence. Unless your character is a professional fighter up against an unsuspecting enemy, a single knockout punch isn't going to be believable.

BLOWS TO THE HEAD THAT CAN...CAUSE AMNESIA

Mema Ree wakes up in a hospital bed, IV lines and tubing poking out of her body like quills on a hedgehog. A man sits beside her bed, his face furrowed with worry. As she stirs, he looks up, his face brightening.

"Mema," he cries, "you're awake!"

She licks her lips, not sure how to respond. She's never seen this man before in her life, and her name isn't Mema…is it?

The man takes her by the hand, tears sliding down his face.

"You were hit in the head by a baseball—John said you didn't see it coming. I've never seen anything like it, you just dropped! But you're awake now, thank God!"

She licks her lips again and blinks. Baseball? John? Nothing sounds familiar. Who is this man? More importantly, who is she?

This trope gets something right: post-traumatic amnesia does exist. In fact, it's pretty common; about 25% of victims with concussions have some sort of amnesia.[6] But it's not the type of amnesia you see on TV.

Post-traumatic amnesia (PTA), also called post-concussive amnesia, comes in two flavors: retrograde and anterograde. In **retrograde PTA**, the victim forgets the events leading up to the injury. Usually, retrograde amnesia is only for the minutes leading up to the injury, but it can rarely wipe out hours or even days. In **anterograde PTA**, the victim has trouble forming new memories *after* the injury. Notice how the victim doesn't forget important biographical information (who they are, family members' names, etc.) in either case. Both kinds tend to get better with time, though retrograde PTA usually improves faster than anterograde PTA.[7]

In doing research for this book, I found one example of a patient who lost his identity after a traumatic brain injury; a 43-year-old Ob/Gyn doctor who, after his injury, didn't know his name or recognize himself in the mirror, and thought he was 7 or 8 years old.[8] He didn't recognize his family, his wife, or even his dog. He also had a laundry list of other ailments, ranging from difficulty speaking to personality and IQ changes. He was also paralyzed on half his body.[8]

Aphasia is the medical term for the loss of ability to speak.

It's a fascinating case study, and I suggest you read it. But that's the point: it's a case study, so rare that doctors who deal with brain injuries daily wrote it up and got it published. It is not the norm. Furthermore, the identity loss didn't happen in isolation—it occurred alongside significant neurologic deficits, such as paralysis and aphasia.

If you need a character to develop generalized amnesia, instead consider dissociative amnesia. Affecting about 1.8% of the population, dissociative amnesia is a poorly understood psychiatric disorder usually brought on by trauma or stress. Most of the time, the amnesia is localized, meaning that your character has amnesia for a traumatic event, or for certain periods of time (months, or even years). Generalized amnesia, in which your character completely forgets their entire life history and/or their personal identity, is extremely rare.

Generalized amnesia is more common in sexual assault victims and combat veterans.

BLOWS TO THE HEAD THAT CAN...FIX AMNESIA

The girl called Mema is sick of being in this hospital bed, sick of people calling her by a name she doesn't recognize. She pulls off the wires on her chest, disconnects the cuffs on her legs and arm, and stands, intending to run away.

But her right leg is weak, and it collapses beneath her. She hits her head as she falls. When she wakes up, she remembers everything.

If a hit to the head can cause amnesia, maybe another hit can cure it! That logic doesn't hold water (though don't tell that to people who practice homeopathy). Your brain is a complicated web of neurons and support cells, interwoven and interdependent; a second hit is likely to cause more damage, not fix it.

A second hit before the brain has had a chance to recover from the first can cause **second-impact syndrome**—severe brain swelling that is often fatal. Repeated concussions can lead to **chronic traumatic encephalopathy.**

13. SPINE & SPINAL CORD INJURIES

Muhammad is trying to get his house clean before his mother-in-law comes over. Balancing a laundry basket on one hip and his six-month-old daughter, Maha, on the other, he doesn't see the cat until it's too late. He steps on its tail, and it yowls, streaking out from between his feet and causing him to lose his balance. He falls backward, the laundry basket forgotten as he tries to keep from falling on top of his daughter. He lands hard, the back of his neck crunching against the hard edge of the coffee table.

BACKGROUND

THE NERVOUS SYSTEM IS BROKEN up into two main components: the central nervous system (CNS) and the peripheral nervous system (PNS). The central nervous system is made up of the brain and spinal cord, while the peripheral nervous system consists of the nerves that connect the spinal cord to the rest of the body. Neurons are a type of cell that use electricity to conduct signals throughout the nervous system. There are several types of neurons—sensory neurons, motor neurons, interneurons—and similar types of neurons run together. In the peripheral nervous system, a bundle of neurons forms a nerve.

The spinal cord is part of the central nervous system, and it connects the brain to the rest of the body. It's like a stupidly complicated highway, conveying electric messages back and forth between the brain and the peripheral nerves. Damage that highway, and there's no way for the brain and body to communicate below the level where the cord was damaged.

The spine is made up of four (technically five) sections. In descending order, they are the 7 cervical vertebrae, 12 thoracic vertebrae, 5 lumbar vertebrae, and 5 sacral vertebrae, which are fused together to form part of the pelvis. The lowest fifth part of the spine is the coccyx or tailbone. Vertebrae are named based on their type and number in order from the top down: C1 is the first cervical vertebra, T10 is the tenth thoracic vertebra, and so on.

Nerves connect to the spinal cord through holes in the spinal vertebrae called *foramen* and each nerve connects to the spine at a specific level. If the spine is injured at that level, then those nerves and *everything below it* will no longer be able to connect to the brain. This means doctors can pinpoint the symptoms that will result from injury at a particular level. This is critically important if you want to give your character a realistic spinal cord injury. Here are some important levels you should know:

IMPORTANT NERVE ROOT LEVELS

Muhammad wakes to the sound of his daughter screaming. His head is pounding, but he doesn't feel hurt, otherwise. He reaches out for her daughter— but his hands don't move. Panic rises inside him as he tries and tries to get up, but nothing is working. Maha crawls towards him, tears clinging to her lashes, but Muhammad feels nothing as his daughter curls up beside him.

Transection at each level will cause the symptoms listed here as well as all the symptoms below it.

C1 & C2: injuries here are almost always fatal.

C3-C5: innervate the diaphragm. If your character is injured above C5, they will not be able to breathe on their own.

Med students learn the rhyme, "C3, 4, 5 keeps the diaphragm alive.".

C5-T1: Innervate the arms and upper chest. Injury above T1 will result in complete paralysis of the arms and legs (*tetraplegia* or *quadriplegia*).

L1-L3: Control bowel function. An injury here will result in loss of bowel control.

L2-S2: Innervate the legs. Injury above this level, but below T1, will result in paralysis of the legs (*paraplegia*) only.

S2-S4: Control bladder and sexual function.

CAUSES OF SPINAL CORD INJURY (SCI)

Muhammad screams until his voice is hoarse, but no one hears. When his mother-in-law finally arrives, she calls an ambulance right away. Muhammad is strapped to a backboard, his neck immobilized by an uncomfortable plastic brace. He wonders if it is a good sign that he can feel the plastic rubbing against his neck.

There are many ways to injure the spinal cord. It can be cut (*transected*), bruised (*contusion*), stunned (*concussion*), or compressed. Injuries can also lead to swelling of the spinal cord (*edema*). Transection (the physical cutting of the spinal cord) is generally due to penetrating injuries, such as stabbings or gunshot wounds, or unstable fractures of the vertebrae. Blunt injuries, such as crush injuries, acceleration/deceleration injuries, and blunt impacts, tend to cause bruising, swelling, and sometimes even stunning of the spinal cord.

Mechanisms of spinal injury range from penetrating trauma (GSWs, knives, shrapnel, etc.) to high-velocity impacts, such as motor vehicle crashes (MVCs) and falls. Because the neck is so delicate, accidents that would cause minor damage to other body parts can cause serious damage to the neck.

> A **c-collar** is a plastic brace used to keep the neck from moving. If your character is concerned the victim's neck might be broken, they can fashion a home-made c-collar using pillows, bedding, or bulky clothes.

COMPLETE SPINAL INJURIES

At the hospital, Muhammad receives first an x-ray, then a CT- scan, of his neck. After waiting for what seems like an eternity, the doctor returns with the results. He fractured a bone in his neck (C6) and a piece slipped forward, pressing on the spine. He needs urgent neurosurgery to relieve the pressure on his spinal cord.

Complete spinal injuries mean the neurons traversing between the body and the brain have been completely severed, interrupting the brain's ability to communicate with the body and vice versa. The symptoms your character will experience depend on where in the spinal cord the transection occurred.

> Complete transection—meaning the spinal cord was cut all the way through—will cause both muscle paralysis and loss of sensation in the affected areas.

Because the cervical spine (*C-spine*) is the closest to the brain, damage to C1-C7 will affect the whole body, causing paralysis of all four limbs (called *tetraplegia* or *quadriplegia*). It is also the most commonly injured part of the spine, as the neck is vulnerable to injury.

The thoracic spine is rarely damaged because it is protected by the ribs. But a well-placed knife or bullet could certainly slice through. The thoracic nerves (T1-T12) mostly innervate the chest, back, and abdomen.

The spinal cord ends at the top of the lumbar spine, somewhere between L1 & L2. It splits off into a graceful array of nerves called the *cauda equina*, which is Latin for "horse's tail." That's why doctors can give epidurals in the lower back—they're injecting medication into the spinal canal low enough down that there's no chance of hitting the spinal cord itself.

CAUDA EQUINA SYNDROME

If the nerves of the 'horse's tail' are injured (a herniated lumbar disc, massive trauma to the lower back, or spinal hemorrhage) it can result in *cauda equina syndrome*. If your character has *cauda equina,* they won't be able to pee on command (urinary retention) and may lose the ability to control their bowel/bladder (*urinary/fecal incontinence*). They'll also have shooting leg pain (*sciatica*) and numbness of the groin and buttocks.

Any one of these symptoms are red flags. Your character needs to hightail it to the doctor, where they'll likely need urgent surgery to prevent permanent nerve damage.

INCOMPLETE SPINAL INJURIES

When Muhammad emerges from surgery, he still can't feel or move anything below the neck, so he's taken for an MRI of the neck. The doctors tell him that there is swelling and bruising around his spinal cord and that only time will tell as to the extent of his injuries.

What if the spinal cord isn't completely transected? What if only part of it is damaged? Hold onto your hats, folks, because this is where things get weird.

Incomplete spinal injuries tend to injure one type of neuron because similar types of neurons (i.e., neurons that control temperature sensation vs. neurons that control movement) run together in a bundle. And these bundles crisscross back and forth across the spinal column like they were designed specifically to confuse medical students. Because of this complicated interplay of neuronal tracts, your character may lose the ability to move their arms and legs, but may still be able to feel them, or vice versa. Some may have partial weakness of their muscles.

> A bundle of neurons in the PNS is a **nerve**.
>
> A bundle of neurons in the CNS is a **tract**.

SPINAL CONCUSSIONS

When Muhammad wakes the next morning, he moves automatically to reach for his daughter, and by some miracle, his hand moves too! It's only a small twitch, but it's something.

A spinal concussion occurs when a severe injury stuns the spinal cord, making an incomplete injury look like a complete injury. Your character will lose all function (movement and sensation) below the level of injury. This usually happens within 30 minutes of the injury.1 But within 72 hours, your character will start to regain function, and will likely recover completely.[1]

A spinal concussion is a great way to keep your character (and your readers!) on their toes, forcing them to come to terms with a life-altering injury, only to recover. It makes for a great reveal or medical miracle, except that your character should have been told it was coming. MRIs of concussed spines show no damage to the spinal cord, so if your character got imaging, they probably knew their symptoms wouldn't last. But if you're writing historical fiction (or if your character can't get imaging for some reason), this is a fun one.

> If your character has bullet fragments in their body, they likely won't get an MRI. MRIs are basically giant magnets and some—but only some—bullet fragments are magnetic. If doctors can prove the bullets are nonmagnetic, your character could get an MRI.

BROWN-SEQUARD SYNDROME

Brown-Sequard is a crazy-weird syndrome that happens when only half the spinal cord is cut. On the side of the injury, your character will become paralyzed and will lose the ability to feel vibration and proprioception (the sense of one's body in space). On the other side, they'll still be able to move, but will no longer be able to feel pain or temperature—if they put their hand on a hot stove, they won't feel anything. Crazy, right?

PENETRATING INJURIES

For the most part, penetrating injuries do their damage at the moment of penetration; bullet and bone fragments don't necessarily need to be removed after the injury has occurred. However, gunshot wounds can fracture a vertebra; if that is the case, your character will need to be immobilized with a collar or brace until the fracture is stabilized.

TREATMENT

After a few days in the hospital, Muhammad is transferred to a rehabilitation hospital, where he works with physical and occupational therapists several times a day. He still can't move his legs, but he can move his arms enough the lift a spoon to his lips. He also no longer needs a urinary catheter, as he can urinate and defecate on his own. His heart breaks as he realizes that he will never again be able to chase his daughter around the backyard, but he is grateful that he can at least feel the warmth of her little hand in his once more.

The best treatment for spinal injury is to prevent it from happening, by immobilizing victims with potentially unstable neck injuries. Once the injury has occurred, the victim may need surgery, either to prevent compression of the cord itself or to stabilize the spine. However, in most cases, there isn't much to do once the damage has been done. Treatment is often focused on preventing complications, such as pneumonia or pressure ulcers. Several different types of rehabilitation—physical therapy, occupational therapy, speech therapy, counseling, etc.—are critical to helping the victim come to terms with their new reality and return to their life.

PROGNOSIS

The old saying among neurologists was "neurons are forever," meaning they don't replicate, and they don't grow back. New science is challenging that dogma, as emerging research in mouse models and stem cells reveals the possibility for neuronal growth and repair.[2] But that research is a long way from being practically applied.

Once the brain or spinal cord is injured, there is very little that can be done. Complete spinal cord transections are very unlikely to improve. In incomplete spinal cord injury, swelling of the cord and spinal contusions can sometimes make your character look worse than they are, and their symptoms might improve with time. However, after a few days, most improvement levels out.

BREAKING DOWN THE CLICHÉ: DEATH BY FALLING OVER

*Jack is up to *here* with his sister Jill, who has once again decided to bail on the evening's plans with their aging mother. They almost made it, they're standing on her porch, for goodness' sake, but Jill just got a text, and Jack can already tell she's gone.*

"Sorry, man," Jill says, eyes never leaving her phone, "my friend needs a ride to the hospital."

Jill always uses that excuse when a drinking buddy hits her up. Somehow, that just makes Jack angrier—can't she even try to pretend she has a legitimate excuse?

Before he knows what he's doing, Jack reaches out to snatch Jill's phone away. She twists out of his grasp, stepping backward off the last porch step. Her arms flail as she falls backward, the back of her neck slamming hard against the bottom step. Jack waits for her to get up, but she doesn't move, her eyes still open. He hurries down the steps, and checks his sister's pulse, finding nothing. Jill is dead.

Falls from standing are a favorite way to kill off or paralyze characters. They don't require much set-up—falls can happen anywhere—and it's very easy to turn an innocent shoving match into murder. No wonder movies, tv, and literature love this trope.

The crazy thing is, it's totally legitimate. Falls, even just from standing, really can cause life-altering injuries and sudden death. I had a patient in his 20s who was paralyzed from the neck down because he slipped on a sock and fell wrong. The height of the fall is obviously important, but the way your character lands—what surface they hit and what body part hits first—is critical. This means you have a lot of flexibility with falls as to how injured you want your character to become.

Water is not a soft landing. If your character jumps from just 20 feet, they'll hit the water at 25 mph, causing an impact strong enough to break bones.[3]

If your character breaks their neck at C1 or C2, they die instantly. If they break their neck at C3-5, they'll suffocate if they don't get prompt medical attention. Falls can also cause fatal brain bleeds, such as epidural or subdural hematomas (See *Ch. 12: Traumatic Brain Injuries*). So, if you're looking to kill or completely paralyze your character, a fall from standing is a totally legit way for you to do so.

However, the thoracic and sacral vertebrae, and to a lesser extent, the lumbar vertebrae, are more protected since they're connected to the ribs and pelvis. This protection means it usually takes higher force impacts—falls from great heights, car accidents, etc.—to crush those vertebrae and sever the spinal cord at the thoracic level. So, keep that in mind if you're looking to paralyze your character from the legs down only, a fall from standing probably won't do the trick.

14. INJURIES TO THE CHEST

Noah is driving home from work when a dog runs out into the road in front of him. He yanks the wheel and slams on the brakes, trying to avoid it. But the road is slick with rain, and he spins out of control. The last thing he remembers is the brick sign of the neighborhood church flashing in front of him.

BACKGROUND

THE CHEST, OR THORAX, EXTENDS from the top of the rib cage to the diaphragm (a thin, horizontal muscle that controls breathing). It contains five main structures: the heart, the great blood vessels (the aorta and the vena cava), the lungs, the trachea, and the esophagus. Damage to any one of these structures can prove fatal.

> The **mediastinum** contains the heart, aorta, vena cava, trachea, and esophagus, along with several smaller arteries, veins, and nerves.

ANATOMY 101

The lungs take up most of the space in the thorax, extending from the diaphragm all the way up past the collarbone. In the middle of the chest, between the lungs, is the space called the *mediastinum*. The heart sits here, just behind the breastbone and extending to the left. The muscular *aorta* arches off the heart, sending off major branches as it runs along the left side of the spine, down towards the abdomen. The *inferior vena cava* and *superior vena cava*—the veins that transport blood from the body and head, respectively—drain into the heart. The *trachea* (or windpipe) runs from the throat along the vertebral column, splitting into two smaller tubes as it enters the lungs. The *esophagus* (the tube connecting the mouth to the stomach) is just passing through, running directly in front of the trachea from the throat to the abdomen, passing through the diaphragm along with the aorta and inferior vena cava.

> The **great vessels** are the giant blood vessels leading into and out of the heart: the aorta, the inferior and superior vena cava, the pulmonary trunk, and the pulmonary veins.

MECHANISMS

The first thing Noah hears when he wakes is the low chanting of a masculine voice. He blinks his eyes open, to see a priest standing over him, wearing a black cassock and a somber expression. Noah groans and the priest nearly jumps out of his skin.

"You're alive!"

Noah looks around. He's lying half out of his car, which smashed straight into the church's sign. Everything hurts, his chest in particular. Every time he breaths, he feels as if he's being stabbed by a thousand knives.

"I am?" Part of him wishes he was not.

The priest frowns but doesn't appear to have heard. Noah wonders if he spoke at all. He can taste blood in the back of his mouth.

"Don't worry, my son," the priest replies, trying to regain his composure, "I've already called 911. The ambulance will be here any moment."

Certain mechanisms of trauma are more likely to result in injury to the chest. If your character was involved in a motor vehicle crash (MVC), they are more likely to experience significant chest trauma if the crash occurred at speeds of more than 35 MPH, if the victim was ejected from the car, or if they were a pedestrian or cyclist that was hit and thrown.[1] Falls from more than 15 ft is also worrisome, as is any trauma that results in a decreased level of consciousness.

EXPERIENCE OF CHEST TRAUMA

By the time the ambulance arrives, Noah can only breathe in fast, shallow pants—and even those are painful. As they cut off his clothes and place him on the gurney, he notices a red mark on the center of his chest. He wasn't wearing a seatbelt, so it must have been where he slammed against the steering wheel. He wonders if he broke something, that would explain why it hurts so much to breathe.

If your character has undergone major trauma, there will be certain signs and symptoms that indicate severe underlying trauma to the chest. The first, of course, is if your character is having trouble breathing. This may mean they feel like they can't catch their breath or that breathing hurts; these symptoms are usually due to rib fractures. They may be breathing fast and shallow, or visibly struggling for breath, their nostrils flaring and the muscles of their abdomen, ribs, and neck contracting with every breath.

The other obvious sign of chest trauma is chest pain. Often, this is due to fractured ribs, but there may also be significant bruising, lacerations, and abrasions. An oblique bruise across the front of the chest—called the "seatbelt sign"—is an ominous sign of significant internal damage.

Other signs of chest trauma include distended neck veins, swelling and purpling of the face and neck, and air bubbles beneath the skin. Paradoxical movement of the chest—one section of the chest moving inward while the rest of the chest moves out—is a sign of a deadly condition called flail chest.

THE DEADLY DOZEN

Trauma to the chest is directly responsible for 20-25% of all trauma deaths and contributes to mortality in another 25%.[2] That's right; almost 50% of trauma deaths are related to chest injuries. On the other hand, nearly 85% of all chest injuries can be treated without surgical intervention. This dichotomy creates an awesome dynamic for writers to exploit potentially deadly injuries that can be treated with gauze and tape, or a needle inserted in exactly the right spot.

Most deaths due to thoracic trauma are part of the "deadly dozen"—twelve life-threatening injuries to the thorax. Six are immediately life-threatening (the "lethal six"), while the other six are considered potentially life-threatening (the "hidden six"). I have no idea who coined these names, but they clearly had an excellent sense for the dramatic. Let's start with the obvious.

THE LETHAL SIX

The lethal six are injuries that can kill in minutes. Luckily for your character, they can also be treated in the field—or at least stabilized so that they don't die on their way to the hospital.

1. **Airway Obstruction**

We've talked about airway obstruction a lot in Chapter 2: Trouble Breathing, so I'm not going to spend much time on it here. If something is completely blocking the victim's airway, they are going to pass out and die within minutes. Anything can block the airway—a chunk of food, throat swelling due to an allergic reaction, a foreign object, even shards of bone due to a seriously smashed skull. Treatment is to clear the airway. This may mean performing the *Heimlich* (if they're choking on a foreign body), positioning an unconscious victim, giving epinephrine to reduce swelling, and/or intubating (See *Ch. 2: Trouble Breathing*).

2. Blood in the Chest (Massive Hemothorax)

Noah feels lightheaded and sick as he's loaded into the ambulance and driven away. The paramedics start two IVs, one in each arm, which makes him feel a little better, but not by much. By the time they arrive at the hospital, Noah is starting to feel cold.

Any penetrating or blunt trauma can cause bleeding in the chest cavity. The blood can come from pretty much anywhere—the lung, the chest wall—the exact source isn't important. What does matter is how much blood there is. Your character will start to go into shock after losing just 30% (~1.5L) of their blood; the thoracic cavity can hold up to 80% of the body's blood. Your character will die of hemorrhagic shock way before the thoracic cavity fills up.

> There are only a few places in your character's body that can hold enough blood for them to bleed out. These include the abdomen, the chest cavity, and the thighs.

This massive amount of blood in the chest cavity is bad for two reasons. First, it means the victim has significant bleeding and will likely go into hemorrhagic shock. Second, the blood compresses the lungs, making it hard to breathe. A victim of a hemothorax is literally drowning in their own blood.

> For more on shock, see Volume 1: Setting & Character, *Ch. 14: Shock.*

As he's rolled into the hospital, Noah is surrounded by a crowd of men and women wearing scrubs. He barely notices as they examine him, listen to his lungs, and roll him over to check his back. He's having too much trouble breathing and being strapped to the backboard isn't helping. There's so much going on he can't keep track of it; machines are rolled in, wires are connected to his chest, finger, and arm, and a plastic mask is placed over his mouth, blowing cool air. A man wearing scrubs tells Noah that the x-ray showed he has multiple rib fractures. Noah doesn't even remember getting an x-ray. The man, Noah thinks he's a doctor, tells him that he's lost a lot of blood and is still bleeding into his chest. They've given him blood and fluids, but he'll need to be taken into surgery to stop the bleeding. Noah barely has the strength to nod his head in agreement.

If your character has a massive hemothorax, they will have chest pain or heaviness, and trouble breathing. They will quickly begin to go into hemorrhagic shock. Their blood pressure will plummet, their breathing and heart rate will become fast, and their skin will become cold, pale, and sweaty. They will probably feel exceedingly anxious, lightheaded, and dizzy. If the bleeding is severe, they could pass out within minutes.

Treatment is to drain the blood using chest tubes (small plastic tubes inserted into the sides of the chest near the armpits) and give fluids and blood transfusions as needed. If the victim continues to bleed, they'll need to be taken for emergency surgery. If the victim is bleeding out super-fast—the chest tubes are running red and the doctors can't transfuse blood fast enough—the trauma surgeons may decide to perform an *emergent thoracotomy*, cutting through the ribs to open up the thoracic cavity so the surgeons can see and stop the blood flow. An emergent thoracotomy is rarely the definitive treatment; it is used to stop the bleeding long enough to get your character into the OR.

> "Cracking the chest" is slang for an emergent thoracotomy.

Noah wakes up after surgery feeling drowsy and confused, but no longer in pain. The surgeon arrives while he's still groggy. She tells him that they stopped the source of the bleeding, but that they needed to put in chest tubes to drain the fluid from his chest. He looks down to see a clear tube inserted near his armpit, a pale pink fluid running through it. Noah, who's always hated blood, passes out at the sight.

3. Collapsed Lung (Tension Pneumothorax)

A penetrating injury to the chest can cause a collapsed lung by creating a one-way valve in the lung. Air that was breathed in through the trachea leaks out of the lung and into the space between the lung and its lining—called the *pleural space*. With every breath, your character sucks air into the pleural space, but the air can't escape when they exhale. As more and more air is trapped inside the pleural space, it pushes on the lung until it collapses.

> Pneumo = air
>
> Thorax = chest cavity

Once the lung collapses, all hell breaks loose. Not only is your character breathing with only half a lung, but the blood gets trapped, unable to pass through the lung to get back to the heart. As blood backs up, the heart can no longer pump blood to vital organs, and your character is suddenly in serious trouble.

If your character has a tension pneumothorax, they'll have chest pain, followed by trouble catching their breath. As the blood backs up in their heart, they'll rapidly descend into cardiogenic shock, with a racing pulse, fast, shallow breathing, cool skin, dizziness, weakness, and plummeting blood pressure. They will also have bulging neck veins, as the blood returning to the heart gets backed up. The doctor won't hear any air flowing through the lungs and she won't need to do any tests after that; she'll proceed straight to treatment.

Treatment of a tension pneumothorax (called "tension pneumo" by those in the know) is to get the air out of the chest to allow the lung to re-expand. This is done with a procedure called a *needle decompression*, and it's remarkably simple. The doctor simply inserts a needle into the middle of the chest, between the first and second rib. Air will gush out, both confirming the diagnosis and treating the condition. A tube will then be inserted into the space to continuously pull out the air and help re-expand the lung. This procedure is called a *tube thoracostomy*. The chest tube usually needs to remain in place for a couple of days while the lung returns to its normal size and shape.

A **simple pneumothorax** is when the lung collapses without trauma, usually due to burst balloon-like 'blebs' in the lung. See *Ch. 1: Chest Pain*.

4. Sucking Chest Wound (Open Pneumothorax)

Another deadly kind of pneumothorax is the open pneumothorax or sucking chest wound. An open pneumothorax is caused by an injury to the chest wall. When your character breaths in, the air enters through the chest wound, not through the trachea. Unable to get air into their lungs, your character will asphyxiate.

To have an open pneumothorax, your character must have an opening in the chest. It doesn't have to be big—the size of a penny will do—but it will make a hissing (or sucking) sound every time they breathe. The wound will likely be bleeding heavily; your observant character may notice pinkish foam forming around the wound. The victim will also be coughing up blood, and one side of the chest may appear bigger than the other. They'll breathe fast and shallow and may have a crackling sound when they breathe. As their condition worsens, their heart will race, their neck veins will engorge, and they may develop a blue tint around their lips and finger (*cyanosis*).

Luckily for your characters, treatment of a sucking chest wound can be performed in the field by anyone with gauze and some tape. The first step is to prevent any more air from getting inside the chest cavity; this means putting a bandage over the wound, then taping it on three sides. Leaving the fourth side without tape allows the wound to "burp" out air as your character exhales. Once in the hospital, a chest tube will be inserted, and your character will be taken to surgery to fix the gaping hole in their chest.

5. Flail Chest

When Noah wakes up, the surgeon is still there, chatting with the nurse. She tells him that the bleeding inside his chest was not his only injury; he also broke three ribs in multiple places when he slammed against the steering wheel. Those broken ribs are now pushing on his lungs with every breath, causing bruising.

Noah immediately tries to breathe more shallowly, but the surgeon shakes her head. She tells him that the most important thing he can do is to breathe deeply to prevent pneumonia and fluid buildup in his lungs. She hands him a device she calls an incentive spirometer, which looks like a tube with a blue plastic ball. She tells him to put the device to his lips and inhale as deeply as he can. He does so, marveling at how little it hurts. When he mentions this thought, the surgeon just smiles and tells him the plan is to make sure his pain is well-controlled so that he can breathe deeply.

> An **incentive spirometer** is a tool to help patients remember to breathe deeply. It is an important component of pulmonary hygiene.

A flail chest happens when your character's ribs break in such a way that there are one or more ribs that are broken in at least two places so that they are completely disconnected from the rest of the rib cage. Since this floating segment of ribs is no longer connected, it doesn't move with the rest of the rib cage. Instead, it's sucked inward when your character breaths in, and pushed outward when they breathe out. This paradoxical movement is problematic for two reasons. First, it makes breathing both difficult and painful. Second, and more importantly, it causes a bruising on the lung that can impair oxygenation.

> In normal respiration, the chest moves outward when your character breathes in. With a flail chest, breathing in sucks the unattached section of rib inwards, resulting in what is called "paradoxical movement."

If your character has a flail chest, they'll have clear bruising and/or abrasions on their chest, particularly around the area of injury. They'll also have chest pain that worsens every time they try to breathe in. They might even feel like they're having trouble breathing.

Flail chest is diagnosed with X-rays and is treated with pain medications, physical therapy, and oxygen. In severe cases, they'll need mechanical ventilation, such as a BVM, or being put on a ventilator. Mechanical ventilation provides a sort of internal splint, forcing the island of ribs outwards with each forced breath, but it's generally considered a last resort.

 NATALIE DALE, MD

6. **Blood Compressing the Heart (Cardiac Tamponade)**

The heart is covered by a thick, fibrous sack called the *pericardium*. Normally, it acts as a mechanism to protect and lubricate the heart. But when the heart is injured and begins to bleed, that blood can get trapped inside the pericardial sack. As the sack fills with blood, it compresses the heart, squeezing it until it can no longer function.

If your character has cardiac tamponade, they'll exhibit many of the symptoms common to the Lethal Six: chest pain, trouble breathing, increased breathing and pulse rate, dizziness, lightheadedness, and fainting. A doctor examining your character will notice a classic trio of signs called *Beck's triad,* characterized by:

- Low blood pressure, particularly with a narrowing of the gap between the first and second number (i.e., blood pressure of 110/90). This phenomenon, called a "narrow pulse pressure," indicates the heart is failing to pump blood properly. This failure leads to…

- Engorged veins in the neck. As the heart fails, blood backs up in the veins. It's backed up in all the veins, but the only ones you can see it in are the veins in the neck.

- Muffled heart sounds. As the pericardium fills with blood, it muffles the sound of the beating heart.

Cardiac tamponade is treated by removing the blood in a procedure called *cardiocentesis*. This procedure is done with a big needle inserted just under the ribcage, pointing towards the left shoulder. The needle penetrates the pericardium and pulls out (*aspirates*) the blood. It is a procedure that is both life-saving and super dramatic.

THE HIDDEN SIX

The hidden six may not be immediately visible upon the primary exam, but they can still kill your character within hours if they don't get treatment. As a writer, the hidden six are where it's at! These diagnoses are easy to miss in the frantic rush of the preliminary survey but missing one can have deadly consequences.

> Myocardial contusions are more common after deceleration injuries (a sudden stop from high speeds), than direct blunt force to the chest.

1. **Bruised Heart (Myocardial Contusion)**

Like any other tissue, the heart can get bruised. When it does, heart muscle dies, and the heart loses its ability to conduct electricity and pump properly. If you think that sounds a lot like a heart attack (or *myocardial infarction*, for those in the know), you're exactly right! A cardiac contusion is basically the same thing as a heart attack. The only difference is that it's caused by trauma, rather than a clogged artery.

If your character has a myocardial contusion, they'll feel like they're having a heart attack: severe chest pain, lightheadedness, shortness of breath, nausea/vomiting, and fatigue. Injuries associated with myocardial contusion include multiple broken ribs, broken breastbone (sternum), and the presence of pulmonary contusion, hemothorax, or torn blood vessels in the chest. Untreated, myocardial contusion can lead to sudden heart failure and cardiogenic shock.

Testing includes an EKG, an echocardiogram, and telemetry monitoring for changes in the heart's electrical rhythm for 24-hours. But because myocardial contusion is relatively rare, and its symptoms can overlap with many other signs of chest trauma (chest pain and trouble breathing, anyone?), its diagnosis can be easily missed. Don't let that happen to your character; unless, of course, you want them to die suddenly within 24-hours of their trauma.

> **Electrocardiogram** (EKG) measures electrical rhythm of the heart. **Echocardiogram** ("Echo") is an ultrasound of the heart.

2. Bruised Lungs (Pulmonary Contusion)

Pulmonary contusions occur when blood and fluid collect in the small sacs of air in the lungs called the *alveoli*. Most common after blunt trauma to the chest, pulmonary contusions are usually found beneath fractured ribs and tend to be particularly severe beneath *flail chest* injuries. They can range in severity from mild and self-healing, to severe enough to require intubation.

> *The next day, Noah is woken before dawn by the surgeon, who scowls as she presses the stethoscope to his back. She asks if he's having any coughing or trouble breathing, but Noah shakes his head. She tells him that she's hearing some worrisome crackling in his lungs, and to let her know if he notices any problems.*

Signs of pulmonary contusion include trouble breathing and worsening hypoxia (decreased oxygenation in the blood). When they first show up at the hospital, your character's symptoms will be similar to most chest trauma: chest pain, trouble breathing, increased breathing and pulse rate, and fatigue. But over the next 24-48 hours, your character will worsen. They may start coughing up blood, have cool, clammy skin, and their lips and fingers may become tinged blue. The doctors will hear wheezing or crackles in their chest and will notice that their blood pressure is dropping.

> **Hemoptysis** is the medical term for coughing up blood.

Pulmonary contusion is diagnosed with a chest CT and monitoring the level of oxygen in the blood (*pulse oximetry*). Mild cases are treated with oxygen and careful monitoring; more severe cases require intubation and ventilation.

3. Torn Aorta (Traumatic Aortic Transection)

A torn aorta is one of the most lethal of all traumatic chest injuries; nearly 40% of all people who experience it die instantaneously.[3] So why is it included in the hidden six instead of the lethal six? Because, of the 60% who survived, their aorta was only partially torn.[3] That partial tear becomes a ticking bomb, just waiting to go off; blood from the muscular aorta acts as the fuse as it pushes into the small tear, expanding it until the damaged aorta finally bursts. Once that happens, your character will bleed out in seconds.

Diagnosing a torn aorta is tricky. Your character will have chest pain, but that's expected after their severe trauma. A cautious doctor will take your character's pulse and blood pressure in both arms; if they're different, it's a bad sign. Your character will then get a chest x-ray, which will show a *widened mediastinum*, basically a sign that the aorta is fat and swollen. The docs will confirm with a chest CT and/or arteriogram, and your character will be swept off to emergency surgery.

Arteriograms use dye injected into the arteries to look for tears in the blood vessel walls..

4. Torn Windpipe (Tracheobronchial Injury)

Injury to the *trachea* (windpipe) or *bronchi* (tubes leading into the lungs) leads to air ending up in the chest, rather than in the lungs. It is usually due to penetrating trauma, though deceleration can also cause this type of injury.

Your character will have trouble breathing and may be able to feel air bubbles beneath the skin of their throat. It's diagnosed with *bronchoscopy* (a camera threaded down the windpipe) and treated with intubation of the uninjured bronchus followed by emergency surgery.

5. Torn Esophagus

Esophageal tears are almost always due to penetrating trauma.[2] If your character has a torn esophagus, they will literally be spilling the contents of their mouth (and stomach if they're vomiting) into the chest cavity. Immediately, the hole will cause chest pain and trouble swallowing (*odynophagia*). But the real fun begins when your character develops a fever around 24 hours after the trauma. This is a huge red flag, but it's easy to miss. After all, your character may have had other injuries that could have become infected, or they could be developing pneumonia from not breathing deeply. But here's the thing; fail to treat a torn esophagus promptly, and the fatality rate shoots skyward.[2] This possibility for a missed diagnosis makes for a great ticking clock; will the doctors recognize your character's symptoms for what they are, or will they be ignored until it's too late?

The keen doctor will recognize the fever for what it is; a medical emergency requiring immediate surgery and antibiotics. Esophageal tears that are treated within 12-24 hours of the injury tend to fare much better than those treated later.[2]

6. Torn Diaphragm (Diaphragm rupture)

Noah quickly improves on the ventilator and is weaned off the next day. He goes home a few days after that. He hopes that's the end of his ordeal, but a month later he starts to feel crampy abdominal pain. At first, it comes and goes, but soon it's nearly constant and severe enough to double him over. He goes back to the ED and when they ask the last time he pooped, he realizes he can't remember. He hasn't even farted all day.

The diaphragm is not only the muscle that controls breathing, but it also serves as the barrier between the abdomen and the thorax. Tear it, and the contents of the abdomen can spill up into the chest.

Noah is given a chest and abdominal CT and diagnosed with a complete bowel obstruction due to a loop of his intestines that are actually in his chest cavity! The doctors tell him it is caused by a tear in his diaphragm, which likely happened during his car accident. He's taken to surgery, where his trapped intestines are freed and the tear in his diaphragm is repaired.

You'd think that a torn diaphragm would cause all sorts of problems, and it definitely can, especially if the damage is severe enough to comprise your character's breathing. But most of the time, the diagnosis is completely missed at the time of hospitalization. Your character may only realize what's happened when a loop of the intestine gets trapped in the hole of the diaphragm, causing a potentially deadly blockage that must be treated with surgery. Yet another way to hospitalize your character days, or even weeks, after the traumatic event.

BREAKING DOWN THE CLICHÉ: COUGHING UP BLOOD

"I have to tell you…" *blood dribbles from his mouth*

"Don't speak. These arrows—I can pull them out. You're going to be OK!"

Shakes head *"You have to—have to find…"* *more blood dribbling* *"Before it's too late."*

Exhales one last breath Head falls to the side, eyes open* *Dead*

In order to cough up blood, there has to be blood in your lungs or trachea for them to come up. Injury to the esophagus can also cause bleeding from the mouth. Conditions causing bleeding outside the lungs won't result in your character coughing up blood. If you want to make your character cough up blood, penetrating trauma is your best shot as it can cause tracheobronchial and/or esophageal injury. A pulmonary contusion can also cause your character to cough up blood, though it probably won't happen until 24-48 hours after the initial injury.

In fact, most of the Lethal Six won't cause bleeding from the mouth. The only exception is massive hemothorax; if paired with a torn esophagus or trachea, your character can cough up blood to your heart's desire.

15. GUT WOUNDS

Octavia took a night off from her family duties to go dancing with friends. She's about ready to go home when a gunman walks into the nightclub and begins shooting. She tries to take cover behind the bar, but she's too slow, a feeling like fire slams through her gut. She collapses to the floor, moaning in pain. The gunshots seem to go on forever, then there's silence.

BACKGROUND

WE TALKED IN-DEPTH ABOUT ABDOMINAL anatomy in *Ch. 3: Abdominal Pain*, so I'm not going to go into detail again here. Instead, I'm going to approach the abdominal cavity as a trauma surgeon might; by thinking about the mechanism of injury and how that could have translated to injured organs.

Unlike the thorax—which is relatively protected by the rib cage—the abdomen is soft, squishy, and vulnerable. About 14% of trauma deaths are due to abdominal injuries, and most abdominal trauma leads to multiple injured organs.[1] Because it is so pliable, the abdominal cavity can hold up to 5L of blood: literally, all the blood in your character's body can fit in that cavity. For that reason, a missed diagnosis of abdominal bleeding can have fatal consequences.

> The only other body cavities that can hold anywhere near that amount of blood are the chest and thighs.

After what feels like an eternity, police and paramedics clamber into the building. Octavia is lifted onto a stretcher—she feels dizzy from pain and blood loss—and taken to the nearest hospital.

> For more on penetrating vs. blunt trauma, see <u>Volume 1: Setting & Character</u>, Ch. 2: *Trauma Center*

When thinking about trauma, the abdominal organs are categorized into two subtypes: hollow organs and solid organs. Hollow organs (the stomach, intestines, bladder, kidney, and gallbladder) are tubes that carry fluids—and solids—through the body. The primary concern in hollow organs is that if they are perforated, they will leak their contents into the abdominal cavity, causing massive irritation and a serious potential for infection. The liver, spleen, and pancreas, on the other hand, are solid organs with considerable blood supply. Damage to these organs is more likely to lead to extensive, and potentially life-threatening, bleeding.

ABDOMINAL TRAUMA BY ORGAN

In the ED, Octavia is surrounded by a crowd of people in scrubs, starting IVs, taking blood, measuring her pulse and blood pressure, and oxygenation. Octavia feels lightheaded and sleepy—the doctor has to shake her gently before she realizes he's asking her a question.

SOLID ORGANS

Liver: The liver is the most commonly injured organ in the abdomen, likely because it is very large and relatively unprotected.[2] Located in the right upper quadrant (RUQ) of the abdomen, damage to the liver is generally characterized by excessive bleeding. Blunt trauma can shatter the liver into pieces while penetrating trauma can slice through the heavily vascularized tissue. Worse, penetrating trauma can also slice through the sizable arteries and veins that run to and from this organ, namely the *hepatic arteries* and the *portal vein*. If your character's liver is damaged, they'll have abdominal pain (diffuse or in RUQ), possibly accompanied by signs of shock.

> A stab wound to the liver can range from a mild annoyance to a life-threatening emergency, depending on the angle and depth of the laceration. In other words, you choose how seriously your character is injured!

Spleen: Located on the upper left side of the abdomen (LUQ), sheltered by the ribcage, spleens are relatively delicate organs. As such, spleens are one of the most commonly injured organs in the abdomen.[1] Blunt force injuries (MVCs, falls, assaults, and sports injuries to the left side of the body) are the most common mechanism for spleen injuries. Enlarged spleens—most commonly due to mono (*infectious mononucleosis*)—are particularly susceptible to rupture.

> A shattered spleen could be an unexpected complication (or even cause of death) in a young character recovering from mono.

While minor injuries to the spleen may heal on their own, a ruptured spleen is a great way to get your character to bleed out, fast. Spleens are the most highly vascularized organ in the body.[1] Minor injuries to the spleen will result in pain along the left edge of the rib cage; more severe injuries will have more diffuse pain, along with signs of shock.

Pancreas: Located just behind the stomach, the pancreas is a solid organ that produces digestive enzymes designed to break down proteins. It isn't injured often—pancreatic injury occurs in less than 2% of blunt trauma—but when it is injured, there are often dire consequences.[3] Injuries to the pancreas are most often caused by penetrating injuries, such as gunshot and stab wounds. Pancreatic injury due to blunt trauma usually occurs due to direct trauma to the epigastric area—the top of the abdomen, just below the breastbone. In adults, that usually means a steering wheel; in children, it's the handlebar of their bicycle.[3]

Pancreatic injuries usually occur alongside other traumatic injuries. Given the archetypal setting of concurrent multi-organ injury, pancreatic injuries can be easy to miss. Furthermore, the only major symptom of pancreatic injury is acute and severe epigastric pain that pierces through to their back, a symptom that could easily be misattributed to their other injuries. But misdiagnosis of pancreatic injury can result in a range of complications, from chronic pain to death. If you have a young character whom you want to suffer from additional complications of an abdominal injury, pancreatic injury is a good option.

Kidney: Located in the *retroperitoneal space* (aka the back portion of the abdomen) the kidneys are particularly susceptible to blunt trauma to the back and flanks. Part hollow, part solid, the kidney can both bleed and leak urine, resulting in mid-back pain (called 'flank pain') and blood in the urine. A worrisome sign of kidney injury is bruising along the flank.

While penetrating traumas can certainly hit the kidneys, the big concern with penetrating traumas are the arteries leading to the kidneys, called the superior and inferior renal arteries. These bad boys carry a LOT of blood. Nick one, and your character can bleed out very fast.

HOLLOW ORGANS

Intestines: The small intestines are where most absorption of nutrients happens, while the large intestines (the colon and rectum) are where fluid is resorbed. When the intestines are punctured, sh*t gets real, literally spilling out into the abdominal cavity. In the abdominal cavity, the small intestine is most commonly affected by trauma, followed closely by the colon.

Untreated, perforated intestines can lead to *peritonitis*—inflammation of the lining of the abdominal cavity—and infection. If your character has a perforation, they will have abdominal pain and rigidity, guarding, fever, nausea, and vomiting.

Stomach: Located in the left upper quadrant (LUQ), the stomach is relatively protected by the ribcage. In fact, the stomach is rarely injured in trauma; less than 8% of people with abdominal trauma experience injury to the stomach. Penetrating trauma is more likely to affect the stomach, though blunt trauma could rupture the stomach as well, particularly if your character recently had a big meal.

Gastric perforation leads to the contents of the stomach spewing into the abdominal cavity. Stomach acid and the enzymes it contains are caustic and can lead to severe peritonitis. A character with a perforated stomach will exhibit all the same signs and symptoms as one with perforated intestines.

Bladder: Situated low and central in the abdomen, the bladder is protected by the pelvis. Most often damaged by penetrating trauma, damage to the bladder results in leakage of urine into the abdominal cavity. Your character will have lower abdominal pain and blood in their urine.

THE BIG PICTURE: MULTIORGAN ABDOMINAL WOUNDS

As the nurses cut off Octavia's clothes, the doctor performs a quick exam, listening to her heart and lungs and examining the gunshot wound in her belly. He presses down on her abdomen, which is painful enough, but when he releases the pressure, Octavia nearly screams in pain.

Now that we've talked about how different organs look when damaged, I'm going to take a step back and emphasize that most abdominal trauma will affect more than one organ. Sure, a single stab wound might only hit the liver, but it could just as easily pierce the gallbladder and diaphragm as well. Gunshot wounds (*GSWs*) are highly likely to injure multiple organs as the bullet passes the body, causing both direct and indirect (*cavitation*) injury. Blunt force trauma and deceleration injuries are also very likely to injure more than one organ. So, if your character has experienced abdominal trauma, it is highly likely that multiple organs will be affected.

This means that your character's symptoms may be rather vague. They'll have severe abdominal pain but may not be able to pinpoint exactly where the pain is coming from. They may begin to show signs of shock (fast breathing rate and heart rate and low blood pressure) and may feel tender when touched or moved. But their symptoms will likely be too general to make a diagnosis without further testing.

For more on shock, see Volume 1: Setting & Character, *Ch. 14: Shock.*

DIAGNOSIS

The doctors place a probe on Octavia's abdomen, she recognizes it as an ultrasound probe like the ones she had during her pregnancy. The doctor's expression is grim as he looks at the tiny, black and white screen. The images keep moving, and Octavia has no idea what on earth he's looking at, but he must have seen what he was looking for. He informs her she has blood in her abdomen and is going to need immediate surgery.

A doctor treating your character will not know what organs have been injured just based on the physical exam. There are a few tests your character may be given if they've had abdominal trauma: FAST, peritoneal lavage, abdominal x-ray, and abdominal CT scan.

The FAST (Focused Assessment with Sonography for Trauma) is an ultrasound used in the trauma room to determine if your character has any fluid (blood) in their abdomen. If your character has a positive FAST, they're wheeled straight to surgery. FAST is a quick and dirty way to figure out if your character is bleeding, but it isn't foolproof. Small bleeds (less than 500mL) won't show up, meaning that your character could have a small bleed that could go undiagnosed. What's that I hear? Yup, that's a ticking clock all right.

The Diagnostic Peritoneal Lavage (DPL) is an older technique, mostly supplanted by the FAST exam. The trauma surgeon sticks a tube into the abdominal cavity and rinses it out with saline, looking for signs of blood (or feces, or urine) in the flushed water. As you might imagine, it takes longer than the FAST, is more intrusive, and can

Stable means your character's condition isn't acutely worsening. But it's a moving target. "Stable" means one thing in the ED, another on the floors, and quite another in the ICU.

only be performed if your character is stable. But it's also much less likely to miss small bleeds.

The **abdominal X-ray** is useless for looking for blood. Instead, it looks for air underneath the diaphragm, a sure sign that a hollow organ (usually the intestines) has been punctured. It's a quick and dirty test; if positive, your character goes straight to the OR. If negative, they may get an abdominal CT to get a better look.

For more on CT and other imaging studies, see Volume 1: Setting & Character, Ch. 6: Outpatient Medicine.

An **abdominal CT** gives the best picture of the abdominal organs and their injuries. However, a CT takes a long time, and can't be performed if your character is circling the drain. Don't forget the CT's nickname: the "donut of death"! An overworked and exhausted resident may kill your character by overlooking a source of bleeding and sending them to the CT unaccompanied.

TREATMENT

After confirming that she hasn't eaten anything in the last few hours, the nurses' prep Octavia for surgery. The pain in her stomach is excruciating, and she's feeling so lightheaded she's worried she might faint. When the doctor returns and tries to explain the procedure—he calls it an "ex-lap"—she's so dizzy that she barely registers a word. She just nods, gritting her teeth against the pain. By the time they roll her into the freezing cold OR, she's shivering all over.

EX-LAP VS. OBSERVATION

Treatment of abdominal trauma depends on the severity of the injuries. Most of the time, the choice is between immediate surgery and careful observation with pain control, with non-emergent surgery performed once the victim is stable. If it's deemed your character needs surgery, they'll have a procedure called an exploratory laparotomy, or "ex-lap." In this procedure, the surgeon will cut open the abdomen to search for and repair sources of bleeding and perforation. In the old days, doctors used to rush all victims of multiorgan trauma straight to the OR, but recent

The lethal triad of trauma—sometimes known by the melodramatic title of the "Trauma Triad of Death"—consists of:

Hypothermia: low body temperature

Metabolic acidosis: acidification of the blood and tissues

Coagulopathy: poor blood clotting

studies have shown that these victims are liable to develop a 'lethal triad' of symptoms that can make surgery very dangerous. To prevent the lethal triad, surgeons prioritize control of bleeding and utilize strategies to keep the victim's body warm.[4]

The OR is bustling, full of people in blue scrubs wearing puffy blue caps matching the one Octavia herself is wearing. They help her onto a cold stainless-steel table, arranging pre-warmed blankets and plastic sheets filled with warm air all around her. Octavia shivers again, glad for the warmth. A woman wearing scrubs introduces herself as the nurse anesthetist, then places a plastic mask over Octavia's face. It smells faintly of plastic. The woman tells her to count backward from ten, but Octavia only gets to 8.

A **nurse anesthetist** (CRNA) is a nurse trained specifically in the administration of anesthesia. They can do most of the procedures an anesthesiologist can. See <u>Volume 1: Setting & Character</u>, *Ch. 10: Advanced Practice Providers.*

Not all victims of abdominal trauma need surgery! If your character is hemodynamically stable (their blood pressure and pulse rate are normal) and they don't have any signs of peritonitis, they'll probably just be observed for a few days in the hospital to make sure they don't go downhill.

ORGAN-SPECIFIC TREATMENT

Spleen and liver injuries are classified by severity; less severe classifications are treated with pain control and observation, while more severe injuries require surgery. Severely ruptured spleens may require a complete *splenectomy* (removal of the spleen). In the liver, severe damage may require a *lobectomy*—removal of one (or more) lobes of the liver.

Gastrointestinal perforations (aka perforations of the stomach, small intestine, colon, and rectum) are treated with surgery. For the small intestines, this may mean cutting out whole segments and reattaching the ends. However, if the colon or rectum was injured, the doctors may need to cut out the injured part of the colon and connect the still-healthy piece to the skin, forming a *colostomy*. If your character has a colostomy, they will no longer defecate normally. Instead, watery stool from the colon will collect in a bag they keep on their stomach, called a *colostomy pouch*. Talk about a major lifestyle adjustment for your character!

COMPLICATIONS

When Octavia wakes up, she's in a small room bounded by curtains. Her throat feels scratchy, and her mouth is bone dry, but she no longer feels the searing pain in her abdomen. She reaches for her belly with hands covered in IV tubing and tape, feeling the thick bandages that wrap around her middle. The nurse anesthetist stands beside her, still wearing her bright blue scrub cap. She informs Octavia that the surgery went well, and that the surgeon will be there to talk to her soon. He arrives minutes later, before Octavia, still woozy from the anesthesia, has the chance to think. He informs her that, unfortunately, the bullet tore through her small intestine and liver. They had to remove sections of her intestine, and an entire lobe of her liver, but she's lucky that the bullet didn't hit any major arteries or her spine. He wants to keep her in the hospital for a few days to monitor her progress. When he asks if she has any questions, Octavia can't think of any, so she shakes her head, and the doctor hurries away. A long while later, a medical transporter arrives to wheel Octavia up to her room on the floor, where her husband and young son are waiting.

The PACU (Post-Anesthesia Care Unit) is where your character will recover from surgery.

Unlike head and spine injuries, abdominal injuries tend to improve quickly. So, if your character survives their abdominal trauma, they'll probably recover pretty well. Even if your character requires a colostomy, there is hope. Many colostomies can be reversed once your character is stable enough for the longer, more intensive reversal procedure. However, if you're looking to re-injure your character after abdominal trauma, you've still got some options.

POSTOP FEVER: WIND, WATER, WALKING, WOUND, WONDER DRUGS

The surgeon gives Octavia an incentive spirometer (a plastic tube with a little blue ball that rises as she inhales) and tells her to practice breathing deep with it. But deep breaths hurt Octavia's stomach, so she doesn't touch the thing.

The 5 W's is the mnemonic every medical student learns regarding postoperative fever. And while any operation can result in a fever, abdominal surgeries are both common and at higher risk of infection, particularly if there was bowel perforation. The mnemonic is used to categorize the likely cause of fever based on when it occurred.

Less than two days after the surgery, Octavia starts feeling winded. The nurses note that she has a slight temperature. The surgeon returns, telling Octavia that her fever is most likely due to collapsed air sacs in her lungs due to her not breathing deeply enough. He promises to increase her pain medications if she promises to use her incentive spirometer, which he calls her "IS," several times an hour. She agrees, and she begins to feel better after a few days.

Wind: If your character develops a fever within 24-48 hours after surgery, it's most likely due to a problem in the lungs. Earlier problems (i.e., in the first 24 hours) are due to *atelectasis,* or the flattening of the air sacs of the lung after surgery. Often, atelectasis doesn't have any symptoms, though your character may notice a slight cough or trouble breathing. Untreated, atelectasis can lead to pneumonia, which usually sets in around 48-72 hours after surgery.

Water: If your character develops a fever 3-5 days after surgery, it's probably a *urinary tract infection* (UTI) due to the indwelling Foley catheter shoved up their urethra during surgery, which is probably still in place.

Walking: A *deep vein thrombosis* (DVT) is a blood clot in the deep muscle of the leg, usually the calf. Your character, stuck in bed due to their recent surgery, could develop one after about 4-6 days after surgery. They'll have a red, painful, and swollen calf. If they're unlucky, a piece of the clot might break off and travel to the lungs, giving them a pulmonary embolism (See *Ch. 1: Chest Pain*).

Wound: When you think of fevers after surgery, your first thought is probably the surgical incision site. But it takes a while for the bacteria that cause wound infections to take root and grow into a problem. Wound infection usually doesn't show up until 5-7 days after surgery. If the surgical site is infected, your character will usually have pain, redness, swelling, and perhaps even oozing pus at the wound site.

After a week in the hospital, Octavia spikes a fever once more. Her surgical site has become red and inflamed, the surgeon believes it has become infected. She's placed on antibiotics and begins to feel better in a few days.

Traumatic wounds can become infected much faster than 5 days.

Wonder Drugs: There are an insane number of drugs that can cause fevers. These fevers can occur at any point before, during, or after the surgery. If you want to bamboozle the docs in your story, give your character a drug fever. Drugs that commonly cause fevers include antibiotics (yup, the drugs the docs gave your character to treat their fever could now be *causing* it), antiseizure meds, blood thinners (particularly heparin), and diuretics (water pills).

ABDOMINAL COMPARTMENT SYNDROME

If your character survived major abdominal trauma, they are at higher risk of *abdominal compartment syndrome.* This syndrome, caused by intestinal swelling after blunt trauma, significant abdominal hemorrhage, or prolonged surgery, results in skyrocketing pressures within the abdomen. These high pressures shut off blood flow to essential organs, particularly the kidney if your character is lying on their back (and after abdominal surgery, they *will* be lying on their back). The kidneys start to fail, followed by the heart and lungs.

> Abdominal compartment syndrome is a great way to kill off (or at least, seriously sicken) your character after their loved ones thought they were in the clear.

LONG-TERM CONSEQUENCES

Surgeons refer to people who've never had surgery on their belly as having a "virgin abdomen." That's because, once that abdominal cavity is cut open, it increases the risk of the formation of thick, stringy tissue called *adhesions*. Adhesions can cause all sorts of problems, ranging from bowel obstruction to infertility, and once they're there, there's little that can be done.

BREAKING DOWN THE CLICHÉS

GUT WOUND REVEAL

> *The battle is won! The rebels gather round, hugging each other, practically dancing up and down with joy. But one does not join in. As the others turn, beckoning him to join the revels, he pulls aside his coat, revealing a bright red stain blossoming across the lower portion of his shirt.*
>
> *"You're hurt!" someone cries.*
>
> *He stumbles forward, then collapses to the ground, dead.*

Having never been shot myself, it seems downright unbelievable that someone wouldn't notice getting shot, but I've heard from some pretty credible sources that people sometimes really don't feel the bullet.[5] That being said, there are a couple of things to keep in mind if you're going to utilize this trope.

1. Gunshot wounds have entrance and exit wounds, and the exit wounds are generally bigger and messier. If your character has a small wound in the front, they probably have a bigger, gorier wound in the back (or vice versa, if they were shot in the back).

2. The amount of blood on the outside isn't a good indicator of the amount of bleeding on the inside. A fun twist on this trope would be to have minimal external bleeding but to still have your character die of internal bleeding.

3. Not all guns are made equal. A wound from a handgun will look very different from a wound from an assault rifle. Make sure that the type of weapon that hits

your character is consistent with the degree of wounds you want them to walk away with.

4. Your character won't be knocked backward by the force of the bullet. It's basic physics: every action has an equal and opposite reaction. If the bullet was strong enough to knock your character backward, it should also have knocked over the person firing the gun.

5. Don't pull out the knife (See *Ch. 11: Head, Neck, & Throat Injuries*), dig out the bullet (see below), or cough up blood (See *Ch. 14: Injuries to the Chest*).

DIG OUT THE BULLET

"We have to get the bullet out," the captain says, kneeling over his fallen comrade, "before infection sets in."

The injured man groans, paling as every face turns towards him. He clutches his gut, gritting against the searing pain. But deep down, he knows his captain is right. Reluctantly, he nods. The captain claps him on the back.

"Let's get this man a bottle of whiskey."

Just like you don't have to pull out the knife, you don't have to surgically remove the bullet. Not only is it painful and unnecessary, but it could kill your character. Just like a knife, a bullet can be lodged in a blood vessel, preventing significant leakage. Pull it out, and your character could bleed out.

Current research indicates that, contrary to previous belief, bullets are *not* sterile and can be a potential source of wound infection.[6] Furthermore, nonsterile clothing can be dragged into the wound with the bullet. Even so, most bullets do not need to be removed. Instead, your character will be given antibiotics and a tetanus shot.

So, when *would* a bullet be removed?

First, if the bullet (or bullet fragments) is in the brain, it needs to be removed to prevent infection.[7] Second, if the surgeon is going to operate on the area anyway, they will probably remove the bullet while they're in there. However, it won't be high on the priority list; if your character is unstable, or the surgery is taking too long, the surgeon might need to close your character back up before the bullet can be removed.

16. INJURIES TO THE ARMS & LEGS

Paolo hasn't had an easy life. He's fallen from rooftops, been kicked in the ribs by a horse, and even crashed his motorcycle when he was younger. But nothing compares to this. Now, he's trapped beneath the rubble of his collapsed apartment building. His throat is raw from screaming, and he can't feel his legs anymore, but he can certainly see the huge slab of cement blocking them from his view. Delirious and exhausted, he starts to daydream about the crazy adventures of his youth.

BACKGROUND

THE ARMS AND LEGS (OR the upper and lower extremities if you're using medical terminology) are common sources of injury. There are 64 bones of the upper extremity, including the scapula (shoulder blade), the humerus, the ulna, the radius, and the bones of the hand (carpals, metacarpals, and phalanges). Joints include the shoulder, elbow, wrist, and finger joints. The lower limb consists of thirty bones, including the femur (the biggest single bone in the body) the patella, the tibia, the spindly fibula, and the bones of the foot (tarsals, metatarsals, and phalanges). Joints include the hip, knee, ankle, and toe joints.

> Doctors refer to the fingers as digits numbered 1 (thumb) to 5 (pinky).

Any one of these bones can be broken; any joint sprained, strained, or dislocated. Giant nerves—like the *brachial plexus* or the *femoral nerve*—can be damaged, causing pain, numbness, tingling, or even paralysis. Damage to arteries like the femoral artery, which runs along the inside of the thigh in the groin, can cause your character to bleed out.

You've probably sprained an ankle or broken a finger at some point in your life. Most extremity injuries aren't immediately life-threatening but can quickly become so depending on the situation. A mountain-climber's broken leg can result in death from hypothermia; an amputated finger can become infected if improperly treated. When it comes to injuries to the extremities, you are limited only by your imagination.

BROKEN BONES

As a child, Paolo used to work on his family's farm, repairing fences and helping his father stack bales of hay in the barn. When he was thirteen, he fell from the hayloft, breaking his left wrist. He hadn't cried—even back then, he'd known crying was a sign of weakness—but he'd wanted to. Instead, he clutched his throbbing wrist to his chest and gotten his mother, who'd driven him to the hospital.

SYMPTOMS

If your character has a broken bone, they'll feel significant pain at the site of the injury. The site will quickly swell and turn red, and they'll have difficulty moving the affected limb. They may even have fragments of bone sticking through the skin, or an obvious deviation where the bone should be straight.

DIAGNOSIS

While doctors can have a pretty good idea that your character broke a bone just doing a history and physical, diagnosis requires an x-ray. Complicated injuries, especially those with potential nerve or vascular involvement, may need a CT or MRI.

TYPES OF FRACTURES

Depending on which bone is broken and how badly, a fracture can range anywhere from a minor (if painful) annoyance to a life-threatening emergency. Generally caused by blunt trauma, fractures come in several flavors; they can be open or closed, displaced or nondisplaced, or they can be described by the morphology of the break itself. You don't have to know all the different subtypes to give your character a broken bone, but there are a few questions you should ask yourself as you write.

First, is your character's fracture open or closed? In open fractures, also called compound fractures, the bone is sticking out through the skin, or there is a wound deep enough to expose the bone. In closed, or simple, fractures the skin remains intact. Open fractures are a limb-threatening emergency; without surgery, your character could lose the limb and possibly even die of infection. Simple fractures are generally less dangerous but still might require surgery to fix. That brings me to the second question.

Is the fracture displaced, or nondisplaced? A nondisplaced fracture is like a crack in the pavement; the bones are broken, but they're still properly aligned. In a displaced fracture, the pieces of bone have shifted so they're no longer aligned.

Displaced fractures generally require reduction (shifting the bone back into place). Depending on the bone involved, the amount of pain and swelling, and the extent of the damage, reduction can be done in the ER with the help of muscle relaxants, sedatives, and pain control; or it may require surgery.

> *The doctors said the growth plate of his radius and ulna were fractured and recommended surgery. But Paolo's parents couldn't afford the surgery. Instead, he'd been stuck in a cast for weeks, and the itching drove him crazy. That arm had stopped growing after that, leaving his left arm a full inch shorter than the right.*

If your injured character is a child, there are a few important types of fractures you should keep in mind. Greenstick, or incomplete fractures, occur when the bone is broken only part of the way through and is more common in young children. Spiral fractures are generally caused by twisting injuries; a spiral fracture in a young child is a red flag for child abuse. If any type of fracture is located in the growth plate (near the ends of the bones) the child will need immediate surgery to prevent that limb from becoming crooked or stunted.

FEMUR FRACTURES

As the biggest single bone in the body, the femur requires a lot of force to break. But once broken, femur fractures can be dangerous, even deadly. The marrow (the inside of the bone) is highly vascularized, so if the femur is fractured, it is going to bleed like crazy. And the thigh is big and fatty enough that it can hold a ton of blood, anywhere from 1-2 liters, enough to send your character into hemorrhagic shock.

Most femur fractures require both traction and surgery. Recovery can take anywhere from a couple of months to a year, so if you're going to have your character break their thigh, make sure you're ready to have them live with the consequences.

> For more on hemorrhagic shock, see Volume 1: Setting & Character, *Ch. 14: Shock.*

TREATMENT

There are several facets of treatment for simple fractures. A splint, cast, or sling for immobilization, ice, and pain medication to help dull the pain (*analgesia*), and rest to prevent further injury. Physical therapy is also essential in many cases to prevent weakening of the muscles (*atrophy*) in the affected area.

Immobilization allows the injury to heal in the appropriate position; when a fracture is not appropriately immobilized, misaligned bone healing can lead to significant deformity. Most simple fractures require a cast for immobilization.

Casts are made of plaster and are individually shaped to your character's hand. Your character will wear their cast for around 4-6 weeks, though this number can jump significantly if your character is older, frail, or has a condition that causes them to heal slowly. It's important to note that the bone is not 100% healed when the cast is removed which will take another 3-6 months.

More complicated injuries, such as compound, displaced, or comminuted fractures, require traction or surgery. Open fractures additionally require antibiotics. The most common surgical technique for fracture repair, *open reduction, and internal fixation* (ORIF) uses rods, screws, and/or plates surgically implanted beneath the skin to keep the ends of the bones aligned. Fractures requiring surgical repair include broken femurs, hips, and shoulders, as well as compound, comminuted, or misaligned fractures. Traction (the use of pulleys and weights to stretch the soft tissue surrounding the bone) is used to help stabilize unstable fractures or realign the broken ends of the bone. It is frequently used to treat long bone fractures (fractures of the legs and arms) and is often used in conjunction with surgery.

> Comminuted fractures occur when the bone has been broken in at least three places, resulting in shards of bone.

Pain medications, as you might expect, are used to alleviate pain. Medication of varying strength can be prescribed. Tylenol, ibuprofen, and even opioids like oxycodone are sometimes prescribed based on the severity of the injury. While mild injuries, like a broken finger or toe, might be effectively treated with Tylenol and/or ibuprofen, more severe injuries, such as a fractured hip or femur, might require IV morphine. Ice reduces swelling and is particularly useful in the treatment of fractured fingers and toes. Physical therapy generally begins after the cast is removed, but certain injuries, particularly those requiring surgical fixation, may begin within a week or two of the injury.

PROGNOSIS

Bones are good at healing, though not so good that they grow back stronger, as some old wives' tales would have you think. Simpler, cleaner breaks of smaller bones heal faster than messy, comminuted breaks or fractures of large bones. Below is a list of APPROXIMATE healing times for fractures; remember, there is lots of variation here due to your character's age, gender, relative health (an elderly chain-smoker with osteoporosis will heal much more slowly than a healthy child), degree of injury, and presence of other injuries.

Body Part	Healing Time
Toes	4-6 weeks
Foot	6-12 weeks
Heel	3-4 months
Ankle	6+ weeks
Lower Leg (*Tibia*)	4-6 months
Lower Leg (*Fibula*)	6-12 weeks
Thigh (*Femur*)	4-6 months
Pelvis	8-12 weeks
Fingers	4-6 weeks
Hand	4-6 weeks
Wrist	2-6 months
Lower arm	4-6 weeks
Upper arm (*Humerus*)	12+ weeks
Shoulder (*Scapula*)	6-12 months
Collarbone (*Clavicle*)	6-8 weeks
Spine	6-12 weeks
Skull	3-6 months

SPRAINS, TEARS & DISLOCATIONS

SPRAINS

Paolo has played soccer ever since he could walk, so by the time he was a senior in high school, he was the star forward of the team. They were getting ready to compete for State when he twisted his ankle during practice. He'd immediately collapsed, the joint unable to hold his weight.

A sprain is the stretching or tearing of the fibrous tissues that hold a joint in place, called ligaments. Ligament tears can range in severity; they can be small and mild, or they can pass through the complete diameter of the ligament, called a full-thickness **tear.** The most common anatomical location for a sprain is the ankle, though knees, elbows, wrists, fingers, and even shoulders can be sprained as well.

If your character has a sprain, they'll have pain, soreness, and swelling at the joint, followed by bruising a day or two later. Mild sprains are just that—mild - resulting in stiffness and swelling that your character will probably find more annoying than actually painful. However more serious sprains can result in severe pain that can prevent them from walking or moving that limb. In fact, ankle sprains can look so similar to ankle fractures that the only way to definitively tell them apart is with an X-ray.

The doctor took a few X-rays, then diagnosed Paolo with a Grade 2 ankle sprain: a partial tear of the ligaments of his ankle. Over Paolo's violent protestations, he prescribed ibuprofen, rest, and total abstinence from soccer for four weeks. Paolo had to watch as his team lost the Championships without him.

Sprains are treated with RICE: **r**est, **i**ce, **c**ompression, and **e**levation. Rarely, sprains are serious enough to require surgery. Sprains can take a long time to heal, though. While mild sprains may take only 2-3 weeks, severe sprains can take upwards of 3 months or more.[1]

TEARS

Tears occur when the soft tissue around a joint is ripped or torn apart, resulting in pain, decreased mobility, and stiffness of the joint. There are a few famous tears you should be aware of.

ROTATOR CUFF TEAR

The rotator cuff is the collection of muscles and tendons connecting your character's arm to their shoulder blade. Rotator cuffs are often torn after a fall on an outstretched hand, or if your character tries to lift something too heavy for them. If your character has a rotator cuff tear, they'll have shoulder pain, particularly when lifting the injured arm, or lying on their injured side. They'll also have weakness in that arm; some may not be able to lift the arm above the shoulder. Finally, they may feel a cracking or popping sensation inside their shoulder joint when they try to move it. Most rotator cuff tears are treated nonsurgically, with RICE, ibuprofen, and physical therapy.

Undeterred, Paolo continued playing soccer, even earning an athletics scholarship for college. But in his sophomore year, Paolo collided with a player from a rival school. He felt his knee pop and give way beneath him. Choking back his tears, Paolo limped off the field with the help of his teammates—he couldn't put weight on the knee.

If you follow sports, you've probably heard of ACL and MCL tears—knee injuries famous for taking down famous athletes like Kevin Durant, Tom Brady, and Alex Morgan.

The ACL and MCL provide stability to the knee. The *anterior cruciate ligament* (ACL) keeps the knee from moving backward and forwards, while the *medial collateral ligament* (MCL) stabilizes side-to-side movement. There are more ligaments than just these two in the knee, but when these, in particular, are injured, it can lead to some serious issues.

If your character has an ACL tear, they'll hear an audible popping sound in their knee, followed by sudden, severe pain at the front of the knee. If they try to walk, the knee will feel unstable and painful—the knee might not even hold their weight. ACL injuries tend to happen when your character is twisting or pivoting.

In contrast, MCL tears tend to be caused by direct collisions with the knee; someone hits your character in the side of the knee, and they fall hard. MCL tears feel a lot like ACL tears (pain, swelling, and joint instability) with the addition of a feeling of locking or popping every time they move their knee.

The doctors felt Paolo's swollen knee, then took him to an MRI—a large, white, donut-like instrument that made clacking and clattering noises so loud that Paolo could hear them through the noise-canceling headphones the technician gave him. When they told him he'd torn both his ACL and his MCL, and that, even with surgery, it was unlikely he'd ever be able to play competitive soccer again, he finally broke down and cried.

Both ACL and MCL tears are diagnosed with an MRI of the knee. They are treated with RICE, physical therapy, and time. Surgery is usually reserved for competitive athletes.

DISLOCATIONS

A dislocated joint occurs when the bones of a joint pop out of alignment. Most often caused by a fall or a direct hit to the joint, a dislocated joint is a painful emergency. The shoulder, the most mobile joint in the body, is also the most likely to become dislocated, but elbows, wrists, fingers, hips, knees, ankles, and even ribs can also become dislocated.

If your character dislocates a joint, the first thing they'll notice is severe pain, trouble moving the affected joint, and a visible disfigurement of the joint. They might also experience numbness or weakness of their hand or foot below the joint, implying that the dislocation is impinging on the nerve. If not treated promptly, the joint will swell and the muscles surrounding the joint will begin to spasm painfully.

The first step to treating a joint dislocation is closed reduction; forcing the joint back into place. Ideally, this should be done by a medical professional who knows what they're doing, but in a pinch, one of your non-medical characters could do it. The pain is relieved as soon as the joint is replaced, though your character may be quite sore and tender for a few days (or weeks!) after, so your character will need to keep the joint immobilized—usually in a sling—for a few days afterward. The final step in treating a joint dislocation is physical therapy to prevent it from happening again.

People with dislocations often skip immobilization and physical therapy, putting them at higher risk of re-injury. It's a great potential for an Achilles heel in your character.

Once a joint has been dislocated, the ligaments holding it in place have stretched, so it's more likely that that joint will be dislocated. Some people dislocate their joints so frequently that they can pop them back in themselves and go on with their day.

AMPUTATIONS & DEGLOVING INJURIES

AMPUTATIONS

Amputations are the removal of a limb or digit. They can be surgical or traumatic, partial or complete. A partial amputation occurs when something—soft tissue, bone, muscle—still connects the severed pieces, while a complete amputation means the two pieces are entirely separated. About 25% of all amputations are traumatic, meaning that the amputation occurred due to an accident—the rest are due to medical issues such as diabetes.[2] Most traumatic amputations involve the upper extremities.

The most common cause of traumatic amputation is traffic accidents, closely followed by workplace accidents. Factories, farms, and construction sites are frequent culprits. But there are lots of different ways to lose a limb, including lawnmowers, firearms, fireworks, doors, and even rings getting caught on things. As a

Proximal = closer to the center of the body.

Distal = further from the center of the body.

i.e., the elbow is proximal to the hand.

NATALIE DALE, MD

writer, you have ample opportunity to get creative if you plan to divorce your antagonist from an appendage.

Amputations are gross, gory, and excruciating. Often, the amputation isn't a neat cut, but a bloody mess of mangled tissue and broken bone. Bleeding is the most immediate problem with a traumatic amputation; the higher up on the limb the amputation occurs, the bigger the bleeding blood vessel and the heavier the resulting hemorrhage. These high-level amputations are life-threatening. To stop the bleeding and prevent imminent demise, a tourniquet needs to be applied proximal to the severed limb as quickly as possible.[3] But even if all your character lost is their hand, they can still bleed out from the wrist in less than a minute.

To treat the amputation, your character should pack the wound as best they can, placing pressure to try and stop, or at least slow, the bleeding. If the bleeding is severe, your character may need to place a tourniquet. Then, they should grab the amputated limb and hightail it to the hospital. Don't put the amputated body part on ice; if your character has time, wrap it in gauze soaked in cold (and ideally, sterile) water. Once in the hospital, they'll be given antibiotics and the wound will be anesthetized, irrigated, and packed with gauze. Then they'll either be brought to the OR for immediate reattachment or taken for further imaging.

See FAQ in <u>Volume 1: Setting & Character</u> for more on using tourniquets.

Not all amputated limbs will be able to be reattached. Clean amputations with sharp edges are more likely to be reattached, while amputations due to crushing or tearing injuries are unlikely to be salvageable. Younger age, smaller limb amputation (aka fingers, toes, and ears), proper preservation of amputated body parts, and a shorter time to treatment increase the likelihood that surgeons will be able to successfully attach the limb.

DEGLOVING

Degloving injuries, also called avulsion injuries, occur when the superficial layers of skin and tissue are ripped off the underlying muscle and bone. Earning its name from the image of the skin being ripped off a hand like a glove, degloving injuries are gory and, unsurprisingly, horrifically painful. Large avulsion injuries can be fatal, usually due to sepsis or hemorrhagic shock.[4]

Treating a degloving injury is both complicated and costly. Once the injury has been stabilized, your character will most likely need skin grafts, and possibly blood vessel grafts as well. There is also a high risk of both infection and tissue death, called necrosis, so they'll need to be on IV antibiotics and will

Skin grafts are the surgical placement of healthy skin—usually taken from your character's back or thighs—over lost or damaged skin. Blood vessels can also be similarly grafted.

likely need multiple surgeries to clean out the dead tissue. Sometimes, the limb may even need to be amputated.

Even once the surgeries are done and your character is free to go home, they will likely have disabilities for life. Nerve damage can lead to numbness, pins, and needles, and even phantom limb pain. Scars from the grafting procedures are not only visibly disfiguring, but they can also cause loss of sensation or even chronic pain in the area. The scar can tighten painfully, forming *contractures)*. If the scar tissue goes all the way around a limb (called a *circumferential injury*), this tightening of the scar tissue can cut off blood flow to the limb and will need to be removed through a painful procedure called an *escharotomy*.

CRUSH INJURIES

Voices above draw Paolo back to the present; he's been found! He calls back, his voice hoarse from screaming. What feels like an eternity later, the rubble is cleared, and Paolo can see his rescuers clearly. Only the slab of cement laying across his thighs stands between him and freedom.

Crush Injuries are exactly what they sound like; injuries caused by your character getting crushed between two heavy objects. Sounds pretty simple, right?

Not so fast. Crush injuries are dangerous for two reasons. The first is obvious; heavy thing squashing bodies leads to broken bones, ruptured organs, and smooshed blood vessels that can no longer pump blood to the places they're supposed to go. That all sounds pretty bad—and it is. But the real reason crush injuries are commonly fatal is because of what happens when your character gets uncrushed.

After much deliberation, the rescuers can lift the cement slab and pry Paolo free. His legs are crushed, the skin mottled white and black, but he doesn't feel pain. He's put on IV fluids and pain meds and then rushed to the hospital.

When the giant rock/spaceship/grand piano crushes your character beneath them, it smooshes the cells, causing them to burst. While your character continues to be crushed, those cells stay smooshed. But when the weight is removed, the broken cells spill their contents out into your character's bloodstream.

At the ED, Paolo is put on a bunch of medications and admitted to the hospital. He's got a bunch of wires on his chest monitoring his heart rhythm, and a tube stuck up his junk to help him pee. Just as he's settling into his new room, he suddenly feels lightheaded. Then, the world goes black.

The chemical composition inside the cell is very different from the outside—and nowhere is this more apparent than in potassium levels. Turns out, that potassium is both very important in the regulation of the heart rhythm and in high concentrations

 NATALIE DALE, MD

inside the cell. When cells start spilling all their potassium into the bloodstream, the heart goes haywire, resulting in potentially deadly changes to the heart's rhythm.

Paolo wakes up in an ICU, covered in wires. The nurse tells him that he went into ventricular fibrillation (a deadly heart rhythm) due to the rising levels of potassium in his blood. There was a Code Blue, and the doctors had to shock his heart back into the correct rhythm. He was transferred to the ICU to stabilize the electrolytes in his blood and to prevent further complications.

But that's not all! Skeletal muscles are full of proteins like CK and myoglobin; when crushed, they spill these proteins into the blood too. This phenomenon, called *rhabdomyolysis* (my = muscle, lysis = breakdown), overwhelms your character's kidneys, which are just trying to filter the blood. Your character's urine will turn brown, and their kidneys will start to fail.

If your character has been crushed, they need to be treated immediately once the rock/spaceship/grand piano crushing your character starts to be moved. This means they need IV fluids and pain meds given *during extrication*. If your character can't be extricated, the limb may need to be amputated on-site. Either way, they'll need to be transferred to the hospital for cardiac monitoring and continued fluid resuscitation.

A crush injury presents a great opportunity to kill off a character after everyone thinks they're safe. What better way to toy with your readers' expectations than to have them survive, maybe even walk away, from a horrific accident, only to succumb to a cardiac arrest (see *Ch. 1: Chest Pain*) a few hours later. If you want to draw it out, have them refuse to go to the hospital, then have their family watch in horror as they die of acute renal failure over the next several days.

BREAKING DOWN THE CLICHÉ: RUNNING ON A BROKEN LEG

He jumped from the two-story building, landing hard. He felt his thigh bone snap beneath him, and he fell to the ground with a scream. The pain was blinding hot, bringing tears to his eyes, even though he was a man who rarely cried. But he couldn't stay down, couldn't risk letting them find her. So, he pushed himself to his feet, gritting his teeth against the pain, and ran out into the night,

Your character will not be able to put weight on a broken bone without significant pain. However, that doesn't mean they can't walk (or run) if their life depends on it. If they've broken their toe or even their fibula, they'll be able to shift the limb so that they aren't putting their full weight on it; they'll limp, but they'll be able to get away. But if your character has broken their femur or tibia, don't even think about having your character make a break for it! I don't care how manly they are, or how much their life depends on a quick getaway; they'll collapse the moment they try to put any weight on that leg.

17. BURNS

Quinn has been married for fifteen years, and in a dedicated relationship for more than thirty. She's raised two rambunctious sons, hosted innumerable cocktail parties for her wife's clients, and in all that time, she has never once let dinner burn. But tonight, after spending hours preparing a celebratory dinner celebrating her wife's final chemo treatment, she allows herself a few moments to rest in the recliner while she finished the bourbon braised, bacon-wrapped shrimp in the broiler.

BACKGROUND

The skin is an organ whose main job is to protect the body. It does so by keeping fluids and heat inside, and germs outside. The top layer of the skin—called the *epidermis*—is a waterproof, protective barrier. At the bottom of the epidermis lies a layer of stem cells; damage this layer, and the skin will not be able to regrow there. Below the epidermis lies the dermis, through which small blood vessels, nerves, hair follicles, and sweat glands run. The deepest layer, called the subcutaneous tissue or hypodermis, contains fatty tissue along with larger blood vessels and nerves.

Stem cells are non-specialized cells that can differentiate into many different cell types. Skin stem cells can become any type of skin cell.

A burn is defined as damage to the skin and underlying tissue by a thermal source. And that thermal source doesn't just mean fire or heat. Burns can be caused by electricity, sunlight, chemicals, hot liquids, and even radiation.

CAUSES OF BURNS

Quinn wakes to the smell of smoke. Leaping from her chair, she races into the kitchen to find smoke pouring from the oven. Fumbling, she pulls it open, only to be greeted by billowing, caustic smoke and heat so intense her eyebrows singed. She coughs, her throat burning with every breath. Inside

     NATALIE DALE, MD

the oven, flames dance where her dinner should be. The fire alarm blares, piercing through Quinn's thoughts like a hot knife. How could anyone think in this noise?

THERMAL

Thermal burns are caused by heat: hot objects (hot stove, branding iron, etc.), scalding liquids, steam, and of course, fire.

Coughing, Quinn grabs the oven mitts and reaches into the oven, trying to pull out the flaming shrimp. She grabs the pan and pulls, but the heat is too intense, even through the mitts. She yelps in pain, and drops the pan to the floor, the hot oil splashing all over the fancy new nylons, then catching the woven kitchen rug on fire. She throws a kitchen towel over the flame, hoping to smother it, but the towel only catches fire too.

ULTRAVIOLET LIGHT

Sunlight, along with other sources of UV such as tanning beds, sun lamps, or even UV light sanitizers, can cause burns. Most of the time, sunlight only causes first and second-degree burns, though it is theoretically possible to get a third-degree burn from UV light.

ELECTRICAL

Electrical burns are caused by a direct current of electricity racing through the body. While only about 4% of all burns are electrical burns, they have a high mortality rate. Because electricity travels *through* the body, it can cause all sorts of damage, particularly to organs that rely on electricity. These include:

- **Heart:** An electric current can cause abnormal heart rhythms and can even cause the heart to stop beating altogether.

- **Brain:** Your character may pass out when the electric current passes through their body, or they may start having seizures. They may become paralyzed, stop breathing or even fall into a coma.

- **Muscles:** Since muscles are stimulated to contract by electricity, a strong electrical current can cause dangerously strong muscular contractions that can break bones and tear a muscle. Then the damaged muscle cells spill proteins into the bloodstream, causing kidney failure and electrolyte disturbances (which can, in turn, lead to heart arrhythmias).

- **Kidneys**: Unable to filter the proteins the muscles are dumping into the bloodstream; the kidneys may shut down.

- **Loss of limb**: due to severe swelling.

If your character has an electrical burn, their doctors won't be able to see the internal damage. Instead, your character will have *contact points*—the electrical equivalent of entrance and exit burns. The first contact point will be where they touched the electrical source (usually their hand), while the second will be at the point where they contacted the ground (usually their foot). These wounds will look just like thermal burns from the outside, but don't be fooled; the electrical charge will have caused damage throughout the path between the contact points.

> Electrical shocks, such as dropping a hair straightener into the bathtub, do not cause external burns.[2]

LIGHTNING

No electrical injury is more dramatic than a lightning strike. Classic injuries associated with lightning strikes include a blown eardrum (*ruptured tympanic membrane*), shoulder dislocation, fractures caused by intense muscle contraction, cold and pulseless extremities, the heart-stopping (*asystole*), and a feathering, fern-like pattern (called *Lichtenberg figures*) along the skin.

RADIATION

Radiation burns occur when high-energy radioactive elements come in contact with your character. The most common cause of radiation burns is in cancer patients undergoing radiation therapy (See *Ch. 24: Cancer*).

> *Quinn's wife, Querida, runs into the kitchen, her silk blouse flapping open to reveal the blistering red skin above where her left breast should be, a souvenir of her radiation therapy. She doesn't hesitate, just grabs the fire extinguisher from the pantry and starts dousing the fire. It's out in less than a minute, leaving the kitchen rug, towels, and oven mitts blackened and covered in a dusting of white powder.*

CHEMICAL

> Chemical burns to the eye cause redness, tearing, pain, and blurred vision. It can result in permanent damage, including blindness.

Chemical burns occur when your character comes in contact with a chemical irritant, such as chlorine, bleach, sulfuric acid, or ammonia. These chemicals can be found in everyday substances, such as battery acid, oven cleaners, drain cleaners, pool cleaners, and paint cleaners. Chemical burns can be *alkaline* (ammonia, lye, potassium hydroxide), or *acidic* (sulfuric acid, hydrochloric acid, vinegar).

The first step in treating a chemical burn is to remove the source of the irritation by taking off all your character's clothes (you never know what could be contaminated) and rinsing the area thoroughly. If you want an idiotic character to make the injury worse, have them try to "neutralize" the agent by pouring an acidic substance over an alkaline injury, or vice versa. That will only cause an exothermic reaction, resulting in even more severe burns!

Querida takes one look at her wife, with blistering burns covering her feet and lower legs, and immediately calls 911. Quinn protests, the burns don't even hurt, but Querida just insists that Quinn wait in the living room until the first responders arrive. While Querida is on the phone, she absently tries to brush away the fine dust covering the countertop, but the powder just aerosolizes at her touch. Her eyes are suddenly burning, her vision blurry. She washes her hands in the kitchen sink, then rinses her eyes with water until the fire truck and ambulance arrive.

Using certain types of fire extinguishers in enclosed spaces can cause mild chemical irritation to the eyes, throat and skin.

While contact with skin can certainly cause major burns, the biggest problem with chemical burns is ingestion and inhalation. Whether the ingestion was intentional (suicide attempt) or unintentional (usually children), chemical burns to the mouth, esophagus, and throat can be both painful and dangerous.

EVALUATION

The paramedics start two IVs—one in each arm—and hang bags of clear fluid attached to them. They place an oxygen mask over Quinn's face that blows air with the ferocity of a winter gale. Querida sits on the narrow bench beside her, clutching Quinn's wedding ring and necklace in both hands.

Minor burns can be treated at home and should heal fully within a few weeks. Major burns need urgent medical care. Any burn where there is a risk of smoke inhalation needs to be treated in the emergency department. And while most people seen for burns in the ED are treated and then released, those with the most serious injuries will need to be treated at a Burn Unit—a section of the hospital devoted to caring for people with burns.

Burn Units require highly specialized care. As such, they are almost always located in Level 1 Trauma Centers.

PRELIMINARY SURVEY

When they arrive at the ED, Quinn is taken straight back to a curtained room. A nurse helps Quinn change into a hospital gown—her dress is easy enough to slip out of, but her nylons seem to have fused to her legs. A phlebotomist arrives, taking blood from the IV site and placing them in little tubes with multicolored tops before vanishing. Finally, the nurse carefully cuts away the nylon, making sure not to disturb the areas that are melted on her legs.

For more on the the preliminary survey, see Volume 1: Setting & Character, *Ch. 2: Trauma Center.*

The first step in treating burn victims' injuries is to get your character away from the fire. Once they're safe, it's back to the ABCs of the preliminary survey. They'll evaluate for signs of imminent airway collapse, such as facial burns or soot in the saliva that indicate there's a chance the airway has been damaged. Next, they'll slap on a facemask (called a *nonrebreather*) and give your character 100% oxygen at a high flow rate while simultaneously monitoring your character's oxygenation through a pulse oximeter. If there's the faintest hint that the airway might be compromised, they'll sedate and intubate your character in a heartbeat.

A character with inhalation injuries will have a delicate airway. While intubation is often necessary to save their life, it can cause devastating complications such as airway perforation.

The next step is circulation. Typically, two IVs will be placed, one in each arm, in order to administer copious amounts of fluids as fast as possible. Finally, they'll "expose" your character, cutting off clothes, rinsing them off, and checking for wounds, as well as removing all rings, watches, and jewelry. Doing so not only prevents further burns (jewelry retains heat, chemicals still on clothing can continue to cause burns) but also prevents damage when the injured limb begins to swell.

Remember: these steps will likely occur simultaneously, especially in the ED where your character will be surrounded by nurses and docs.

WORKUP

If your character had a major burn, or if there is a risk of inhalation injuries, your character will need a chest X-ray to evaluate their lungs, a pulse oximeter to check how much oxygen is in their blood, and several blood tests, including a *Carboxyhemoglobin* level to determine how much carbon monoxide (CO) is in

NATALIE DALE, MD

their blood. They might also need a test called an *arterial blood gas*, or ABG, which evaluates the blood from your character's arteries, rather than the veins. To get that blood, a doctor will have to stick a long needle into your character's wrist. It's more painful than drawing blood from a vein (where most blood is drawn from), and it can be a scary and uncomfortable experience that often takes more than one attempt. How would your character react to a needle being shoved repeatedly into the tender skin of their wrist?

GRADING BURNS

Burns are graded based on both the depth of the skin they penetrate, and the amount of body surface burned. Burns can be partial or full-thickness. Partial-thickness burns involve only the epidermis and/or part of the dermis, while full-thickness injuries damage the entire dermis.

BURN SEVERITY

> *Once the nylons are gone—at least, the non-melted part—Quinn can see the extent of her injuries. She has small, pink spots along her legs and upper arms, probably from where the oil spattered. Some of them are pink and shiny, others deep red and starting to blister; those hurt like hell. But the larger burns, the ones covering her entire right foot and part of the left are yellowish white, the edges charred. Strangely, she feels barely any pain in the left foot and absolutely none in the right.*

FIRST DEGREE BURNS (SUPERFICIAL BURN)

Superficial burns are those that affect only the top layer of skin (the *epidermis).* They look like sunburns because most sunburns are first-degree burns. Your character's skin will be red, painful, and dry. It will turn white when pressed, a phenomenon called *blanching.* There won't be any blisters and the skin may start to peel off after a few days. After 5-10 days, the burn should heal completely without any scarring.[1]

> Burns can become more severe with time. What may initially look like a first-degree burn may start to blister, becoming a second-degree burn within a few hours.

SECOND DEGREE BURNS (PARTIAL-THICKNESS)

Second-degree burns are called a *partial-thickness injuries,* meaning that they involve the top layer of skin (the epidermis), as well as part of the underlying structure, called the dermis. There are two subtypes of second-degree burns: superficial partial-thickness and deep partial-thickness.

Superficial partial-thickness burns look like first-degree burns (red, blanching, swollen, and painful) with the addition of fluid-filled blisters that form after injury. These types of burns are often the most painful, as the burn did not penetrate deep enough to damage the nerve endings. If your character has a superficial partial-thickness burn, it'll take several weeks for them to heal, but they probably won't have any major scars.

Deep partial-thickness burns, on the other hand, appear yellow or white and do not blanche. Your character will have decreased sensation, as the nerves have been slightly damaged. Deep partial-thickness burns take longer to heal—3-8 weeks—and will likely cause scarring.[1]

THIRD-DEGREE BURNS (FULL-THICKNESS)

A third-degree burn is a full-thickness injury. If your character has a third-degree burn, it means they have completely damaged both their epidermis and their dermis. Your character's skin may look white, brown, or even black and charred. The burn will not hurt, as the nerves that run through the dermis will have been damaged. This nerve damage means that your character won't be able to feel anything at the burn site at all and may even experience weakness in the injured limb.

Full-thickness burns can't heal on their own. If your character has a third-degree burn or greater, they'll require skin grafts and healing will take several months.

> Many full-thickness burn victims develop neuropathic pain—burning, stabbing, or shooting pain—as the injury starts to heal.

FOURTH, FIFTH, AND SIXTH-DEGREE BURNS (FULL THICKNESS)

Full-thickness burns can be further categorized by the depth of underlying tissue involvement. A character with fourth-degree burns will have charred skin and significant damage to underlying structures, such as nerves, blood vessels, and bone. Fifth-degree (charred skin, bone exposed) and 6th-degree burns (complete loss of skin, revealing charred deep tissue and bone) are the most severe levels of burns.

Full-thickness burns are totally numb, as the nerves running through the area have been completely destroyed. A fourth-degree or higher burn is a catastrophic injury that will likely leave your character with disabilities and disfigurements that will last the rest of their life.

BURN DISTRIBUTION

When the doctor arrives, she looks carefully at Quinn's burns, prodding them gently. She asks if Quinn needs any painkillers, but Quinn waves her away; the burns barely hurt at all.

Querida stands beside her wife, one hand on her shoulder. Once the doctor is finished with her exam, she tells Quinn that she has a variety of first, second, and third-degree burns over her face, arms, hands, lower legs, and feet. All in all, the burns cover about 10% of her body. Because the worst of the burns, the third-degree burns, are on her feet and ankles, she will need to be admitted to the hospital for further care.

The second important factor when considering the level of care that your character will need after a burn is what body parts were injured and how much of their *body surface area* (BSA) was burned. Requirements for admission to a burn unit include[3]:

- Burns over a large area of the body (>15% BSA)

- Major 3rd-degree burns (over >5% BSA)

- Burns in worrisome locations: face, eyes, ears, hands, feet, groin, and over joints

- Chemical or electrical burns

- Burns associated with major trauma

- Burns with the possibility of inhalation injury (more on this later)

- Burns that might be related to abuse (child abuse, elder abuse, and/or domestic violence)

> Doctors estimate BSA using the Rule of Nines:
>
> Head = 9% of body
>
> Front of trunk = 18%
>
> Back of trunk = 18%
>
> Arms = 9% each
>
> Legs = 18% each
>
> Groin = 1%

SUMMARY: MAJOR VS. MINOR BURNS

When trying to decide how seriously you want to injure your character, it may be helpful to classify their burns as either major or minor.

- **Minor burns** are all first-degree burns and small second-degree burns that cover less than 10% of your character's body. They should heal on their own in a few weeks.

- **Major burns** are any full-thickness (third-degree or higher) burns, large second-degree burns, and burns to sensitive areas, such as the hands, groin, or face. Major burns take longer to heal (months) and require surgical treatment such as skin grafting and wound debridement.

> **Wound debridement** is the surgical removal of dead tissue from a wound.

SMOKE INHALATION INJURIES

Signs that your character is suffering from an inhalation injury can be subtle, a bit of soot at the corner of their mouth, a hoarse voice, or even singed nose hairs. To the observant medical professional, these are red flags indicating that your character needs immediate intubation. But those surrounding your character might have no idea. Your character might even skip going to the hospital, only to have their airway swell up hours later.

> No one wants to be intubated, especially if they aren't feeling ill. How would your character react to being told that they need to have a tube shoved down their throat when their only complaint is a cough?

Other red flags indicating your character may have an inhalation injury include burns to the face or inside the cheeks, sooty-looking saliva, soot inside the mouth, cough, wheezing, or trouble breathing.[4] If your character exhibits any of these signs, they may need to be intubated in order to prevent their airway from swelling shut.

As the doctor is turning to leave, Quinn begins to cough. Her throat is still sore from whatever smoke was coming out of the oven, and her voice sounds hoarse. The doctor turns back and asks Quinn to cough into a tissue. The thin white fluid she produces is flecked with soot.

Not all burns result in smoke inhalation and not all smoke inhalation is associated with burns. But if your character has been in a house fire, they've probably inhaled some smoke. If they did, that's bad news for them; smoke inhalation injuries increase the risk of death after a fire by more than twenty times![4] There are three main ways smoke inhalation can injure your character: irritating the airways, airway swelling leading to asphyxiation, and carbon monoxide poisoning.

UPPER AIRWAY INJURY

The doctor asks Quinn to open her mouth. Quinn does so, though she feels like coughing again. The doctor's face grows grim as she shines the penlight back and forth. Finally, Querida can't stand the uncertainty.

"What's going on?" she asks. "What's wrong with her mouth?"

The doctor looks like she's trying to think. "Quinn, you have burns in your mouth, on your face, and soot in your sputum. These are all signs that point to smoke inhalation injury. We're going to have to watch you carefully. If your breathing gets worse, I may need to put a tube down your throat to help you breathe."

The upper airway (the throat and windpipe down to the voice box) is most likely to be injured due to heat. This can cause all sorts of damage, such as burns and blisters. Your character may experience a burning in their mouth or throat, trouble swallowing, or cough. Or they may not feel anything at all. The danger with an upper airway injury is that the damaged tissue will swell up, closing off the airway. Once that happens, it becomes very difficult to intubate, and your character may asphyxiate. For that reason, medical professionals should be watchful of the possibility of inhalation injuries.

Quinn refuses point blank to be intubated. She's breathing just fine, thank you. But Querida has noticed that her voice sounds hoarse, that it looks like she's not quite breathing normally, though Quinn will never admit that, of course. Finally, the doctor suggests a diagnostic test—called fiberoptic bronchoscopy— to determine if Quinn needs intubation.

LOWER AIRWAY INJURY

Injury to the lower airways is usually due to the chemicals present in the smoke. As such, they tend to show up hours after your character's exposure. Your character may develop increased fluid in their lungs (*pulmonary edema)* or the collapse of the air sacs in the lungs (*atelectasis*). A *fiberoptic bronchoscopy* (a camera threaded down the windpipe) can definitively show damage in both the upper and lower airways.[7]

But when the doctor returns with the supplies, Quinn is struggling to breathe. She's leaning forward, the muscles of her chest and neck flaring as she gasps for breath. The doctor moves quickly, calling out for medications and intubation supplies. Someone takes Querida by the arm and escorts her from the room. Sometime later, Querida couldn't say if it was a few minutes or a few hours, the doctor returns. She tells Querida that the intubation was successful, but Quinn will need to stay on a ventilator to help her breathe.

CARBON MONOXIDE POISONING

If your character has inhaled smoke, the next concern is for Carbon Monoxide (CO) poisoning. CO is produced by incomplete combustion, and it binds strongly to a molecule in red blood cells called hemoglobin. Normally, hemoglobin binds oxygen and delivers it to the tissues. But when CO is bound instead, oxygen can't be delivered to the rest of the body. Without oxygen, your character's tissue—particularly high-energy tissues like the brain and heart—will die, and your character will asphyxiate while still breathing.

Because blood is still flowing, and your character is still breathing, CO poisoning can be easy to miss. Your character won't go blue around the lips (*cyanosis*) and the pulse oximeter may show full oxygenation levels because the hemoglobin is bound to oxygen, just the wrong type. Instead, they'll exhibit vague symptoms, like headaches, poor concentration, chest tightness, and anxiety. If your character doesn't know what to look for, they could fall into a coma.

Symptoms of CO poisoning vary by how much CO is bound to the hemoglobin. Mild CO poisoning presents with a headache, chest tightness, and trouble concentrating. As more and more CO binds to the hemoglobin, the headache will become severe, and your character will become confused or tired. They may even start to have seizures. Severe CO poisoning results in a coma, a slow and weak pulse, and, eventually, death.

Mild CO poisoning can be treated with 100% oxygen through a nonrebreather mask (or ventilator if your character was intubated. More severe CO poisoning requires treatment with a pressured chamber of oxygen, called *hyperbaric oxygen therapy*.

TREATMENT

After a few days, Quinn is extubated. She then begins a seemingly endless cycle of debridement and skin grafting, along with several different types of therapy. A physical therapist helps her regain strength and balance in her legs, while an occupational therapist helps her relearn to use her scarred hands. She even has a speech therapist, who helps her relearn how to talk and eat while the painful burns in her throat and mouth are healing. After two weeks, the doctors say she is finally ready to go home.

Treatment of burns depends on the extent of the injuries, the presence of other trauma, and how ill your character looks. If they're circling the drain, they'll be rushed to the ICU for intensive management, including respiratory and blood pressure support. Mainstays of burn treatment include:

Fluid resuscitation: Prevent organ dysfunction (particularly the kidneys) by giving mondo doses of fluids.

Pain control: Burns are painful, but treating burns is even worse. Your character is going to need IV pain medications (such as IV morphine) once they start surgical management. But oversedation is dangerous, so doctors will need to walk a tightrope between adequate pain control and completely snowing your character.

Wound Cleansing & Debridement: The dead tissue must be cleaned out so that healthy tissue can take its place. It's exceedingly, horrifically painful.

Skin Grafting: The main surgical treatment of full-thickness burns is skin grafts: placing healthy skin tissue from one part of the body over the damaged skin. Most of the time, the healthy skin comes from your character's thigh, abdomen, back, or butt.

Antibiotic: Burns are treated with an antibiotic ointment called *silver sulfadiazine* to prevent infection. Oral and IV antibiotics are only used if your character develops an acute infection.

Feeding: Many burn patients can't eat on their own, so a *nasogastric tube* (NG tube) will be dropped down their throat so that they can be fed. Talk about a liquid diet!

> IV feeding doesn't work long-term. If your character is going to be out of it for a while, they'll need an NG tube to get the food into their gut.

Monitor Urine Output: Your character will have a urinary catheter placed, and the nurses will closely monitor how much urine comes out. Too little urine output is a sign that your character isn't getting enough fluids.

COMPLICATIONS

FLUID LOSS

You've probably heard the "3 Rules of Real Estate" (Location, Location, Location!). If there were "3 Rules of Burns" they would probably be "Fluid Resuscitation, Fluid Resuscitation, Fluid Resuscitation!"

The skin is an organ, and one of its main jobs is to keep the inside of the body moist. If your character has 20% or more of their body covered in burns, they will be leaking fluids like a boat made of Swiss cheese. Fluid loss leads to kidney failure and other organ damage. So, replacing those fluids becomes paramount.

At the hospital, doctors will calculate how much fluid is needed in the first

24-hours based on your character's weight and how much of their body is burned. As a writer, you don't need to know the formula (it's called the *Parkland formula* if you're interested), but you do need to know that it's an absurd amount of fluid. An average-sized (200lb) man with 50% of his body burned will need EIGHTEEN liters of fluids, given over 24 hours. That's more than 3 times the average human's total blood volume. But your character is going to need every drop of that fluid to survive.

HYPOTHERMIA

The skin's other main job is to keep your body's warmth inside. Disrupt it, and the heat loss can spell hypothermia. For that reason, burn units are kept exceedingly warm, somewhere between 82 and 86°F. But until your character makes it to the burn unit, doctors will use other methods to prevent heat loss. These include covering your character with warm blankets or a Bair Hugger (plastic contraptions filled with warm air) giving warm IV fluids, or simply blowing warm air over them.

INFECTION

The third job of the skin is to keep out invaders, particularly bacteria. With the skin damaged, your character is at high risk for infection. One species of bacteria, in particular, *Pseudomonas aeruginosa*, is famous for infecting burns. These bacteria became famous because they make your character's wounds smell like rotten grape juice. Of course, *Pseudomonas* aren't the only germs that can infect wounds; plenty of other bacteria, viruses, and even fungi can infect wounds. But the wounds aren't the only infection your character needs to worry about.

If your character has severe burns, they are going to be hospitalized for a long time. As such, they are at risk of all the fun hospital-acquired (*nosocomial*) infections, most commonly pneumonia, and urinary tract infections. Sepsis (See *Ch. 5: Fever*) is one of the most common causes of death in hospitalized burn patients.

CONTRACTURES

Quinn knows she looks different. Despite the best efforts of her surgeons, her legs and feet are pockmarked with scars, and her ankle will never move the same way again, stiffened by the healing scar tissue over the joint. When she brings up her fears, that she now looks and walks like an old woman, Querida just kisses her and tells her she loves her anyway.

As scar tissue matures, it contracts. This contracture can cause several problems, including pain, limited mobility, and deformity. If the scar tissue is over a joint, contracture can lead to limited mobility of that joint. Circumferential burns (burns

     NATALIE DALE, MD

running the entire way around a limb, neck, or trunk) are even worse. When they contract, they can cut off blood flow to the limb or even impair your character's ability to breathe.

Contractures are treated by cutting away the scarred flesh. The procedure, called an *escharotomy*, prevents scar tissue from tightening over time. This procedure requires local anesthesia; even though the scarred tissue won't feel any pain, the incision will extend down into the healthy tissue.

REAL TALK: QUALITY OF LIFE OF BURN VICTIMS

In 1973, Dax Cowart suffered severe burns on over 85% of his body. He was in such horrific pain that he repeatedly begged the doctors and nurses to let him die. His pleas were ignored, and he survived, severely disfigured and disabled. He went on to become a lawyer and patient rights advocate, arguing that no one should be forced to undergo the torture he suffered during the fourteen months he was hospitalized. Up until he died in 2019, Mr. Cowart maintained that even knowing that he would go on to live a full and happy life, he would still have chosen to end his life in order to escape the horrific pain of treatment.[7]

I bring this up not for the ethical conundrum it sparks, but as an example of how horrible and painful treatment of burn victims can be. Treating burns is a long, excruciating process that can be quite traumatic. And that's on top of the disability and disfigurement those burns might cause. So, if you're going to give your character major burns, make sure you're ready to dive into the thorny ethics of burn survival.

BREAKING DOWN THE CLICHÉ: RUNNING INTO A BURNING BUILDING

"Snowball!" the little girl cries. "Snowball is still in there."

Blaise turns to her husband, clutching her daughter in her arms. "Don't you even think—"

But he's already gone, racing towards their house. He leaps over a burning pile of wood—the remains of their front door and disappears into the flames. Seconds pass, or hours, Blaise can't tell. Then she sees something—movement in the flames. It's her husband, running back towards them, a soot-covered kitten cradled in his arms.

I get it; saving someone (or something) from a burning building is a cliché for a reason. It's heroic, it's tense, it's the ultimate save-the-cat moment. But there are two main problems with this cliché (other than the fact that it's been done to death). Let me burn it down.

HEAT

House fires are insanely hot. The average house fire reaches 1100-1500 degrees Fahrenheit. The highest temperatures are near the ceiling, so it will be cooler in your character's vicinity. But even the floor—the coolest point—will easily top 100 degrees. Your character will begin to feel pain when the ambient temperature hits ~110°F. At 131°F, your character's skin will begin to blister, resulting in 2nd-degree burns. At 162°F, your character's skin will burn all the way through the dermis, causing the numbness of 3rd-degree burns. Once temperatures near 500° F (remember, this is still less than halfway to the AVERAGE temperatures house fires can reach), your character's clothing will catch fire (cotton) or melt (synthetic).[6] And that's only with a few seconds of exposure. Sticking around long enough to find and save Snowball is simply not an option.

> Personal example: When it hit 119°F last summer, it was painful to be in direct sunlight for more than a few moments. Growing up in the PNW, I'd never experienced anything like that before.

SMOKE INHALATION

Do you remember the first time you tried a cigarette? How the fiery material burned all the way down your lungs, and you coughed and coughed and coughed until you thought you might throw up? Smoke from house fires is like that but on steroids. When a building burns, everything inside burns with it; not just wood, but carpet and plastic and dishwashing soap. All those chemicals become aerosolized, making for smoke so potent it can bring experienced firefighters to their knees. If your character gets a good lungful, they won't be running anywhere.

Of course, not all smoke inhalation damage is this overt. Your character could very well escape from a burning building, with only a bit of soot at the corner of their mouth to hint to your readers that something direr is about to happen. Remember, inhalation injuries to the airway can result in potentially deadly airway swelling.

   NATALIE DALE, MD

PART III: CHRONIC DISEASES

18. LIFESTYLE DISEASES

LIFESTYLE DISEASES ARE NONCOMMUNICABLE CONDITIONS that are linked to *modifiable risk factors*, such as unhealthy diet, physical inactivity, tobacco use, drug/alcohol use, and unsafe sexual practices. However, I hate the term "lifestyle diseases." It feels like victim-blaming, and it completely ignores the very real effect that genetics, environment, and even our microbiome (the bacteria living inside us) have on our health. Yet it is impossible to write off the mountains of data showing that certain diseases are closely tied to the Western—and particularly, the American—lifestyle.

In this chapter, I'll quickly go through some of the most common of these lifestyle diseases, focusing on their symptoms and how they might impact your characters' quality of life.

HIGH BLOOD PRESSURE (HYPERTENSION)

A medical assistant calls Rose's name and takes her back to the office. He wraps a cuff around Rose's arm, which tightens uncomfortably. As the pressure loosens, he glances at the screen, then raises his eyebrows.

"Let's try that again."

He repeats the exercise, but the number flashing on the screen is the same: 160/92

"Are you nervous?"

Rose manages a small nod. She hates how being in this place makes her feel. The medical assistant smiles sympathetically.

"It's probably just white coat syndrome. I'll let the doctor decide what he wants to do with that."

Then he leaves, rolling the machine out with him.

High blood pressure is an asymptomatic lifestyle disease that puts your character at risk of other conditions. Normal blood pressure is about 120/80mmHG; high blood pressure is anything that is routinely over 140/90mmHg. One high measurement isn't enough to diagnose; your character needs to hit that 140/90mmHg mark at least twice, and ideally when they're home and relaxed. *White coat syndrome* is a common condition of high blood pressure that occurs only at the doctor's office; your character's blood pressure is normal when taken at home. White coat syndrome does not count as hypertension.

SYMPTOMS

Most of the time, high blood pressure is asymptomatic. The exception is if your character's blood pressure gets super high—more than 180/120mmHg. This extremely high blood pressure causes damage to the blood vessels and leads to symptoms of organ dysfunction. This is called a *hypertensive emergency*. Symptoms include coughing and trouble breathing due to fluid buildup in the lungs (*pulmonary edema*), chest pain due to lack of blood flow to the heart muscle (*cardiac ischemia*), blurry vision due to swelling in the eye (*papilledema*), and headaches or confusion due to swelling in the brain (hypertensive *encephalopathy*). A hypertensive emergency requires admission to the hospital for rapid lowering of the blood pressure and monitoring.

COMPLICATIONS

Longstanding hypertension can have very real consequences for your character. Since high blood pressure doesn't have any symptoms, it would be very easy for a character to ignore their disease (refuse to see a doctor, to take their medications, etc.), setting them up for disastrous consequences down the line. The most common complications occur in the heart, brain, eyes, and kidneys.

Chronic, untreated hypertension is a great way to set your character up for heart diseases, such as angina or myocardial infarction (See *Ch. 1: Chest Pain*). High blood pressure also forces the heart to work harder, which can lead to *congestive heart failure*, or CHF (See *Ch. 20: Chronic Breathlessness*). Most deaths due to hypertension are due to these heart conditions.

High blood pressure in the brain can

> CHF causes fluid buildup in the body due to the heart's inability to keep up. Symptoms include trouble breathing, cough producing pink/white sputum, and swelling of the legs and feet.

cause blood vessels to burst blood (*intracerebral hemorrhage*), leading to stroke (See *Ch. 7: Stroke*). In the eyes, chronic hypertension causes swelling of the blood vessels that can cause visual disturbances such as blind spots or blurry vision. *Papilledema* swelling at the back of the eye—is an ominous sign of a hypertensive emergency. Kidney damage is subtle and often seen only on urine tests, but chronic untreated hypertension can eventually lead to kidney failure.

WHO GETS IT?

Like high cholesterol, high blood pressure is more common in characters who are older, obese, sedentary, male and use tobacco or alcohol. In addition, if your character is black or consumes large amounts of sodium (usually found in highly processed foods), they're at even higher risk.

TREATMENT

The first step in the treatment of hypertension is lifestyle changes, such as decreasing sodium intake, losing weight, regular exercise, decreasing alcohol intake, increasing intake of fresh fruits and vegetables, and stress management. There are also a bunch of different blood pressure-lowering medications, such as beta-blockers, ACE-inhibitors, and thiazide diuretics.

HIGH CHOLESTEROL (HYPERLIPIDEMIA)

When the doctor finally arrives, twenty long minutes later, Rose has sweated through her blouse. The doctor introduces himself, then tells Rose that she is indeed due for a few vaccines today, but that he wants to talk to her about her bloodwork and her blood pressure first.

Cholesterol is a type of fat that your body uses for energy. Too much cholesterol in the blood causes the formation of plaques (fatty deposits) on the walls of the blood vessels. This plaque formation, called *atherosclerosis,* causes the arteries to become narrow and stiff.

SYMPTOMS & COMPLICATIONS

On its own, high cholesterol is almost always asymptomatic. However, having high cholesterol will put your character at higher risk of:

- Heart diseases such as angina, myocardial infarction, and aortic stenosis

- High blood pressure

- Stroke

The doctor tells Rose that the last time she was in, nearly a decade ago, her LDL cholesterol, the bad cholesterol, was significantly elevated. He asks if anyone else in her family had high cholesterol, but she doesn't know. All she knows is that her dad died of a heart attack at 55, and her mom of a stroke at 61. At 64, she has now outlived them both.

Cholesterol levels increase in the blood up until age 65; the older your character is, the more likely they are to have high cholesterol. Obesity, male gender, tobacco use, heavy alcohol use, and inactivity (*sedentary lifestyle*) are also risk factors. Genetics also plays an important role, as can the presence of other diseases, such as diabetes or thyroid disease. If you need a young, relatively healthy character to die of a heart attack, consider giving them a family history of high cholesterol (*familial hypercholesterolemia, familial hyperlipoproteinemia,* etc.).

TESTING & TREATMENT

The doctor tells Rose he wants to recheck her cholesterol levels. If they're still elevated, he'll start her on a cholesterol-lowering medication. He also wants her to take her blood pressure once a week at home or the drug store—somewhere she feels more comfortable. If her blood pressure continues to be elevated, she may need to be started on a blood pressure-lowering medication.

Starting at age 35 for men (45 for women) your character's regular doctor will test the cholesterol levels in their blood. If it's elevated, they'll recommend weight loss and exercise, and perhaps start your character on a class of cholesterol-lowering medication called *statins.*

OBESITY

Obesity is a disease of being significantly overweight. The WHO defines obesity as having a Body Mass Index of more than 30.

Obesity is a multifactorial disease, meaning that it is caused by both modifiable and non-modifiable risk factors. Some modifiable risk factors, such as healthy eating and exercise, can be heavily influenced by non-modifiable risk factors, such as poverty. One study found that in the US, obesity and poverty are closely linked.[1] Impoverished individuals are more likely to have poor diets, as many live in food deserts without access to fresh food. They are also more likely to be sedentary, as they can't afford gym memberships or exercise equipment, and may even live

> BMI = weight in kg over height in meters^2
>
> Healthy = 19-24.9
>
> Overweight = 25-29.9
>
> Obese = 30-39.9
>
> Severely obese >40

in neighborhoods where it is not safe to exercise outdoors.[1] In other words, some of these "modifiable risk factors" may not be so modifiable after all.

SYMPTOMS

Rose waits, wondering if the doctor is going to get on her case for being overweight; her daughter certainly does. Her knees have begun to ache, as does her back. Her husband says she snores and sometimes stops breathing in the middle of the night—maybe that's why she always feels tired. She knows she should exercise more, and should probably stop counting fries as vegetables, but she's made it this far, hasn't she? But the doctor just notes that her weight today is 201, putting her BMI at 32. Is that something she would like to discuss today?

Unlike the previous diseases, obesity is not a silent disease. Anyone looking at your character will know they have it, and your character will feel it. Physical symptoms of obesity include:

- Back pain

- Joint pain, particularly in the knees

    o Often results in arthritis

- Fatigue and trouble sleeping

- Shortness of breath with minimal activity

- Heat intolerance or excessive sweating

- Skin infections

Sleep apnea: a sleep disorder that causes your character to snore and even stop breathing during the night, is closely linked with obesity.

Obesity can also take a mental toll on your character. There is a massive stigma surrounding obesity and many people with the disease also suffer from depression.

COMPLICATIONS

Rose shakes her head no. Her brain is already swimming with the news of her cholesterol and blood pressure. She expects him to argue, but he just tells her that's ok and that he looks forward to seeing her in a month. After he leaves, a nurse comes in and administers the shots. Rose looks away the whole time.

Weight is a highly stigmatized topic that needs to be handled carefully.

Being obese will put your character at higher risk of a host of diseases including:

- Certain cancers

- Depression

- Diabetes (Type 2)

- Gallbladder disease

- Heart disease

- High blood pressure

- Infertility

- Pregnancy complications

- Reduced mobility

- Sleep apnea

- Stroke

ALCOHOLIC LIVER DISEASE

Alcoholic liver disease is a range of liver conditions caused by excessive alcohol use, in both quantity and duration of use. The risk of your male character developing some sort of alcoholic liver disease increases at 40g of alcohol per day, or around 3 drinks per day, for ten years.[2] More than 80g of alcohol, or about 6 drinks a day, severely increases the risk that your character will develop cirrhosis. If your character is female, she may need as little as half that amount.[2] However, it's important to note that not all chronic alcohol abusers will develop this condition.

> For more on alcohol and alcohol use disorder, see Volume 1: Setting & Character *Ch. 17: Drugs & Addiction.*

Hepatic steatosis, also called fatty liver disease, is a reversible condition of excess fat storage in the liver, causing it to enlarge. It is generally asymptomatic and diagnosed with blood tests, though your character may notice a bit of pain/swelling in the right upper quadrant (RUQ) of the abdomen. Hepatic steatosis is sometimes reversible if your character is able to quit drinking and lose weight.

Alcoholic steatohepatitis is inflammation of the liver caused by excessive alcohol intake. Symptoms include nausea/vomiting, RUQ abdominal pain and tenderness, fatigue, and fever. Your character may also exhibit characteristic yellowing called *jaundice* that starts in the whites of the eyes and spreads to the skin. Severity ranges from mild to potentially life-threatening.

Alcoholic cirrhosis is permanent scarring of the liver due to alcohol. It is irreversible. When it first starts, cirrhosis can be asymptomatic. Your character may also have symptoms similar to alcoholic steatohepatitis—fatigue, fever, nausea/vomiting, jaundice, and RUQ abdominal pain. If the cirrhosis is severe, they may experience:

- *Portal hypertension* is the liver equivalent of congestive heart failure (see *Ch. 20: Chronic Breathlessness*). Since large swathes of the liver are too scarred to function properly, blood can't make it through the liver, so it backs up. This causes veins in the gastrointestinal system to enlarge (called *varices*) and even burst, causing your character to vomit blood (*hematemesis*), or poop out blood (*melena* if it's old and black, *hematochezia* if it's bright red). These bleeds, called *variceal* bleeding, can be life-threatening.

- *Ascites* is the buildup of fluid inside the abdomen. Your character's belly will look swollen as if he/she is heavily pregnant. It can be diagnosed/treated with a procedure called a *paracentesis*, which uses a big a$$ needle to pull fluid out of the abdomen. If your character has severe ascites, they may need regular, therapeutic paracentesis to keep the fluid from building up to badly.

Other signs of chronic alcohol consumption include loss of sensation in the hands and feet (*peripheral neuropathy*), pancreatitis, spidery collection of veins on the skin (*spider telangiectasia*), and a unique thickening of the palm of the hand, called *Dupuytren's contracture*, that causes the third and fourth fingers to involuntarily curl inwards.[2] Men may also develop small testicles (*hypogonadism*) and enlarged breast tissue (*gynecomastia*).

OTHER LIFESTYLE DISEASES

There are several other diseases associated with lifestyle, but since I talk about them in-depth in other chapters, I won't go into too much detail here.

Chronic obstructive pulmonary disease (See *Ch. 20: Chronic Breathlessness*), or COPD, is a lung disease that is very closely associated with cigarette smoking.

Stroke (See *Ch. 7: Stroke*) and **coronary artery disease** (See *Ch. 1: Chest Pain*) are considered lifestyle diseases as many of their underlying causes—high blood pressure, plaque formation, etc.—are associated with the western lifestyle.

Type 2 Diabetes (See *Ch. 19: Diabetes*) is considered a lifestyle disease, particularly since it can often be controlled with changes to diet and exercise.

Certain types of cancer are closely linked to lifestyle factors (See *Ch. 24: Cancer*). The obvious example is **lung cancer**, which is associated with cigarette smoking, including second-hand smoke, and exposure to environmental factors such as asbestos, radon, and even air pollution.[3] **Breast cancer** is associated with being overweight and inactive, **cervical cancer** is associated with smoking and poverty, and both **prostate cancer** and **colon cancer** are associated with unhealthy diets and lack of physical exercise.[3] But remember, even these so-called "lifestyle cancers" have important risk factors that are non-modifiable, such as age, race, genetics, and family history.[3]

BREAKING DOWN THE CLICHÉ:
FAT IS SYNONYMOUS WITH LAZY, RUDE, OR EVIL

> *The woman in line in front of me—a total Karen—screamed at the poor manager, her three chins wobbling independently with every screech.*

I read a book recently I won't say which one—that relied on this stereotype. I absolutely adored everything else about the book. But I could always tell when a character was going to end up being a bad guy because they would inevitably be described as fat. Major characters, minor characters, it didn't matter. If they were fat, they were going to somehow pose an obstacle to the protagonist. Conversely, characters who were fit and trim were nearly always helpful.

Don't fall into this trap. For one, it's lazy writing. For another, it isn't true. Obesity is a multifactorial disease, not a character flaw.

19. DIABETES

Simone hasn't been feeling well lately. She's bone-tired, and it always feels like she's thirsty, hungry, or both. Her friends said they feel the same way too—junior year is stressful, especially when you're taking four AP classes—but they aren't falling asleep on their textbooks during homeroom. Simone squints at the clock; the tiny lines marking the minutes are strangely blurred. It's been less than twenty minutes since her last trip to the bathroom, but she already has to go again. She wonders if she can hold it until class gets out; she doesn't want her teacher, Mrs. S, to think she's skipping class.

BACKGROUND

DIABETES GETS ITS OWN CHAPTER because it is a common disease with all sorts of interesting complications (for the writer, not so much for the people suffering from it). Untreated or undertreated, it can lead to fainting, ulcers, infections, nerve damage, kidney damage, heart disease, depression, blindness, hearing loss, and even death. And yet, there are millions of people walking around with the disorder, living completely normal lives. As a writer, diabetes offers you the opportunity to write a character that appears totally well one minute and within inches of death the next—provided you do it correctly.

CAUSE

Diabetes mellitus is a disease caused by the dysfunction of the hormone insulin, which is produced by the pancreas. Insulin's job is to move sugar into the cells to provide fuel for all cellular functions. If the sugar can't get into the cells, they run out of fuel and stop functioning. Meanwhile, the sugar has nowhere to go, so it circulates in the blood, causing high blood sugar.

Sugar is sticky. When there's a lot of it in the blood, it causes changes to the lining of the tiny blood vessels, called capillaries. This *microvascular dysfunction* is the source of many of the complications of diabetes, ranging from eye changes to nerve and kidney damage. *Macrovascular disease*—namely increased plaque formation in the large arteries—leads to heart disease and stroke. Chronic inflammation, too much insulin in the blood, and increased cholesterol production also play a role in the many complications of diabetes.

TYPES OF DIABETES MELLITUS (DM)

There are two main types of diabetes mellitus: Type 1 DM and Type 2 DM. A third type, gestational diabetes, is diagnosed during pregnancy—and will be discussed in further depth in subsequent volumes. Prediabetes is a prequel to type 2 DM; it means your character's blood sugar is abnormally high, but not quite high enough to diagnose diabetes…yet. For many people, prediabetes is a wake-up call for them to improve their eating and exercise habits. Prediabetes is reversible; diabetes is not.

Diabetes insipidus is an unrelated kidney disease causing frequent urination and thirst.

	Type 1	Type 2
Onset	Sudden & often an emergency	Gradual
Typical Patient	Young & thin	Older & Overweight
Insulin Production	Low	Low, normal, or high
Diabetic Ketoacidosis (DKA)	Common	Rare

TYPE 1

Type 1 Diabetes occurs when your character's pancreas is unable to make insulin. It's an autoimmune disease caused by your character's own immune cells attacking and killing the cells in the pancreas that make insulin. Since your character can't make their own insulin, they are reliant on an external source of insulin—without it, they will die.

Type 1 Diabetes used to be called juvenile onset diabetes because the vast majority of people are diagnosed before their twentieth birthday. However, because it is an

Insulin can be given as an injection or as a wearable insulin pump that is programmed to dispense the proper dose.

     NATALIE DALE, MD

autoimmune disease, your character can be diagnosed later in life. Talk about a creative way to play with your readers' expectations!

Diagnosis of Type 1 DM often occurs in the emergency department, due to a life-threatening complication called *diabetic ketoacidosis,* or DKA (don't worry, I'll get there, I promise). When diagnosed in a non-emergent situation, it's usually because of the telltale symptoms of increased urination (*polyuria*), increased thirst (*polydipsia*), fatigue, weight loss, and blurry vision. Type 1 DM is treated with insulin and close blood sugar monitoring.

TYPE 2

Svetlana Shevchenko, Mrs. S to her students, was diagnosed with Type 2 diabetes when she was in middle school. The other kids made fun of her, calling her a cow, and telling her that she deserved diabetes for being so fat. She tried to tell them that everyone in her family—fat, thin, and in between—had it, but no one believed her. So, when she notices Simone, one of her best students, excusing herself to go to the bathroom for the third time that period, she wonders if she should say something.

> Type 2 DM has a stronger genetic component than Type 1 DM.

Type 2 DM is by far the most common type of diabetes, accounting for more than 90% of all diabetes diagnoses in the US.1 While Type 1 DM is caused by a lack of insulin, Type 2 DM is caused by insulin resistance, meaning that more and more insulin is required to transport sugar into the cells. It's as if your character's cells have developed a tolerance to the hormone, requiring more and more insulin to do the same job. Though the exact mechanism of insulin resistance remains unclear, obesity, genetics, and older age increase your character's risk.

When the bell rings, Mrs. S asks Simone to stay behind. The poor girl looks uncomfortable, fidgeting with her necklace, and she understands why—already, the girl's supposed friends are giggling behind their hands. She asks Simone if she's feeling all right; she was going to the bathroom an awful lot. Simone blushes a deep scarlet from the base of her neck all the way up to the roots of her ink-black hair. She shoots a look back at her friends, then shakes her head. Mrs. S restrains a sigh but lets her go. Maybe she'll try to corner her before class tomorrow before the other girls arrive.

> The prevalence of Type 2 Diabetes diagnosed in childhood is increasing worldwide.

Diagnosis of Type 2 DM tends to be more gradual. If your character has been getting regular checkups, they'll likely have been told that they are prediabetic, and will be getting blood tests that will reveal their diagnosis before your character shows any symptoms.

If your character isn't being closely followed, they'll eventually go to the doctor with signs of hyperglycemia. The typical trio of increased thirst, urination, and fatigue are common, but so are increased hunger, dry mouth, and even blurry vision. If your character hates going to the doctor, they may end up with some of the chronic signs of Type 2 diabetes, like yeast infections, cuts and scrapes that take forever to heal, and numbness or pins and needles in their feet.

Type 1 DM can also present with signs of hyperglycemia, rather than full-blown DKA.

Type 2 DM is treated first with diet and exercise, then with oral medications to reduce blood sugar. If your character is able to reduce their blood sugars and improve their overall health, they may be able to go off medications altogether. However, this doesn't mean that they're "cured"—it just means they're doing a good job of holding it at bay. On the other hand, if your character has severe Type 2 DM, they may need insulin.

TREATMENT

Type 1 diabetes is treated with insulin, as are women with gestational diabetes and some people with type 2 diabetes. There are several different types of insulin, depending on how quickly they start to work and how long they last. There are four main types of insulin:

- Rapid-acting insulin starts working in less than 20 minutes and can last up to 5 hours.

- Short-acting insulin starts acting in 30 minutes and lasts for up to 8 hours.

- Intermediate-acting insulin starts working 60-90 minutes and lasts up to 24 hours.

- Long-acting insulin is a slow-release insulin that lasts up to 24 hours.

Insulin regimens are complicated, and every character will have a different regimen. Rapid-acting and short-acting insulins are usually taken with meals, and the dosage varies depending on the level of their blood sugar. Long-acting and intermediate-acting are generally given at the same time each day and provide a stable, baseline level of insulin so your character's blood sugars aren't shooting all over the place.

Treatment of type 2 diabetes is a little more complicated. Mild cases can sometimes be treated with diet and exercise alone. If that doesn't work, your character may be given oral hypoglycemic agents, such as Metformin or sulfonylureas. They may also need to be started on insulin.

DIABETIC DISASTERS

DIABETIC KETOACIDOSIS (DKA)

Simone glances at the clock, and her heart nearly stops; it's past midnight. Her essay is due in less than eight hours! It's a big one, worth fifty percent of her grade, but she just can't seem to concentrate long enough to put words on paper. Her stomach hurts, and she's feeling nauseated—she even threw up half an hour ago. If she could just concentrate, but her brain feels like it's made of oatmeal.

DKA is a high blood sugar emergency caused by too little insulin. It can occur due to physical or emotional stress, such as after surgery or during a big life change, or it can come out of the blue. While the exact physiology is complicated, the basic gist is that DKA occurs when there is so little insulin that your character's cells can't absorb sugar and the body begins to think it's starving. To rectify this perceived problem, the body starts breaking down fats at an alarming rate, causing the production of acidic compounds called *ketones*. The blood acidifies, and your character becomes volume-depleted, leading to shock.

> For more on the different types of shock, <u>Volume 1: Setting & Character</u>, *Ch. 14: Shock.*

There's a knock on the door, and moments later, Simone's dad walks in.

"Oi mô! It's time for—"

He stops midsentence. Simone knows how this looks, she's curled up in her study chair, holding her stomach against the pain. She vomited again a few minutes ago, and some of it missed the trash can, leaving droplets of yellow bile on her bright purple carpet. She's breathing hard and fast, like she just ran a race, though she has no idea why.

"I just have to finish this paper," she croaks, "then I'll sleep, promise."

Her dad shakes his head. "We're going to the hospital."

A character in DKA will typically have nausea and vomiting, as well as abdominal pain, particularly on the upper side, where the liver sits. They'll be drinking a lot, peeing a lot, and will feel hungry and weak. The buildup of ketones in their blood causes their breath to smell fruity—a sure sign that your character is in DKA. Other symptoms of DKA include dehydration, fast heart rate, and fast, deep breathing, called *Kussmaul respirations*. If left untreated, your character will become drowsy and may even slip into a coma.

Simone is brought straight back into the ER. They poke and prod her, sticking IVs into the crook of her arm and hanging bags of fluid from the pole at the head of her bed. A nurse hands her a silver, bean-shaped tray; Simone doesn't have to ask what it's for, she just vomits into it. Then the nurse pricks the side of her index finger and puts a droplet of blood onto a slip of paper that she then slips into a handheld machine.

"Honey, your blood glucose is over 300," he says. "Do you have diabetes?"

DKA is diagnosed with blood tests showing high blood pressure, acidification of the blood, and the presence of fatty acids called *ketones*. It is treated with insulin, IV fluids, and potassium. Your character will need to be admitted to the hospital for further monitoring.

A few minutes later, a man wearing scrubs and a white coat arrives. He tells her that her symptoms and the results of her blood tests are consistent with diabetic ketoacidosis, which means that she has diabetes Type 1 as if that means anything to her. He says that she's going to be admitted to the hospital so that they can get her blood sugar under control.

While people with either type of diabetes can develop DKA, it is much more common in people with Type 1 DM. But don't worry—there's a hyperglycemic emergency that is more common among those with Type 2.

Simone leaves the hospital with a mountain of paperwork instructing her how to measure her blood sugar and take her insulin. Her insulin regimen is stupidly complicated—there's long-acting insulin and short-acting insulin, insulin she takes at bedtime, and extra doses of insulin given when she eats. She has to prick her finger after every meal and give herself shots into the stomach five times a day. It sucks.

> In the hospital, insulin is given on a sliding scale, meaning the nurse calculates the dose of insulin based on blood sugar levels.

HYPEROSMOLAR HYPERGLYCEMIC NONKETOTIC SYNDROME (HHNS)

Say that ten times fast! HHNS is a true high blood sugar crisis, with blood sugars reaching over 900mg/dL (FYI, normal is somewhere between 80 and 200mg/dL, depending on the last time your character ate).[1] In HHNS, there's just enough insulin around that your character won't make ketones. Instead, your character's body will try to pee out the excess sugar, and pee they will. They'll urinate so much, both in volume and frequency, that they won't be able to drink enough to replace all that water they're losing. All that water loss leads to severe dehydration and concentration of blood, called *hyperosmolarity.*

If your character has HHNS, they'll be incredibly thirsty and peeing practically nonstop. They'll have low blood pressure and a fast heart rate. But the real problem is the increased concentration of glucose and electrolytes in the blood. This increase in electrolytes leads to neurologic changes, such as seizures or involuntary movements. They might even slip into a coma.

Treatment of HHNS is with mondo doses of IV fluids and a little bit of insulin. Your character will need to be monitored in the hospital and their medication regimen altered.

LOW BLOOD SUGAR (HYPOGLYCEMIC) EMERGENCY

A few weeks after her hospitalization, Simone's crush asks her to prom. Not wanting to give herself a shot in front of him, she decides to take a double dose of her insulin right before he picks her up. They're supposed to go out for dinner, but instead, they just make out in the back of his car. As they're walking hand-in-hand up the cobblestone walk leading to the mansion where Prom is being held, Simone realizes she's feeling a bit lightheaded but shakes it off.

NPH insulin—the most used insulin—starts to take effect after 2-4 hours.[1]

When your character's blood sugar is low, the first organ to notice is the brain. Because of this, the symptoms of hypoglycemia revolve around neurologic changes, such as irritability, sudden changes in behavior, weakness, and headache. They'll sweat profusely and have tremors in their hands, as well as increased blood pressure and intense feelings of anxiety. Without treatment, your character will become confused and have convulsions before slipping into a coma.

They walk into the ballroom, full of upperclassmen in beautiful dresses and tuxedos. Simone's hands are shaking, her palms slick with sweat as they walk onto the dancefloor. She feels anxious for some reason, her pulse pounding in her ears. The loud music makes her head hurt. As she puts her arms around her date's neck, her heart flutters, skipping a beat. It's just nerves, she tells herself, but a part of her wants to run out of the room and crawl into bed.

Luckily, hypoglycemia of this magnitude is relatively hard to come by without taking a blood sugar-lowering medication. Your character's body—even a diabetic one—has hormones in place that prevent the body's blood sugar from dropping too low. To develop true hypoglycemia, something has to be wrong with the balance of insulin and other hunger hormones.

> Colloquially, some people call themselves "hypoglycemic" when they're hangry. And while they may be sensitive to drops in blood sugar, a true hypoglycemic emergency is hard to come by without a blood sugar lowering drug, like insulin, on board.

After the slow dance, Simone's legs are so wobbly she has to sit down. Her date offers to go get her…something. Did he say he was going to punch someone? Punch, lunch, crunch? She giggles, and her date frowns. He says something else, but he sounds like he's talking underwater, so she just nods, sinking gratefully into the folding metal chair. Her eyes slide shut.

The most common reason hypoglycemia occurs is because your character took too high a dose of their insulin. It's a major reason for diabetics to visit the emergency department. If your character only takes oral anti-diabetes medications, one class of drugs called *Sulfonylureas* can cause hypoglycemia if your character takes a high dose.

Mrs. S is standing by the punch bowl, watching closely to make sure no one spikes it with vodka like they did last year when a student approaches her. He's not one of hers, but she noticed him dancing with Simone earlier.

"Umm, teacher?" he begins, "my date is acting weird."

Mrs. S straightens, following his gaze to Simone, slumped in a chair in the corner. The girl never told her why she was hospitalized, but she's seen her surreptitiously checking her blood sugar during class. Mrs. S wastes no time, practically running across the room, pulling out the packages of honey she keeps in her purse for exactly this reason.

Another reason your character could become hypoglycemic is if they, or someone else, is injecting them with insulin, a phenomenon called *factitious hyperglycemia*. Other potential causes of hypoglycemia include an insulin-secreting tumor (*insulinoma*), severe alcoholism, liver failure, severe illness, and certain rare genetic diseases.

Mrs. S shakes Simone and, to her relief, she opens her eyes.

"Eat this," she says, pouring, squeezing the honey into Simone's mouth. "How much insulin did you take?"

Simone shrugs. "Dunno. Lots?"

"Do you have your glucometer on you?"

Simone shakes her head. Even with the honey, she still looks like she's about to pass out. Mrs. S pulls her own glucometer from her purse, and tests Simone's blood sugar; it's only 40mg/DL. She gives her another packet of honey; this time, Simone is able to squirt it into her mouth herself.

Hypoglycemia is diagnosed with a blood test showing a glucose level of less than 70 mg/dL. It's treated by giving your character a sugary drink, like orange juice or soda—along with a starch, like bread or crackers. Of course, this only works if your character can eat. If not, try putting honey or sweet syrup into their mouth. Retest their blood sugar after 15 minutes— if it's improved, make them eat a meal. If not, it's time to call 911. In the hospital, if your character is unconscious, they will get IV sugar water until their blood sugar is at least 100mg/dL.

> If you want an idiot character to fail at helping, have them administer low-calorie, sugar-free syrup. It happens way more often than you'd think.

Fifteen minutes later, Mrs. S checks Simone's blood sugar again—it's up to 80mg/dL.

"All right," she tells the girl, who looks mortified, "let's go get you some food."

COMPLICATIONS

There are many long-term complications of diabetes. If you're looking to write a character in poor health, who is constantly ending up in the ER with one complication or another, a diabetes diagnosis is a safe bet. Of course, this isn't true of all diabetics; there are millions of people who lead healthy lives with their diabetes well under control. But in writing, giving your character a disease like diabetes is a noticeable detail; if you include it, your readers will expect that it will come into play at some point.

> Hemoglobin A1C is a blood marker used to track overall blood sugar control. Ideally, the A1C level is below 6%, though new recommendations for Type 2 DM aim for an A1C below 7-8%.[2]

Simone struggles for years to control her blood sugar; her AIC is consistently above 7%. One day, as she's sitting cross-legged on her bed in her dorm when her roommate asks what happened to her foot. Simone looks down to see what looks like an ulcer on the bottom of her foot, a red, raw circle surrounded by thick yellow skin. It looks horrible, but Simone doesn't feel a thing.

Since there are so many different complications, I'm only going to touch briefly on each of them. People with diabetes are at higher risk of

- Heart disease

    o People with diabetes are 2-4 times more likely to have a heart attack.[4]

- Stroke

- Nerve damage

    o Death of nerves in the hands and feet, leading to numbness and pins and needles.

    o Hypersensitivity of nerves, leading to burning pain with a light touch.

- Kidney disease

    o Diabetes is the #1 cause of end-stage renal disease (ESRD), the most severe form of kidney disease.

- Eye disease

    o Seventy-five percent of people with long-standing diabetes develop swelling in the blood vessels of the eye (*diabetic retinopathy*) that can cause blindness.[3]

    o Increased risk of cataracts and glaucoma

- Poor wound healing

- Increased susceptibility to infection

- Diabetic foot

    o Repeated injuries to the foot with poor healing and increased risk of infection.

    o Can result in severe bone and blood infections.

o   May require amputation.

Simone goes to see a podiatrist, who diagnoses her with a diabetic foot ulcer. He tells her that she's in luck; the ulcer is still superficial. If she stays off it, keeps it clean and dry, and cleans the area daily to prevent infection, it should improve. Simone isn't happy to be on crutches, but it serves as a wake-up call; she needs to do everything she can to keep her blood sugar under control, otherwise, she risks losing a foot—or worse.

BREAKING DOWN THE CLICHÉ: INSULIN AS A MURDER WEAPON

The man is fast asleep in his hospital bed, the corners of his lips crusted with drool. It's hard to believe that this is the man who ordered the murder of her son. Nurse Nefarious steps forward, syringe in one hand. She checks behind her, but the curtain is closed. In one smooth motion, she pulls aside his hospital gown and injects the syringe full of insulin into his abdomen, under a roll of fat. No one will notice a tiny pinprick—not there. He doesn't even snort. She withdraws the syringe, depositing it in the locked sharps container, then hurries from the room. Minutes later, she smiles as she hears a "Code Blue" called over the loudspeaker.

What better way to murder someone than with a hormone produced by their own body? Foolproof, right? Not so fast. If there is any indication of foul play, the victim will undergo a forensic autopsy, which will include a blood test that will prove your character did not die of natural causes.

When your body makes insulin, it also produces a protein called C-peptide. Store-bought insulin doesn't produce this protein. All the forensic pathologist has to do is get a blood test on the victim looking for the presence of C-peptide in the blood and voila! If C-peptide is present, they'll know if the insulin was *endogenous* (made by the body). If there is no C - peptide, or if the c-peptide is much lower than the level of the insulin, they'll know that the insulin was *exogenous* (made in a lab).

For more on potential poisons, see *Ch. 10: Poisons.*

Of course, this doesn't stop people from trying. A Google search of "insulin murders" comes up with a horrifying list of high-profile murders using insulin as the murder weapon. Then again, if they're on Google, it means they got caught.

20. CHRONIC BREATHLESSNESS

TROUBLE BREATHING ISN'T ALWAYS AN emergency. There are lots of people in the world who deal with shortness of breath daily. If you have a character who needs to struggle with exertion, giving them one of these common chronic causes of breathlessness could help.

Tim is a healthy guy. He may be almost eighty, but he still plays 18 holes of golf every morning. At first, he doesn't worry when he feels his heart occasionally start to pound—he just assumes it's part of getting older. But when he notices that he's out of breath and coughing up thin white sputum after the 7th hole, he begins to wonder if there is something wrong.

ASTHMA

Asthma is a disease that causes inflammation of the airways. While most cases are mild, asthma can occasionally be severe enough to cause complete airway obstruction and death (See *Ch. 2: Trouble Breathing*). It is usually, though not always, provoked by certain triggers, ranging from exercise or viral infections to environmental triggers like pet dander or pollens. If your character encounters their asthma trigger, they'll usually have symptoms within 30 minutes.

Symptoms of asthma include shortness of breath, chest tightness, and cough. These symptoms often get worse at night. Anyone listening may hear an audible wheezing sound as they try to breathe. Your character may also feel as if they can breathe in but can't breathe out.

Treatment depends on the severity of symptoms, but usually includes some combination of a rescue inhaler (Albuterol inhaler) and a steroid medication to prevent flare-ups. A severe asthma exacerbation may need to be treated at the hospital (See *Ch. 2: Trouble Breathing*).

ATRIAL FIBRILLATION

At the doctor's office, the medical assistant frowns as she puts her fingers on his wrist to take his pulse. When the doctor comes in, she too feels for his pulse. She tells him that his pulse feels irregular, and she writes an order for him to get an electrocardiogram (EKG).

Atrial fibrillation, nicknamed "A-fib," is a common heart arrhythmia that occurs when the top chambers of the heart, called the atria, aren't contracting as they should. Symptoms include exertional dyspnea along with fatigue and palpitations. If someone takes their pulse, the rhythm will feel irregular and erratic. If your character is older and has a history of heart disease, alcoholism, cancer, or even just stress, atrial fibrillation is a great reason for them to have shortness of breath.

> The pulse in A-fib is described as "irregularly irregular."

> While shortness of breath is a common symptom, most people with A-fib have no symptoms.

He gets the EKG done the next day, but it is normal. He's sent home with a little monitor that clips to his chest, which he wears for a week straight. After he turns the device in, the doctor calls and tells him that his heart is going in and out of normal rhythm. He has a condition called atrial fibrillation. Tim's heart leaps to his throat—is he going to need heart surgery?—but the doctor reassures him that it isn't unusual for a man of his age. She wants to get some further testing and, since he's at elevated risk of stroke, start him on a blood thinner.

> Stroke risk in atrial fibrillation is calculated using the CHAD-VASC score. A score >2 is an indication for blood thinners.

Unlike many arrhythmias, A-fib isn't immediately dangerous; many people walk around with the condition. The main concern is that clots forming in the atria can then break off and spread to the rest of the body, particularly the brain (which causes stroke). For that reason, if your character is walking around with A-fib, they may need to be on a blood thinner.

> Putting your character on blood thinners is a great way to injure them. Blood thinners can turn a minor injury into a major problem. This is particularly true of head wounds.

CANCER

While nearly all cancers can cause fatigue and breathlessness, certain cancers are more likely to cause chronic difficulty breathing.

Lung cancer tends to cause a chronic cough; often, that's its only symptom. As the cancer grows, your character may begin to feel out of breath and may have pain in their chest when coughing, laughing, or just breathing deeply.

Cancers of the neck and throat, like **esophageal cancer** and **thyroid cancer,** can also cause trouble breathing. As cancer grows, it impinges on the trachea, closing off the airway. If your character has one of these cancers, they'll probably also have difficulty swallowing.

Finally, if your character has Stage 4 cancer that has metastasized to the lungs, they may also develop trouble breathing. Cancers that commonly metastasize to the lungs include breast cancer, colon/colorectal cancer, and prostate cancer. Cancer that is metastatic to the lungs will have similar symptoms to lung cancer: chronic cough, shortness of breath, and chest pain.

CONGESTIVE HEART FAILURE (CHF)

Heart failure occurs when the heart is unable to pump blood adequately to supply the body. There are many causes of heart failure, ranging from diseases of the heart valves to long-standing high blood pressure. The heart's job is to push fluid against gravity. As it fails, blood pools in the dependent (lower to gravity) parts of the body. The primary symptoms of heart failure are due to this backup of blood, which causes fluid to leak into the tissues. Symptoms of CHF include:

- Trouble breathing (*dyspnea*) due to fluid backup in the lungs

- Cough that is worse at night/laying down

- Swelling in the legs and feet

- Increased urination at night

- Bulging neck veins

Difficulty breathing in heart failure is usually worse when lying down (**orthopnea**) and can wake your character from sleep (**paroxysmal nocturnal dyspnea**).

If the CHF is severe enough to limit blood flow to the brain, your character may also be confused, act delirious, or suffer from memory problems.

CHF is treated with diuretics; water pills to reduce the fluid load on the heart. Lifestyle factors, such as limiting sodium intake, losing weight, exercising, and stopping smoking, are also important. In severe cases, they may need a drug to help their heart beat more strongly.

COPD (CHRONIC OBSTRUCTIVE PULMONARY DISEASE)

If your character smokes, they might get COPD. COPD is a cluster of two intertwined diseases—*emphysema* and *chronic bronchitis*—caused by chronic inflammation in the lungs that blocks airflow and making it difficult to breathe.

Symptoms of COPD include a chronic cough, particularly one that produces a lot of phlegm (*sputum*). If you give your character COPD, they'll get breathless easily, even just with normal activities like walking up one flight of stairs. Their breaths may sound wheezy and the beds of their fingernails and skin around their lips will develop a bluish tinge (*cyanosis*). They'll get a lot of respiratory infections, like colds and pneumonia, and will tire easily. They may "tripod" (lean forward with their hands on their knees as they try to catch their breath) whenever they find themselves out of breath. They may also cough a lot, bringing up copious, thick sputum.

The first step in the treatment of COPD is to stop smoking. Your character will also be given inhaled medications to help open up their airways and decrease inflammation. If their disease is severe, they may need oxygen, meaning they'll have to carry around a portable oxygen tank for the rest of their life. Quitting smoking prevents flares and further damage to the lungs, improves symptoms, and decreases the risk of heart disease, but it does not reverse the damage that has already occurred.

Like with asthma, your character can have an acute exacerbation of their COPD. Often, exacerbations are due to respiratory infections. If your character has an exacerbation, they'll feel more breathless and fatigued than usual. They'll also be coughing more and bringing up sputum that is thicker, more profuse, or a different color than usual. COPD exacerbations can be very dangerous and may require hospitalization.

For a review on the parts of the heart, see *Ch.1: Chest Pain.*

HEART VALVE DISEASES

A week after he's diagnosed, Tim goes into the office for an echocardiogram—an ultrasound of his heart. The doctor shows him the results. His heart valve isn't completely shutting, allowing blood to flow backward from the left ventricle into the left atrium. This "regurgitation" has caused blood to back up in the left atrium, causing it to stretch and dilate.

Diseases of the heart valves can also cause chronic breathlessness. **Mitral stenosis, mitral regurgitation**, **aortic stenosis,** and **aortic regurgitation** are valve diseases that can cause heart failure and all the symptoms that go along with it: exertional dyspnea, orthopnea, night-time cough and awakenings, and palpitations.

Stenosis = valve narrowing

Regurgitation = valve insufficiency leading to backflow of blood

Mitral stenosis (the narrowing of the valve between the heart's left chambers) is almost always due to rheumatic fever, a disease caused by the same bacteria that causes strep throat (See Ch.5: Fever). If you're playing the long game, you could have your character have untreated strep throat as a child, only to have it cause heart failure (and the chronic dyspnea that comes with it) when they're older. Symptoms of mitral stenosis include symptoms of CHF, plus palpitations, chest pain, and a cough that produces specks of blood (*hemoptysis*).

Aortic stenosis (the narrowing of the valve leading out of the left ventricle and into the aorta) is usually due to old age. It usually doesn't cause any symptoms until the blockage is severe. At that point, symptoms include chest pain on exertion (*angina*) and symptoms of CHF. But the big red flag is that your character will pass out whenever their heart has to beat really hard, either from exertion or sometimes just when going from lying down to standing. This occurs because the heart cannot force enough blood through the narrow opening, so your character doesn't get the blood flow to their brain.

Aortic regurgitation and **mitral regurgitation** occur when the valve in question allows the backflow of blood. Both cause symptoms of heart failure and are associated with rheumatic fever and Marfan syndrome, a genetic condition causing increased elasticity of connective tissue.

> *The doctor asks Tim if he had strep throat or rheumatic fever as a child—he replies that he thinks so, but that his family was too poor growing up to go to the doctor. He's had a heart murmur his whole life, but never bothered to get it checked out. The doctor tells him that he has a condition called mitral regurgitation, likely caused by rheumatic fever. The mitral regurgitation is causing blood to back up into his lungs, and the dilation of the left atrium is likely what is causing the atrial fibrillation. He's going to need surgery to replace the valve.*

Severe valve disease is treated with surgical valve replacement. Mild disease is treated with medications that decrease the fluid load on the heart.

CYSTIC FIBROSIS

Cystic fibrosis (CF) is a genetic disease that causes thickened bodily secretions. People with CF have a chronic cough productive of thick mucus, recurrent lung and sinus infections, trouble gaining weight, and stinky, high-volume diarrhea. They also have very, very salty sweat.

A few decades ago, people with CF could expect to die in their twenties.[1] Their lives were difficult, with numerous hospital visits and time-consuming treatment plans. But all that is changing. New medications and advances in medical care have more than doubled the life expectancy of people with CF. One of these medications, Trikafta, is so powerful that children who start the medications young may never experience some of the symptoms of cystic fibrosis.[2] However, Trikafta costs over $300,000 per year. Since not everyone can afford the new therapies, many people still suffer from what are now treatable symptoms. Welcome to the United States healthcare system.

If you're looking for a condition to give your character that will give them recurring, nasty lung infections, CF might be a great tool. However, people with CF often have a lot of restrictions in their life—they often need daily physiotherapy, have to maintain rigorous *pulmonary toilet,* are more susceptible to infections, and must take daily medications. Often, they can't even be in the same room as someone else with CF without risking becoming infected with the other person's uniquely deadly microbiome of bacteria. If you're going to give your character this disorder, you're going to have to do a lot of research. I'll leave it at that.

> **Pulmonary toilet**, or pulmonary hygiene, is a daily practice, consisting of exercises and/or procedures, used to keep the airways clear of mucus.

LOU GEHRIG'S DISEASE (AMYOTROPHIC LATERAL SCLEROSIS)

Lou Gehrig's Disease, or ALS, is a degenerative disease of motor neurons (the cells that relay signals from the spinal cord to the muscles) that causes progressive muscle weakness. ALS is progressive, incurable, and fatal. Symptoms of ALS usually start with muscle cramping and twitching, often in the hand or arm. As the disease progresses, your character will have more and more trouble controlling their muscles. Their speech will become slurred, they'll have trouble swallowing, and they'll eventually become wheelchair bound. As their muscles become weaker, they'll have more and more trouble breathing, until eventually, they're unable to breathe on their own. At that point, they face a terrible choice: suffocate to death now or live out the rest of their life on a ventilator.

> Every Note Played by Lisa Genova does a beautiful job of describing ALS.

LIFESTYLE FACTORS

If your character is obese, they may chronically feel like they're out of breath, especially when exercising. The same goes if they're a smoker. Pregnancy can also cause feelings of breathlessness; in the first trimester, it's caused by raging hormones, while in the third trimester, it's usually due to her giant, beachball of a uterus squishing abdominal organs up against her diaphragm. If your character is vegan or vegetarian, their breathlessness might be caused by anemia—low red blood cells due to an iron deficiency.

Certain professions increase your character's risk of lung disease. If your character is a coal miner, they may develop black lung disease (*coal worker's pneumoconiosis*), with symptoms of shortness of breath, chest tightness, and coughing up black mucous. If they're a construction worker, shipyard worker, or industrial manufacturing worker, they may have come in contact with asbestos. Asbestos can cause lung scarring and shortness of breath. It can also lead to lung cancers, such as adenocarcinoma and mesothelioma.

Other professions—miners, construction workers, glass manufacturing, foundry workers, welders, machinists, and even dental hygienists—can be exposed to substances like asbestos, silica, and beryllium dust. These substances cause damage to the lung and can cause chronic shortness of breath and cough. If your character is a farmer or spends a lot of time with birds, they may develop an allergic lung reaction, called *hypersensitivity pneumonitis*, that causes cough and trouble breathing, alongside fever and chills. Exact treatments for these conditions vary, but the common thread is to get your character away from the offending agent.

BREAKING DOWN THE CLICHÉ: BATTLE BADASS BREATHING HARD

Breath whooshing

"Oh no! The Wicked Wheezer is here! How shall we fight him off?"

From Darth Vader to Immortan Joe, there are a lot of bad guys out there whose breathing can be heard for miles. Honestly, I don't mind that part. It's ominous, creepy, and kind of great. What I do have a problem with is that they are also totally bada** when it comes to a fight.

If a character is breathing hard at baseline, they are going to struggle to breathe with even a mild increase in exertion. The greater the exertion, the more oxygen the muscle tissue needs, and the harder the lungs will have to work. But if the lungs are already working as hard as they can just to sit or walk around, they aren't going to be able to keep up with the demand.

This is especially if they need to be on oxygen, as Vader and Immortan appear to be. If your character is reliant on an oxygen tank, it means that their lungs are so weak that they need help getting enough oxygen into their blood even just sitting down. I've seen lots of patients who rely on oxygen; they aren't going to win a light saber fight anytime soon.

21. AUTOIMMUNE DISEASES

BACKGROUND

THE IMMUNE SYSTEM IS THE body's defense against disease-causing pathogens such as viruses, bacteria, and fungi. Also known as white blood cells, the cells of the immune system work together to fight off pathogens. There are three main types of immune cells: lymphocytes, neutrophils, and macrophages.

Neutrophils, the most common immune cell, are the first responders of the immune system. Their job is to ingest and kill bacteria. **Macrophages** are the garbage-collectors, eating not only bacteria, but also dead red blood cells and damaged cells. **Lymphocytes** are the memory cells of the immune system and have two main subtypes: B-cells and T-cells. **B-cells** are a type of memory cell that produce *antibodies*—proteins designed to recognize and target foreign material (*antigens*). Many vaccines, including the COVID vaccine, work by stimulating B-cells to make antibodies against the virus or bacteria. **T-cells** are also memory cells. Their job is to upregulate the immune system when a pathogen is detected. Some T-cells, called *cytotoxic T-cells* can also directly kill invading cells. Immune cells communicate through a complex sequence of secreted proteins called *cytokines*.

Autoimmune diseases occur when the immune system mistakes some part of the body—self proteins—as foreign and mounts an immune response.

> *Unique isn't feeling very well. She's been feeling under the weather for months now—gaining weight, sleeping poorly, headaches—but has always brushed it off as stress from trying to balance her job as a paralegal with the night classes she's taking at the law school. But now her muscles feel weak, so she decides to go to the doctor.*

No one really knows why people get autoimmune diseases. The *hygiene hypothesis* posits that autoimmune diseases are a symptom of a bored immune system attacking the body because there are no "bad guys" to attack due to our hygienic lifestyle.

However, the truth is a bit more complicated. Rather than exposure to disease-causing pathogens, newer data show that early exposure to "good bacteria" in early life helps to properly train the immune system to recognize self.[1] Lack of training, due to lack of exposure to these good bacteria, results in the immune system mistakenly mounting an attack against the body because it doesn't understand how to recognize, and therefore spare, the self.

Regardless of the cause of autoimmune diseases, there are a few important trends. The vast majority of autoimmune diseases occur in women ages 20-40.[2] Women are much more likely to have autoimmune diseases than men. When men do get autoimmune diseases, they tend to be older. If your character has one autoimmune disease, they are more likely to develop another. Autoimmune diseases also tend to run in families, though there's no single gene that will make your character more likely to get an autoimmune disease.

> 90% of people with lupus are women of childbearing age.[2]

Autoimmune diseases are a good option looking to give a character a chronic illness, particularly if that character is a woman in her childbearing years. While conditions range widely in severity, most are chronic illnesses that are more likely to slow your character or impede her ability to do certain things, than to kill her outright.

In this chapter, I'll go through a few of the most common autoimmune diseases and how you might use them in your story.

DIABETES

Type 1 diabetes is an autoimmune disease caused by immune cells attacking the pancreas and destroying the cells that produce insulin. Since I've already dedicated a chapter to diabetes (*Ch. 19*) I won't say more here.

MULTIPLE SCLEROSIS (MS)

At the clinic, the doctor tests the strength in Unique's arms and legs; her muscles feel tender, but not weak. She tells him that her vision gets blurry sometimes. He performs an eye exam, looks in her eyes and tells her that everything looks normal. She might have dry eyes, so he prescribes eye drops. Then he asks about her mood and sleep. When she responds that she feels blue often and always feels sleepy, he tells her that she is depressed and prescribes an antidepressant.

Multiple sclerosis is an autoimmune neurologic disease. If you're looking for a chronic illness that will impair your character's vision or mobility, MS is a good choice.

MS is caused by immune cells attacking the fatty coating around neurons, called *myelin*. Without the fatty coating, the electrical signal doesn't work, and the neurons can't communicate with each other. When the immune system attacks the neurons, it leaves scarring, which shows up on an MRI as visible *lesions*. Your character's specific symptoms will depend exactly where in the brain or spinal cord these lesions occur.

SYMPTOMS

Because MS is an autoimmune disease of the central nervous system, symptoms can be just about anything neurologic, ranging from vision changes to paralysis. Because the changes are happening in the brain and spinal cord, the symptoms are usually one-sided. However, there are a few symptoms that are very common.

- **Sensory deficits**, such as numbness and tingling and/or the loss of the ability to feel touch, temperature, or pain, are usually the first sign of MS. These symptoms are one-sided and usually occur in either the arm/hand or leg/foot. They also tend to be transient, meaning that they can come and go without warning.

- **Motor symptoms** generally start as *spasticity*—abnormal muscle tightness—that can be quite severe and may impede your character's ability to walk. As the disease progresses, the spasticity may progress to weakness and even complete paralysis.

- **Eye changes** come in two main flavors. *Optic neuritis* is the inflammation of the optic nerve. It can cause pain with eye movements, a black spot at the center of your character's vision, or even complete vision loss in the affected eye. *Internuclear ophthalmoplegia,* or INO, is a disorder caused by a lesion in the part of the brain where the nerve inputs from the eyes cross, resulting in the weird combination of trouble looking sideways with one eye and a rhythmic movement of the pupil (*nystagmus*) in the other. These strange eye movements often cause double vision. INO is a weird diagnosis and can be hard to explain, but it is strongly suggestive of MS.

- **Coordination difficulty:** Lesions in the cerebellum (the part of the brain that helps coordinate movement) can result in trouble walking (*ataxia*), tremors, and slurred speech.

- **Generalized symptoms** such as fatigue, nerve pain, trouble concentrating and remembering things, anxiety, or depression, and even personality changes.

DIAGNOSIS

MS is most common in women and Caucasians. It is also a disease that targets younger adults; most people receive their first diagnosis in their 20s-30s. The initial presentation of MS is due to an attack causing a lesion in the brain. The most common presenting symptoms include optic neuritis or one-sided weakness and/or loss of sensation. To receive a diagnosis of MS, your character will get a thorough neurologic exam, including an eye exam, and an MRI looking for lesions in the brain and spinal cord.

COURSE

After their diagnosis, your character will probably travel one of three paths: silent, relapsing/remitting, and progressive.

- A **silent**, or stable course means that, after the first attack, your character doesn't have any further symptoms. In fact, the symptoms from their initial presentation may improve with time. However, after many years of a stable course, your character's disease may transition and become secondarily progressive (see below).

- A **relapsing/remitting** course is the most common course for people struggling with MS. If your character has relapsing/remitting MS, they will experience a series of attacks with exacerbation of symptoms, followed by remission and even improvement of symptoms. This course results in a stepwise degeneration of function.

- A **progressive** course is a steady decline in function. **Primary progressive** MS causes steady, relentless decline right from the beginning. It is more common in older individuals (Age > 40) and has a worse prognosis. **Secondary progressive MS** is diagnosed if your character previously had relapsing/remitting or stable MS, but then starts to steadily decline in function. The transition to secondary progressive MS usually indicates that your character is in the final stages of the disease.

TREATMENT

MS treatment has come a long way in the last few decades. During acute attacks, your character may be admitted to the hospital for IV steroids to mitigate the damage. In between attacks, your character will be placed on disease-modifying therapies (DMTs for short) to try and prevent further attacks.

Interferons—the most commonly used DMTs—are effective at preventing relapse. They also make your character feel like they have the flu.

Finally, they'll be given medications to help with the symptoms—muscle relaxants for muscle spasticity, antidepressants for depression, and certain antiseizure medications for nerve pain.

As your character's condition worsens, they may require assistive devices, ranging from rocker knives to Velcro tabs on clothing. Within 15 years of their diagnosis, your character will probably need some sort of mobility assistance ranging from a cane or leg braces to a wheelchair or scooter.[3]

MYASTHENIA GRAVIS

Myasthenia gravis is another neurologic autoimmune disease. Instead of attacking the central nervous system, myasthenia gravis targets the *neuromuscular junction*—where nerve cells communicate with muscle cells. It's hard to describe without going into the specifics of neurotransmitters and receptor proteins, but basically, the immune system targets the protein that is supposed to bind the neurotransmitter called acetylcholine, causing muscles to fatigue too easily. If you need a character who loses strength throughout the day, or if you need your otherwise healthy character to have a respiratory crisis (see *myasthenic crisis* below), the myasthenia gravis is a good option.

SYMPTOMS

In myasthenia gravies, muscles become fatigued increasingly quickly. The more your character uses those muscles, the faster they fatigue. This results in symptoms of skeletal muscle weakness without any loss of sensation or reflexes. Your character will feel strongest at the beginning of the day, weakening the more they use their muscles, and will be the most fatigued/weak in the evenings. Muscles that are used most often, particularly the muscles of the eye, face, and jaw, weaken the fastest. For this reason, the most common initial presentation is double vision (*diplopia*), drooping eyelids (*ptosis*), blurry vision, and slurred speech.

DIAGNOSIS & TREATMENT

Diagnosing myasthenia gravis may require a few different tests, including an antibody test, a nerve-conduction test (*electromyography,* or EMG), and a CT scan of the chest to look for swelling of the thymus, and a specific

> The thymus is a small organ in the chest that is responsible for the maturation of the immune system during fetal development.

test called the Tensilon test. Treatment can be symptomatic—give acetylcholine—or it can proactively try and diminish the immune response with steroids and other immunosuppressive agents. Interestingly, surgery to remove the thymus is often curative.

A myasthenic crisis is a rare but life-threatening emergency. It happens when the muscles of the respiratory system, particularly the diaphragm, become fatigued. The more your character tries to breathe, the more fatigued their respiratory muscles become, until they are no longer able to function. Without treatment, your character will asphyxiate.

Around 20% of people with MG will experience a myasthenic crisis.[4] These crises can be triggered by a variety of situations ranging from physical stressors—pain, pregnancy, extreme temperatures, sleep deprivation, etc.—to psychological. Even certain medications, such as antibiotics, magnesium, and steroids, can trigger it.

Once triggered, your character will enter a downward spiral of respiratory distress; the harder they breathe, the harder it becomes to breathe. The only treatment is to breathe for them, giving their respiratory muscles time to rest. Most of the time, this means they'll be intubated and put on a ventilator until their muscles recover. If the crisis isn't too severe, doctors may be able to use non-invasive respiratory assistance, such as CPAP and BiPap machines (See *Ch. 2: Trouble Breathing*).

SYSTEMIC LUPUS ERYTHEMATOSUS (SLE)

A few months later, Unique returns to the clinic. She stopped taking the antidepressants because they made her constipated and didn't help anyway. Plus, her hair has started falling out in patches, and her skin is scaly and dry. Since her mother has lupus, the doctor decides to run some blood tests.

Lupus (medical professionals call it SLE) is an autoimmune disease that targets the connective tissue of the body—the skin, the joints, and the coverings of organs. Unlike myasthenia gravis and multiple sclerosis, the immune system in SLE targets a wide variety of proteins throughout the body. This means that:

1. Many different organs can be affected.

2. Every person will have slightly different symptoms.

Most people with SLE are women of childbearing age, with the first symptoms usually appearing during adolescence. If your character is a person of color (particularly if she's African American), she is at higher risk than a white woman.[2]

SYMPTOMS

The symptoms of SLE vary by the organ that is being affected. In early SLE, skin, joint, and constitutional symptoms are most prominent. As the disease progresses, organ damage—particularly to the kidneys, lungs, heart, and brain—becomes more problematic.

- **Constitutional:** Fatigue, low-grade fever, weight loss, feeling generally crappy (malaise)

- **Skin:** Butterfly rash (malar rash), discoid rash, skin sensitivity to light (photosensitivity), patchy hair loss (alopecia), poor circulation

- **Gastrointestinal:** Ulcers in the mouth & nose, trouble swallowing, stomach ulcers, nausea & vomiting

> A **butterfly rash** is a symmetrical red rash over the cheeks and nose that looks like a butterfly. A **discoid rash** is a scaly, red, circular rash on high sun areas (mainly nose, cheeks, and ears).

- **Joints & Muscles:** Arthritis, joint pain, muscle pain

- **Heart:** Inflammation of the sack around the heart (pericarditis) or inflammation of the heart valves (endocarditis) (See Ch. 1: Chest Pain),

- **Lungs:** Inflammation of the lining of the lungs (pleuritis)

- **Brain:** Seizures, depression, headaches, psychosis

Blood tests may also reveal low numbers of red blood cells (*hemolytic anemia*). Urine tests may show increased levels of protein and even blood in the urine due to kidney damage.

DIAGNOSIS

Unique's ANA comes back negative. Since she doesn't fulfill the criteria for SLE—she doesn't have a rash and all her labs are normal—the doctor says it is unlikely she has lupus.

Diagnosis of SLE is a bit tricky, as there isn't one test that can 100% diagnose it. Most people with SLE are misdiagnosed with something else first.[4] It takes an average of six years for people with lupus to receive the correct diagnosis.[4] How much of that is due to the US medical system's bias against women and POC, versus how much is due to the challenge of the actual diagnosis? I'll leave it up to your imagination. Just know that if you're writing a female character (particularly if she's a woman of color) and you're looking for a disease that will force her to battle the healthcare system in order to be taken seriously, SLE is a perfect fit.

> Fun fact: SLE can cause a false-positive syphilis test.[2]

If your character has any of the characteristic combination symptoms of SLE, such as butterfly rash plus arthritis plus fatigue, their doctor will order a screening blood test. If that's positive, they'll order some additional blood tests. But while the blood tests can rule out SLE, or suggest causes, they can't 100% confirm it. So, in the end, SLE is a clinical diagnosis, meaning that the doctors will make the final diagnosis based on your character's overall constellation of symptoms.

TREATMENT

Mild episodes of SLE are treated with mild anti-inflammatory drugs called NSAIDs, like ibuprofen and aspirin. Your character should also stay out of the sun, as the sun worsens the skin rashes. If the episode is severe, your character may need oral steroids. To prevent worsening, your character will be put on hydroxychloroquine—a medication traditionally used to prevent malaria.[2]

PROGNOSIS

While SLE is generally considered a chronic disease, it can certainly be fatal. About 10-15% of people with SLE will die due to complications.[5] Fatalities are usually due to complications arising within the heart, lungs, and kidneys. If your character is from a racial or ethnic minority, they're more likely to develop the disease earlier in life, experience more complications, and have a higher fatality rate than if they were white.[6]

DRUG-INDUCED LUPUS

Not all SLE is autoimmune. Your character could develop lupus symptoms after exposure to certain medications. Medications notorious for causing this include:

- **Isoniazid** used to treat tuberculosis

- **Hydralazine,** a blood pressure medication often used in African Americans

- **Procainamide**, an antiarrhythmic medication used for atrial fibrillation

If your character has drug-induced lupus, their blood will test positive for *anti-histone antibodies*. Treatment is similar to the regular treatment of SLE—NSAIDs and hydroxychloroquine—and stopping whatever drug caused the outbreak in the first place.

RHEUMATOID ARTHRITIS (RA)

RA is a chronic autoimmune disease that targets the joints. If your character has RA, they'll have pain and swelling in their joints that is worse in the mornings and improves as the day goes on. Just about any joint in the body can be affected—except for the very last joint on the toes and fingers, called the *distal interphalangeal* (DIP) joint. They'll also have joint stiffness. As the disease progresses, the swelling in the joints can become severe and even disfigured. The hand and fingers are often greatly impacted, resulting in characteristic deformities:

- *Boutonniere deformity* causes the middle joint of the finger (or toe) to remain straight. Only the furthest joint (the DIP joint) can bend.

- *Swan's neck deformity* means the finger bends down at the first joint, then upwards at the second, so that it looks like the long neck of a swan with the last part of the finger as the head.

- *Ulnar deviation* means that the fingers bend outward at the first joint, deviating towards the pinky finger.

But joint disease in RA isn't limited to the hands and feet. Other joints commonly affected include the knees, wrists, ankles, hips, and shoulders. Even the spine is often affected, particularly the first and second cervical vertebrae (C1 & C2). If these joints become unstable, it is potentially life-threatening, and your character will need neurosurgery to stabilize the joint.

SYSTEMIC MANIFESTATIONS

RA is also associated with symptoms beyond the joints, called *extra-articular manifestations*. These include:

- Generalized fatigue

- Weight loss

- Low-grade fever

- Thin skin that bruises easily

- Dry eyes

- **Rheumatoid nodules** are nonpainful lumps that form under the skin. They can also form in the heart, causing potential arrhythmias, and lungs.

- Fluid buildup around the lungs (*pleural effusion*) and heart (*pericardial effusion*).

- Inflammation of the sack lining the lungs (*pleuritis*) and heart (*pericarditis*).

- Anemia

DIAGNOSIS & TREATMENT

RA is diagnosed by the presence of arthritis in several joints, plus X-rays showing joint breakdown typical of RA and blood tests showing elevated levels of inflammation. Treatment of RA is two-pronged: minimize symptoms and prevent further damage.

NSAIDs like ibuprofen are the first medications your character will take to try to minimize their pain and swelling. If that doesn't work, they may take oral steroids. Surgery, such as joint replacement, is the last resort to treat your character's severe pain. To prevent further joint damage, your character will take disease-modifying antirheumatic medications (DMARDs), such as methotrexate. These medications take a long time to work, but they can prevent the disease from worsening.

THYROID DISEASE

The thyroid is a soft, butterfly-shaped organ located at the front of the throat that is responsible for regulating the body's metabolism. Two different types of autoimmune diseases target this organ.

GRAVES' DISEASE

Graves' disease is an autoimmune condition that results in the overstimulation of the thyroid, called *hyperthyroidism*. Symptoms include weight loss, despite increased appetite, feeling hot, sweating excessively, decreased need for sleep or trouble sleeping, irritability/anxiety, diarrhea, and muscle weakness. Someone observing your character might notice that they have a fine tremor of the hands and that their eyes seem to be popping out of their head, a condition called *exophthalmos* that is caused by swelling of the muscles around the eye. They will also have exaggerated reflexes, and they may have a swelling at the front of the neck where the thyroid is.

Unintentional weight loss and decreased need for sleep might sound like a dream come true to your character. Many people with Graves' Disease are hesitant to seek treatment because it makes them feel great. But without treatment, Graves' Disease can cause all sorts of problems.

One big problem with Graves' Disease is that it can cause heart problems. Their blood pressure will rise, and they'll have heart arrhythmias, like atrial fibrillation. Your character may feel palpitations—like their heart is pounding or skipping a beat. Without treatment, they can go into heart failure (See *Ch. 20: Chronic Breathlessness*).

But it gets worse. Untreated, Graves' Disease can lead to a rare complication called **thyroid storm**, a condition of rampant hyperthyroidism. Symptoms include high fever, fast heart rate, nausea/vomiting, and diarrhea. Your character will also exhibit psychiatric symptoms ranging from agitation and confusion to outright psychosis. A thyroid storm is highly lethal; 20% of people with it will enter a coma and die.[2]

The most common treatment for Graves' disease is radiation to kill the thyroid. Since the thyroid is practically the only organ in the body that absorbs iodine, your character will be given radioactive iodine to swallow. Your character's excretions will be radioactive for a few days—they'll need to sleep in a separate bed, wash/launder their clothes separate from their family, avoid close contact, and even use a separate toilet. After the therapy, they will have low thyroid (*hypothyroidism*) and will need to take supplemental synthetic thyroid hormone.

HASHIMOTO'S THYROIDITIS

Unique returns to the doctor a month later. She is cold all the time, and her hair is falling out in patches. Even her voice sounds different. She feels like she's walking through peanut butter; everything feels slow and gray. Her grades are dropping—probably because all she wants to do is sleep—and she hasn't pooped in almost a week.

Hashimoto's is an autoimmune condition that causes low thyroid hormone production (*hypothyroidism*). Symptoms of Hashimoto's are usually chronic and insidious and are caused by a slowed metabolism. As such, they are almost the polar opposite of the symptoms of Graves' Disease, including:

- Fatigue despite sleeping more than usual

- Feeling cold all the time

- Dry skin

- Constipation

- Hair loss

- Slowed thoughts or trouble concentrating

- Hoarse voice

- Hearing loss

If the hypothyroidism is severe, it can mimic severe depression: low mood, slow movements, oversleeping, lethargy, and weakness. This condition is called *pseudodementia*.

The doctor runs yet another blood test, but this time it comes back positive. Unique's TSH is high, meaning that she has hypothyroidism. He prescribes a synthetic thyroid hormone and tells her to come back in a month for further testing.

Both Hashimoto's and Grave's Disease are diagnosed with blood tests showing the levels of the hormone TSH. In Hashimoto's TSH is high, while in Graves' Disease, TSH is low. Hashimoto's is treated with synthetic thyroid hormone.

It takes a few months to get the right dosage, but soon, Unique is back to feeling like herself again.

"The ANA is negative for Lupus."

"Of course, it is."

"What do you mean?"

"It's never lupus."

There's a grain of truth to this trope. There isn't a one-size-fits-all presentation of SLE. Different characters will have different constellations of symptoms. And there also isn't one single test that can positively make the diagnosis. There is, however, more concrete testing that can be done than certain television shows would have you believe. Here's a quick overview.

- **ANA** stands for *antinuclear antibodies*. Almost all people with SLE will have them, but many other conditions can also cause a high ANA. So, a negative ANA rules out SLE, but a positive result just means your character has some sort of autoimmune thing going on.

- Certain lab markers, such as **CRP** and **ESR**, are just markers of inflammation. They'll be high if your character's body has any type of inflammation, ranging from autoimmune disease to infection. High CRP and/or ESR are not diagnostic of anything, but if they're negative, they can help rule out inflammatory conditions.

- Other lab markers, such as a false-positive syphilis test or antibodies against specific proteins (anti-Sm antibody, anti-histone antibody, etc.), are considered immunologic manifestations. They are positive in some people with SLE, but negative in others.

So, what does this mean for diagnosing SLE? There are eleven basic criteria used for diagnosing SLE.

1. Butterfly rash

2. Discoid rash

3. Ulcers in the mouth or nose

4. Skin sensitivity to light (*photosensitivity*)

5. Arthritis

6. Inflammation of the sack around the heart (*pericarditis*) or lungs (*pleuritis*)

7. Breakdown of blood cells (*hemolytic anemia*)

8. Seizures or psychosis

9. Positive ANA

10. Positive lab markers (antibodies, false-positive syphilis test)

If you want your character to be diagnosed with SLE, they should meet at least four of these criteria. It is possible to have a negative ANA and still have SLE, though it is rare.

ANA is also elevated in rheumatoid arthritis.

22. HEADACHE

BACKGROUND

Vera is sitting at her desk when she notices a small dark spot in the center of her computer screen. She reaches up to rub it away, only to realize that the spot isn't on her screen—it's her vision.

You've probably had a headache at some point in your life. Headaches are so ubiquitous that they're understood to be just another part of life. Because of this, lots of characters get headaches. But they're usually just described as a "headache" and left at that. I consider that a wasted opportunity.

Headaches can be disabling. They can be a sign of an underlying problem. They can mimic other conditions. They can even drive your character to suicide.[1]

Don't underestimate the humble headache.

TENSION-TYPE HEADACHE

Vera frowns and reaches up to rub her neck. She's been so tight lately. Between her job at the library and the hours spent writing her thesis, she spends most of her time in this chair. Maybe her eyes are strained from spending so much time at the computer?

People with tension-type AND migraine-type headaches often have tender muscles in their neck and shoulders.

Tension headaches are incredibly common. They're the most commonly experienced type of head pain. Though anyone can get a tension headache, women get them more often than men. The headaches usually start when your character is a teenager and peak during middle age.

Despite its name, the cause of tension headaches is unknown. Though they're associated with chronic muscle tension, no studies have been able to show a causal relationship between muscle contraction and headache.[2] Stress, anxiety, depression, and poor posture also contribute.

SYMPTOMS

Tension headaches are usually described as a steady, vise-like pain or pressure around the head. Usually, it affects the whole head, but may be worse at the back of the head. It's often accompanied by sore/tender neck muscles. Tension headaches are often exacerbated by stress, and they tend to get worse throughout the day.

TREATMENT & PREVENTION

Tension headaches are self-limited, meaning they'll go away on their own. Treatment is with mild pain relief (ibuprofen or Tylenol). Prevention is regular meals, sleep, and exercise along with stress reduction techniques. Avoiding caffeine and quitting smoking can also help.

MIGRAINE

The black spot in Vera's vision gets bigger and bigger. It fills the center of her vision—no matter where she looks, that black spot is right in the center. After half an hour, she gives up and packs up her backpack—no point in trying to write if she can't see the screen. Plus, she's starting to feel nauseated. Was the sushi she had for dinner last night bad? She's been feeling kind of gross ever since she woke up.

Scotoma is the medical term for a blind spot. They are a common migraine aura.

Migraines are recurrent, severe headaches. Their exact cause is unknown. Migraines tend to run in families, but there isn't one single gene that causes them.

Familial hemiplegic migraine is a type of migraine that is linked to specific gene mutations.

SYMPTOMS

By the time Vera gets to her room, the black spot in her vision is gone. Vera debates going back to the library, but she kind of feels like she's going to throw up. Plus, her head is starting to hurt. Not her head, really. Her forehead. It feels like someone has jabbed a screwdriver behind her eyeball.

The headaches caused by migraines are usually one-sided, often located behind the eye, and are often described as throbbing or pulsating. Migraine headaches are quite severe and can last anywhere from 4-72 hours. They are also usually associated with sensitivity to light/sound (*photophobia/phonophobia*), nausea and/or vomiting, and increased sensitivity to smell. Migraines tend to get worse with activity and bending over.

Vera pulls the curtains closed—it's a cloudy day, but even the overcast afternoon hurts her eyes—pops a couple of Tylenol and lies down on her bed. She grabs her computer and turns on her favorite TV show. But even with the brightness turned down, the light is too much. She rolls over and presses a pillow over her head, blocking out all light as she listens to the familiar voices.

There are three phases to a migraine, though not everyone gets all of them. The **prodrome** precedes the migraine by up to 24-hours, and consists of nonspecific signs such as irritability, nausea, fatigue, heightened emotions (elation, depression, irritability, etc.), and yawning.

Next comes the famous **aura**—changes in sensation that occur right before the "true" migraine starts. Auras are temporary and short-lived, lasting from a few minutes to an hour. Most auras are visual. Your character may see spots or flashing lights in their vision, or they may have a giant black spot in the center of their vision, called a *scotoma*. They may even lose vision altogether. But not all auras are visual. Your character could also experience numbness/tingling on part of their body or may even lose the ability to speak. Some auras are so striking they may even be confused for a stroke (See *Ch. 7: Stroke*).

> Most people with migraines don't get auras. In fact, only 15% of people with migraines will ever have an aura.[1]

The headache, which started behind her left eye, has spread to her entire head. Waves of nausea wash over her, and Vera has to run to the bathroom more than once to throw up. As the pain increases, Vera starts to cry. She's had headaches before, but never anything like this.

The third phase of the migraine is the headache itself, which can last hours to days. If your character gets a migraine, they probably won't be able to do much of anything except curl up in a dark room and wait for it to pass.

Finally, after several hours, Vera manages to fall asleep. When she wakes up the next morning, she has a mild headache, but nothing like the day before.

The fourth phase of a migraine is the **postdrome**, sometimes called a migraine hangover. If your character has a postdrome, they'll feel drained and may have trouble concentrating. They may also have nausea, diarrhea, light sensitivity, and a stiff neck.

Vera makes an appointment at the doctor, where she's diagnosed with a "migraine with aura." The doctor gives her a medication called Sumatriptan to take next time she gets a migraine. Vera hopes she never gets another one again.

Like tension headaches, mild migraines can be treated with NSAIDs or Tylenol. More severe migraines are treated with a class of medications called *triptans*, which can be given orally, intranasally, or even injected. But watch out; your character can't take more than three triptans a week, or else they risk getting a stroke! If your character has severe nausea with their migraines, they might also be prescribed an anti-nausea medication.

If your character has frequent migraines, more than 2-4 per month, they might need to be put on a preventative medication. Preventative medications include blood pressure medications, antiseizure medications, and certain antidepressants. Botox can also be used to prevent migraines.

CLUSTER HEADACHE

Cluster headaches are excruciating, one-sided headaches that crop up in—you guessed it!—clusters. These headaches last for anywhere from a few minutes to a few hours. They occur in episodes of frequent attacks that occur daily (or several times a day) for weeks or even months on end. These are called episodes, or cluster periods. Outside of cluster periods, your character may have no headaches for months or even years at a time.

SYMPTOMS

The pain of a cluster headache usually occurs behind the eye and is described as stabbing or burning. Cluster headaches tend to occur at night, waking your character from sleep, though they can happen during the day as well. The headaches are also associated with tearing and redness of the eye, a runny nose, facial swelling, and eyelids all on the same side as the headache. Your character may also feel restless and might pace, rock back and forth, or bang their head against the wall due to the severity of the pain. The headaches are so severe that your character may become suicidal.[1]

TREATMENT

Luckily, cluster headaches can both be treated and prevented. Treatment is with a triptan drug called *Sumatriptan* coupled with high flow, 100% oxygen. Prevention, particularly with a blood pressure medication called *Verapamil*, can quickly reduce the number and severity of your character's headaches.

SECONDARY HEADACHES

Sometimes, headaches are just a symptom in the larger picture of a disease. Lots of things can cause secondary headaches, from hangovers to post-concussive syndrome. Here are a few I think writers will enjoy:

- **Brain bleeds** (*intracerebral hemorrhage*) are headaches caused by burst blood vessels in the head, resulting in a sudden, severe headache called a *thunderclap headache.* These headaches are often described as "the worst headache of my life," and are generally followed by a loss of consciousness (See Ch.7: Stroke).

- **Brain tumors** are a great cause of secondary headaches. If you want to foreshadow your character's upcoming brain tumor, a new, relentless headache is the way to go. Headaches due to brain tumors are usually due to increased pressure; there's only so much room in the skull and tumors take up space. For that reason, headaches due to brain tumors tend to be worse at night and in the early morning, when your character is lying down. They also tend to cause nausea and vomiting which is also more severe when lying down or bending over. Other "red flags" for brain tumors include seizures and focal neurologic changes, such as difficulty with balance (*ataxia*), weakness/paralysis/loss of sensation in one arm or leg, vision changes, language problems (*aphasia*), and trouble hearing in one ear.

- **Brain infections**, such as meningitis or encephalitis cause headaches, along with neck stiffness, sensitivity to light/sound, confusion, decreased level of consciousness, and seizures (See *Ch. 5: Fever*). Other infections, such as COVID-19, ear infections, influenza, and sinus infections can also cause headaches.

- **Giant cell arteritis** causes headache, fever, vision problems, jaw pain, and scalp tenderness. It is caused by inflammation of the arteries in your temple. Without prompt treatment, it can lead to blindness.

- **Idiopathic intracranial hypertension (IIH)** causes a severe headache along with changes in vision and hearing. It's caused by too much spinal fluid inside the skull, putting pressure on the brain and the nerve that leads to your eye called the *optic nerve.* IIH is a fun one because it mimics all the symptoms of a brain tumor. But unlike a tumor, it doesn't require neurosurgery to treat. If you're looking to give your character a brain tumor scare, diagnosing them with IIH instead could work quite well.

> IIH is treated with weight loss and a medication called acetazolamide that decreases CSF production. A lumbar puncture showing high CSF pressure is both diagnostic and therapeutic.

"I do declare, my head is aching from all this stress! Better go lie down and let y'all figure it out."

Another cliché that is quite true. Stress can trigger both tension-type and migraine headaches. However, headaches are often used as a version of the "sickly sidekick" trope; a character gets a headache, and they just can't even. Most of the time, the character with the headache is a wealthy woman. Despite, or perhaps because, of all the stress going on, the affected character goes to her room to lay down, and everyone else now has to figure out how to deal with the problem without her.

This is the part that doesn't ring true with my experience with headache patients. First, chronic stress tends to cause headaches, not necessarily acute events. Second, people who suffer from regular headaches learn to deal with them. Often, this means pushing through a headache, knowing that it will only get worse. My experience working with headache patients is that, like any other chronic pain patient, they figure out coping mechanisms that allow them to work, even with a headache, when it matters most. Only after, once the acute threat/stressor is gone, does the headache come roaring back. Usually, this is the point at which a headache sufferer would have to go lie down; after the crisis has passed.

23. MENTAL ILLNESS

ENTAL ILLNESS IS A HUGE and enormously important topic. I could probably write a whole book on it. In fact, I plan to dedicate a whole volume to mental illness further down the road. But the topic of mental illness is relevant for many writers, so it seems appropriate for me to briefly touch upon the topic here.

In this chapter, I'll briefly go over the signs and symptoms of a few of the most common (and most commonly written about) mental illnesses, as well as some possible treatments. But please remember; mental illness is a broad field and if one of your main characters is experiencing mental illness, you're going to need more in-depth research than I can provide in this chapter.

Willow can't believe how selfish and spoiled she is. Her parents spent so much money to take the family on vacation for her graduation present, and she isn't even enjoying it. All she feels is tired and numb, as if the whole world—even here, on this beautiful beach—has been painted in grayscale.

DEPRESSION

Let's start with one of the most common mental illnesses of all: depression. Turns out, depression isn't a complete diagnosis; there's a whole subset of depressive illnesses, ranging from seasonal affective disorder (also known as SAD) to premenstrual dysphoric disorder, a form of depression that occurs around a woman's menstrual cycle. But when most people say "depression," they're talking about major depressive disorder or MDD.

SIGNS & SYMPTOMS

Willow is exhausted, but she can't sleep. She's hungry, but nothing tastes good. She tries to read—she brought five different books—but can't concentrate long enough to finish even the first chapter. Instead, she spends her days walking the beach alone, staring out at the waves, and wondering what it would feel like to drown.

MDD is a depressive disorder characterized by a daily low mood or lack of interest in life that lasts for at least two weeks. But MDD is about a lot more than just feeling sad. Many people with MDD don't feel sad at all. Instead, they feel gray, blah, or completely numb. In children and adolescents, irritability and anger can be the predominant moods.[1] To be diagnosed with MDD, your character will also need to exhibit key characteristics that distinguish it from the garden-variety blues.

The symptoms of a depressive episode include:

- Feeling guilty, hopeless, or worthless

- Lack of interest in the things that used to make them happy

- Low energy or fatigue, despite getting enough sleep

- Sad or low mood

- Trouble thinking, concentrating, or making decisions.

- Recurrent thoughts of death or suicide

- Some signs of depression that others might notice include:

    o Eating too much or too little

    o Lack of attention to personal hygiene

    o Slowed movements (*psychomotor retardation*) or restlessness (*psychomotor agitation*)

    o Sleeping too much or too little

    o Significant weight gain or weight loss not caused by dieting

    o Tearfulness

> **Retardation** just means slowing. While the term "mental retardation" is no longer used because of its derogatory connotations, other forms of retardation (growth retardation, psychomotor retardation, etc.) are commonly used medical terms.

If your character has MDD, they may lose interest in things they used to enjoy, like gardening or playing with their grandchildren. They might feel worthless, hopeless, or overcome by guilt for things they cannot change. They may feel fatigued, have unexplained body aches, or a heaviness to their limbs like they're filled with lead. Concentrating can become difficult and your character may become completely paralyzed by low stakes, everyday decisions, like what movie to watch on Netflix.

> Even little decisions—like which brand of peanut butter to buy—can be completely overwhelming to someone suffering from MDD.

But MDD is not just in your character's thoughts and feelings. There are observable physical changes that a psychiatrist, or your character's loved ones, might notice. Psychomotor retardation (the physical slowing of your character's movements) can be as subtle as reduced facial expressions or as overt as a slow, shuffling walk. Other characters might notice that your depressed character isn't sleeping much or eating enough. Conversely, they might be sleeping and eating too much, a phenomenon known as *atypical depression*. They may notice that your character has begun to smell, as they've stopped bothering to take showers or brush their teeth. And if your character is having significant difficulty concentrating, others may notice that they are not following conversations or are repeating questions they'd already asked.

Recurrent thoughts of death and suicidal ideation are also key features of MDD. Since Ch. 9 is devoted entirely to suicide, I won't say more here. But please remember; the vast majority of people with MDD will never attempt suicide.[1]

> **Psychomotor agitation**—pacing, hand-rubbing, the inability to sit still—can also be an observable sign of MDD.

TREATMENT

Major depressive disorder is a biological disease caused by an imbalance of neurotransmitters. But it is also greatly affected by social, economic, and cultural factors. For these reasons, the most effective treatment of MDD is a combination of antidepressant medications and therapy.

While there are a wide variety of antidepressants, the most commonly used are a class of medications called *selective serotonin reuptake inhibitors* or SSRIs. And while SSRIs can be life-saving medications, they can also have some nasty side effects, including weight gain, trouble sleeping, nausea, dizzi-

> Antidepressants take up to 6 weeks to start working. Some episodes of MDD can self-resolve in that time, casting a shadow over the true efficacy of the medications.

ness, and restlessness. They can also negatively impact your character's sex life; SSRIs are notorious for not only causing lower sex drive, but also erectile dysfunction and inability to orgasm. If you're looking to make your formerly depressed character go off their meds, hit them with one or two of these side effects, and their decision to go off their potentially life-saving medications will suddenly feel more believable.

> *The Prozac makes Willow feel like she's going to pass out; she actually does faint once, while moving into her dorm room at college, much to her horror. She goes to see the on-campus doctor, who tries her on another antidepressant, then another. But they all give her side effects. And she's feeling better, anyway. After all, she's doing well in her new classes and making new friends. She doesn't need the medications now, so she stops taking them.*

Getting side effects from one SSRI does not mean your character will get them from another one. If a patient has side effects from a medication, their psychiatrist will transition them to a new med that will hopefully work better and not cause side effects. Stopping psych meds cold turkey is dangerous.[1]

Another mode of treatment for MDD is the oft-vilified *electroconvulsive therapy*, or ECT, a procedure that creates electrical currents in the brain triggering a controlled seizure. It is an incredibly effective treatment that can alleviate symptoms in as little as six sessions, or about three weeks. By comparison, most medications for depression take at least six weeks to take effect. While early iterations of ECT were quite barbaric, modern ECT is performed under the effect of anesthesia and muscle relaxants. The main side effect is mild anterograde amnesia, or inability to form new memories, (See *Ch. 12: Traumatic Brain Injury*).

Not everyone with MDD will need treatment for the rest of their life. Your character may be able to receive treatment for a few months, then taper off and never have a depressive episode again. However, if your character has recurrent episodes, they may need treatment for the rest of their life.

ANXIETY

Like depression, anxiety is actually a cluster of disorders, ranging from phobias, such as agoraphobia or social phobia, to panic disorders and generalized anxiety disorder. And while each diagnosis has its own unique traits, anxiety disorders are linked by the common thread of excessive and overwhelming fear,

Worry, also called **apprehensive expectation**, is the expectation that something is about to go terribly wrong.

anxiety, and worry. Sometimes, those feelings of anxiety can translate into physical symptoms, in a phenomenon called *somatization.*

It is important to note that almost all anxiety disorders, from GAD to specific phobia, have a high comorbidity with other psychiatric illnesses.[1] This means that if you give your character an anxiety diagnosis, consider that they may have at least one other comorbid condition.

GENERALIZED ANXIETY DISORDER (GAD)

Generalized anxiety is probably what you're thinking of when you write a character with anxiety. It's a condition characterized by excessive worrying and anxiety that is both difficult to control and negatively impacts your character's life. GAD is a chronic, daily burden that is above and beyond the normal worries of daily life. For your character to be diagnosed with GAD, they'd need to experience this overwhelming, distressing worry and anxiety nearly every day for at least six months.

> GAD is only diagnosed when the anxiety is not better explained by your character's life stressors. If your character is worried and anxious about a loved one undergoing a dangerous surgery, that's not GAD, that's normal human emotion.

GAD is more than just feelings of fear; your character will feel its effects on their body. They may feel restless, on-edge, or irritable. Conversely, they might feel exhausted despite adequate sleep or may have trouble sleeping. Difficulty concentrating, sudden blanks, and racing thoughts can make it difficult to fully engage in work or school. Muscle tension is another symptom commonly experienced by people with GAD. Though anyone with GAD can experience somatization, children with GAD are more likely to experience somatic symptoms, particularly headaches and stomachaches.

Treatment of GAD is with a combination of medications and therapy. The most commonly prescribed medications are antidepressants, such as the SSRIs described above. If your character has certain situations that make their anxiety worse, they may also be prescribed a benzodiazepine—more about these in the next section.

PANIC DISORDER

During her second semester of college, Willow starts feeling rushes of sudden fear. They're small at first—her heart pounding, palms sweating, a horrible feeling like she's forgotten something important—but each one seems to get stronger. She starts checking and rechecking her planner, making certain she hasn't missed anything. Before exams, she arrives an hour early and brings at least five spare #2 pencils. When her friends ask her to go out with them, she declines, fearing that she'll get scared and embarrass herself in front of them. But the more she tries to prevent the attacks, the more often they seem to happen.

A panic attack is an abrupt and unexpected surge of fear that happens totally out of the blue. The fear may be so extreme that your character may believe they're dying, losing control, or going crazy. If your character has a panic attack, in addition to extreme fear, they may also experience overwhelming bodily sensations such as:

- Chest pain or tightness

- Feel like they're choking, can't breathe, or are being smothered

- Nausea

- Numbness or tingling in their extremities

- Shaking or trembling in the extremities

- Sweating, chills, or a rush of heat

- Their heart racing or pounding out of their chest

The medical term for the feeling of the heart pounding out of the chest is **palpitations**.

Panic disorder is characterized by recurrent, unexpected panic attacks. These attacks are so unexpected that your character worries constantly about the next panic attack, when it will hit, what will happen when it does, and even changes their behavior in the hope of avoiding the attacks.

One day, in the cafeteria, it hits her hard: a rush of heat and nausea followed by a tidal wave of fear. Her hands start shaking so hard that she drops her tray, splattering pudding, and soup all over her jeans. Tears stream down her cheeks as she gasps for breath. She wonders if this is what dying feels like. Her friends are talking to her, probably asking what's wrong, but they sound like they're talking underwater. Willow can't speak, can't move, can barely even breathe. Finally, her friends coax her to a booth far from prying eyes and hold her hands as she shudders out her breaths. After several minutes, the fear passes, replaced by mortification. Did she really just lose it in the cafeteria?

Like GAD, treatment for panic attacks is therapy plus antidepressant medications. The antidepressants help prevent the occurrence of panic attacks, while therapy helps your character learn to live their life

For more on addiction and withdrawal from benzodiazepines, see <u>Volume 1: Setting & Character, Ch. 17: Drugs & Addiction.</u>

despite the attacks. However, a class of sedative medications called benzodiazepines can help to stop the panic attack in its place.

Benzodiazepines, such as Xanax, Klonopin, and Valium, are a double-edged sword. They work fast—Valium can take effect in as little as 30 minutes—and can quickly quell both the physical and emotional effects of a panic attack. However, they are also highly addictive. Benzodiazepine dependence can develop in as little as 1-2 months, and your character may develop a tolerance (meaning they need a higher dose to get the same effect) in as little as four months of regular use.[2] And while most instances of withdrawal from benzodiazepines result only in an increase in anxiety, benzodiazepines are one of the few medications from which withdrawal can be lethal.

> Alcohol, benzodiazepines, and barbiturates are the three substances that can cause deadly withdrawal seizures.

PHOBIAS

Phobias are an extreme fear reaction to an object or situation. For it to be a phobia, your character's fear must be out of proportion to the real danger presented, they must be afraid of the object/situation in all instances, and they must actively try to avoid the phobic object whenever possible. When avoidance isn't possible, endurance is met with intense fear and anxiety. Finally, your character's phobia must negatively impact their life and daily functioning; a fear of orangutans isn't going to rise to the level of a phobia unless they're living in the jungles of Borneo.

There are lots of different types of phobias; some are prevalent enough to get their own diagnosis in the DSM-V, while others are simply categorized as a "specific phobia."

Agoraphobia: Agoraphobia is the fear of certain places, such as public transportation, open spaces, enclosed spaces, crowds, or even just leaving the house. Your character does not need to be afraid of all these places in order to be diagnosed with agoraphobia, but they need to be afraid of more than one. Similar to panic disorder, agoraphobia is rooted in the fear that your character may end up panicking in a situation from which they cannot escape or get help.

Social Anxiety Disorder (Social Phobia): Social anxiety disorder is characterized as a phobia of social situations and interactions. It is characterized by intense fear that your character will somehow humiliate themselves, leading to rejection. Performance anxiety is a subtype of social anxiety disorder.

Specific Phobia: A specific phobia is the fear of a specific object or situation, called a phobic object. Examples of common phobic objects include spiders, heights, flying, injections, blood, snakes, and dogs. Anything can become a phobic object; you're limited only by your creativity.

BIPOLAR DISORDER

Bipolar disorder is, as the name suggests, a disease of two poles: depression and mania/hypomania. A character with bipolar disorder will vacillate between episodes, sometimes over a period of years, other times over weeks. In rapid cycling (a subtype of bipolar disorder) characters can shift between depressive and manic episodes in a matter of minutes, while in mixed episodes (another subtype) your character may experience both depressive and manic symptoms simultaneously. However, it is most common for characters to experience sequential episodes: a manic episode followed by a depressive episode.

> Depression in people without bipolar is sometimes referred to as **unipolar depression.**

DEPRESSIVE EPISODE

Two weeks after the incident in the cafeteria, Willow starts feeling gray and numb once more. The panic attacks are happening less often, but Willow is finding it hard to care. She stops going to classes and stays in bed, staring up at the ceiling. Her counselor—whom she told about her depression last summer—pushes her to go back to the doctor and start on medications. She does so reluctantly and is started on yet another SSRI.

Since the symptoms of bipolar depression are almost identical to that of major depressive disorder, I'm not going to spend a lot of time discussing it here. Instead, I'm going to focus on the other pole: mania or hypomania.

MANIA/HYPOMANIA

After just a few days on the new SSRI, Willow is feeling great. Amazing, really. Motivated to catch up on all the classwork she'd fallen behind on, she stays at the library until it closes each night and is there each morning when it opens. When she finishes the backlog of essays and reading, she starts working on projects that aren't due for months. On a whim, she joins her friends when they go out to a frat party. Willow doesn't usually party, so her friends are surprised when she drinks the jungle juice and spends most of the night dancing suggestively with a guy from her biology class. When campus police shut the party down, she ditches her friends and hangs out with biology boy under the bridge, smoking weed.

Mania is defined as a period of elevated mood and energy. Your character might feel happy, elated, or overjoyed, or they might feel irritable and anxious. They may have a falsely elevated sense of self-esteem and a sincere belief that they can do absolutely anything. Other symptoms of mania include:

- Being easily distracted

- Being more talkative, talking over others, or feeling unable to stop talking

- Constant fidgeting or inability to sit still (psychomotor agitation)

- Hyper-focused on a particular goal, such as a project for work or studying for a test

- Participation in activities with potentially harmful consequences, such as excessive spending, cheating on a partner, or doing illegal drugs

- Racing thoughts or feeling like their thoughts are going in all directions at once

- Sleeping less but having more energy

Mania is diagnosed when your character exhibits several of the above symptoms for at least two weeks AND the symptoms are severe enough markedly impact their life. If the symptoms aren't severe enough to impair functioning, or if they don't last the full two weeks, then the episode is considered *hypomania*. But if there are any psychotic symptoms, such as delusions or hallucinations, the episode is manic, no matter how long it lasts.

> *Over the next few days, Willow is the happiest she's ever been. She's never had sex before, but she's determined to change that. She sleeps with biology boy, a guy from her Calc II class that she thought might be married, and a girl she met in the elevator in her dorm. But she doesn't let her studies flag; she keeps going to class and studying late into the night. She's feeling so good that she considers skipping her appointment with the campus physician, but her friends convince her she should go anyway.*

Mania (and hypomania) can feel amazing; imagine the happiest you've ever felt, then imagine feeling that way for absolutely no reason, for days or at a time. But it can also be horribly uncomfortable; instead of elated, your character might feel irritable, agitated, or anxious. They could experience akathisia, an uncomfortable feeling of restlessness that makes sitting still, or sleeping, nearly impossible.

If your character is manic (or hypomanic), they might not have any idea that something is wrong. After all, they may be feeling extremely happy and productive. But the people around them will notice. Your character may talk endlessly about some new project they're excited about, interrupting often, and showing very little interest in anyone else. They might flit from topic to topic with very little warning or be so focused on a task that it becomes impossible to pull them away, even for necessities like food and sleep. They may begin to dress provocatively, imbibe drugs or alcohol, or act inappropriately familiar with casual acquaintances, strangers, or coworkers.

Often, mania or hypomania will precede depression. Your character will have a week or two of elevated symptoms, followed by a depressive crash. While this is the most common pattern, it is not the only one. If your character has *rapid cycling*, they may vacillate quickly between different episode types, sometimes as fast as within the hour. Mixed episodes occur when your character experiences the symptoms of depression and mania *at the same time*; your character may feel all the hopelessness, guilt, and suicidal ideation of depression while having the energy, anxiety, and restlessness of mania. Needless to say, a mixed episodes can be exceedingly dangerous.

TREATMENT

> *The doctor talks with Willow for less than five minutes before telling Willow that she is currently hypomanic. She informs her of her new diagnosis—bipolar disorder—and recommends she stop the SSRI. Instead, she starts her on two new medications: a mood stabilizer called lithium and an antipsychotic called Quetiapine. Willow is horrified that she's being put on an antipsychotic; she isn't psychotic! But the doctor reassures her that it is to help her through this episode; she is not psychotic, and this medication does not mean she's crazy. Willow only half believes her, but she agrees to take the new meds anyway.*

The treatment for bipolar disorder is therapy plus medications (are you noticing a trend yet?). Medications for bipolar disorder are split into two main categories: mood stabilizers and antipsychotics. The most common mood stabilizer is Lithium; it's been around for a long time, and though no one knows exactly how it works, it is extremely effective at treating bipolar disorder. It also decreases suicidality. Unfortunately, it takes a few weeks to kick in. Atypical anti-psychotics are used to bridge the gap until lithium takes effect, breaking your character out of their episode.

After four years on the lithium, Willow starts to wonder if she really needs it. After all, she hasn't had any episodes—hypomanic or depressive—since that big one her first year. The meds have made her gain weight, and sometimes she feels like she doesn't feel things as deeply as she used to. So, one week before graduation, she stops taking her meds.

Because bipolar disorder is a lifelong illness, your character will need to be on mood-stabilizing medications for the rest of their lives. But your character might have trouble sticking to their treatment regimen. After all, once they're no longer in a mood episode, they'll probably feel pretty normal. They might even miss the highs of mania and hypomania, or they might feel like the mood stabilizers have taken away their ability to feel. This numbness, combined with the nasty side effects of the drugs, may lead your character to decide they don't need the drugs after all.

Her symptoms come back within days. To her surprise, she starts getting panic attacks again. She isn't sleeping, but it isn't feeling the joyous, elated feeling she had when she was first diagnosed either. Instead, she feels restless and anxious, unable to sit still for more than a few minutes at a time. Not wanting to feel this way any longer, she goes to see the campus doctor, who puts her back on the lithium and quetiapine. Willow can't help but feel as if she's failed.

And your character won't be alone! A 2021 study found that nearly half of people with bipolar disorder don't take their medications as prescribed.[3] This poor adherence, while exceedingly common, leads to an increased risk of further episodes, strained interpersonal relationships, hospitalization, and even suicide. In real life, it's a troubling and intransigent cycle. In your writing, it can open up opportunities for conflict.

SCHIZOPHRENIA

Schizophrenia is a psychotic disorder, meaning it causes hallucinations and/or delusions. It tends to affect younger people - the average age of diagnosis is early, around 15-25. The earlier your character is diagnosed, the more severe their disease is likely to be. Symptoms of schizophrenia fall into three main categories: positive symptoms, negative symptoms, and disorganized symptoms.

POSITIVE SYMPTOMS

Positive symptoms are the abnormal presence of something that shouldn't be there. In this case, it is the presence of psychotic symptoms: delusions and hallucinations.

Contrary to popular belief, schizophrenia has absolutely nothing to do with multiple or split personalities.

Delusions: Fixed, false beliefs. Examples include your character thinking they are Marilynn Monroe or believing that aliens are listening to their thoughts.

Hallucinations: Seeing, hearing, touching, smelling, or tasting things that are not there. Examples include hearing disembodied voices (*auditory hallucination*), seeing flashing lights (*simple visual hallucination*), or feeling bugs crawling over their skin (*tactile hallucination*). Hallucinations are not unique to schizophrenia. Lots of conditions, from migraine to epilepsy to dementia, can cause hallucinations. But there are a few characteristics of hallucinations in schizophrenia that are important for writers to know.

Not all hallucinations are scary. One patient claimed he heard a voice telling him jokes all day.

Auditory hallucinations are most common, occurring in 60-80% of people with schizophrenia.[4] Complex visual hallucinations, such as seeing a face or a religious icon, are more often seen in specific conditions, including schizophrenia and Lewy Body dementia (See *Ch. 25: Dementia and Delirium*). Multimodal hallucinations—hallucinations that utilize multiple senses, such as if your character hallucinates a person talking to them—are also extremely common in schizophrenia; one study found that people with schizophrenia are twice as likely to experience multimodal hallucinations than any single unimodal hallucination.[4]

Abnormal movements: Such as tremors, repeated, rhythmic movements, facial tics, muscle rigidity, and slowed movements. Catatonia (a condition of reduced reactivity to your character's surroundings) is another type of abnormal movement.

NEGATIVE SYMPTOMS

Negative symptoms are the abnormal absence of normal functioning. Negative symptoms include:

Avolition: A lack of motivation. Your character may show no interest in social interactions or may have trouble keeping up with their commitments. Avolition can be so strong your character may lose interest in the daily tasks of living, such as eating and sleeping.

Diminished emotional expression: Your character may lack normal facial expressions, hand gestures, and inflection in their voice. They may also stop making eye contact.

Lack of normal intonation in speech is called **aprosody**.

Reduced movement: Your character might move less or more slowly than normal.

Disorganized Thoughts and Speech: Disorganized thinking means your character is having difficulty maintaining a train of thought. From an outside character's POV, these changes in thought manifest as strange speech patterns. If you're writing a character with disorganized thinking, here are some speech (and thought) patterns you can use to give them a distinct and authentic voice.

- **Circumstantiality:** Speaks in a roundabout manner and takes forever to get to the point. Remember: lots of people speak circumstantially, so if you're trying to show your character's disorganized thinking, they'll probably need to have other signs of disorganization as well.

  o "I went to the park today—well - I took a walk around the neighborhood, looking at all the beautiful trees. We have so many maples here, I've never lived in a place with so many beautiful trees. Anyways, I was crunching on the fall leaves as I was walking and thinking to myself how lucky I am to live in such a beautiful neighborhood when I found myself at the park."

- **Clang associations:** Your character speaks in rhymes. Generally, rhymes that don't make any sense.

  Watch "The Brain as explained by John Cleese" for a beautiful example of word salad.[5]

  o "I went to the park in the dark. Bark, stark, lark."

- **Incoherence:** Your character speaks fluent but completely unintelligible sentences, a phenomenon sometimes called *word salad.*

  o "I went contributor every tissue wasn't quite emotion."

- **Loose associations (Derailment):** Your character's thoughts are easily derailed; they jump from topic to topic, with only loose connections between the thoughts. The topics of conversation may be tangentially related or loosely associated with one another, or they can be completely unrelated.

  o "I went to the park to play on the swings, but have you ever seen a monkey swing from a tree? I like going to the zoo to watch the penguins."

- **Neologisms:** Your character speaks in made-up words or phrases. Often, this happens because they are unable to remember the word they're looking for. Note that neologisms are not uncommon in everyday language; lots of characters have made up catchphrases or nonsensical words. Furthermore, people with dementia, strokes, and other neurologic disorders often use neologisms, so their presence alone is not enough to portray a thought disorder.

o "I went to the park with my friends to watch the orangeballers."

- **Perseveration:** Excessive repetition of certain words or phrases, or inability to talk about anything else.

o "I went to the park—park, park, park—today."

- **Thought blocking:** Long pauses in the middle of a sentence or being unable to finish a thought. Suddenly stops in the middle of a sentence.

o "I went to the park because…"

- **Word approximations**: Incorrect use of words in the middle of a sentence.

o "I want to the dark today."

A character with disorganized thinking will have these exceedingly strange thought and speech patterns. As the author, this is your opportunity to write a character with a truly strange and unique voice.

DISORGANIZED BEHAVIOR:

Disorganized behaviors occur in schizophrenia because your character's brain isn't properly regulating their behavior. Signs of disorganized behavior include:

- **Inability to perform normal activities of daily living,** such as eating, sleeping, and basic hygiene.

- **Difficulty performing goal-directed activities**, such as going to work or doing their homework.

- **Inability to control emotions**, leading to unpredictable emotional outbursts.

- **Poor impulse control** leading to outbursts and poor life choices.

- **Bizarre behaviors**, such as laughing at inappropriate times, walking in circles, going out into freezing weather without proper clothes, or talking to themselves.

TREATMENT

Schizophrenia is treated with a combination of medications, therapy, and social support. Antipsychotics are the first line of medical treatment. In addition, certain types of therapy, such as cognitive-behavioral therapy, have been shown to be successful. Often, though, medications and therapy are not enough to help someone; that's where social support comes in. If your character has schizophrenia, they may need life skills training and employment services to help them get back on their feet. Their family may need therapy as well, both to deal with the grief of such a life-changing diagnosis and learn to effectively provide assistance and support to their loved one.

POSTTRAUMATIC STRESS DISORDER (PTSD)

PTSD is a cluster of symptoms that occur after a traumatic incident. But it's so much more than just having flashbacks and nightmares. There are four main components to PTSD: the presence of trauma, intrusive symptoms, avoidance of the trigger, and increased reactivity.

THE TRAUMA

To have PTSD, your character needs to have experienced a major traumatic event. And that event can't be something minor, like getting shoved in a locker by the school bully. In order for your character to develop PTSD, the experience needs to involve perceived exposure to death, extreme violence, serious injury, or sexual violence. But while your character can certainly develop PTSD from experiencing the traumatic event themselves, they do not necessarily need to be the victim.

> If your character legitimately believed they might die in that locker—say they had a coat stuffed over their face so they couldn't breathe—then even something as seemingly minor as getting stuffed in a locker could be a trigger.

For example, your character could develop PTSD from witnessing another person be the victim of violence. They don't even need to witness the event; just learning that a loved one (family or close friend) was the victim of a violent event could be enough to trigger it. PTSD can also be triggered if your character is repeatedly dealing with firsthand experiences of trauma, such as an ED nurse who treats victims of sexual assault, or a detective who routinely investigates grisly murders.

Some of the most common traumas that trigger PTSD include car accidents, war (particularly exposure to combat), sexual assault or abuse, childhood or domestic abuse, and physical assault, particularly if they were threatened by a gun.

SIGNS & SYMPTOMS

To be diagnosed with PTSD, your character will need to exhibit a constellation of symptoms associated with the trauma. These symptoms need to have started (or started getting worse) around the time of the trauma. In general, your adult character will need at least one symptom in each of the following categories.

Re-experiencing

Re-experiencing, also called symptoms of intrusion, forces your character to relive their trauma. They can be memories, dreams, flashbacks, or even physical reactions that intrude on your character's life.

In a flashback, also called a **dissociative reaction**, your character feels like they're back at the moment of the trauma.

They are usually distressing, involuntary, and recurrent. Types of intrusion include:

- Frightening or distressing memories of the trauma

- Dreams or nightmares related to the trauma

- Flashbacks of the traumatic event

- Physical symptoms, such as profuse sweating or a pounding heartbeat that harken back to the trauma

Avoidance

If your character has PTSD, they will go out of their way to avoid things that remind them of the trauma. This might mean avoiding places, situations, or people they associate with the trauma, but it can also mean avoiding thoughts and feelings related to the event. For example, if your character was in a car accident while listening to angry music, they might avoid driving and listening to that band, but they might also refuse to allow themselves to feel anger. But remember, while avoidance certainly can be a conscious choice your character makes, it may also be something they are doing without realizing it.

Changes to Mood and Cognition

Negative changes can affect your character's thoughts, memories, and mood. Your character may even be unable to remember the traumatic event at all—a phenomenon called *dissociative amnesia*. Other examples of negative changes include:

- Always feeling negative or like they can't feel anything positive.

- Feeling detached from the world.

- Lack of interest in the things they used to love.

- Persistent, negative, and exaggerated beliefs. Your character might believe that there is something wrong with them or that they can never trust anyone again.

Note how many of these negative changes overlap with the symptoms of depression.

- Wrongly blaming themselves or others

<u>**Increased Reactivity (Hyperarousal)**</u>

Also known as "arousal," your character may feel as if they're constantly on edge, stressed, or irritable. They may have trouble relaxing and sleeping or may feel as if they must constantly be on their guard against an external threat, a condition called *hypervigilance.* Increased irritability may lead to unpredictable outbursts of temper, which are often violent and may be directed at other people or objects. Reckless or self-destructive behavior can also signal hyperreactivity. An increased startle reflex (jumping, gasping, yelling, or even lashing out when startled) is a common sign of hyperarousal.

TREATMENT

PTSD is mainly treated with psychotherapy and medications. Mindfulness training, cognitive behavioral therapy (CBT), and exposure therapy (a treatment that gradually introduces your character to their triggers) are commonly used modalities of psychotherapy. Eye movement desensitization and reprocessing (EMDR) is a relatively new therapy that uses eye movements to treat PTSD. So far, it is achieving incredible success.

Medications for PTSD include antidepressants, such as those used for anxiety and depression. Medical marijuana, where legal, is often used to treat PTSD, particularly to manage the symptoms of hyperarousal. It's important to note that benzodiazepines (the highly addictive meds prescribed to treat panic attacks) are rarely used in PTSD due to their addictive nature.

BREAKING DOWN THE CLICHÉS:

MENTALLY ILL = VIOLENT

> *"Captain! Evil McMasterplan has released the inhabitants of the insane asylum. They're flooding into the city now!"*

> **Horrified silence**

> *"Call in the National Guard. They're our only hope now."*

In fiction, insanity is often synonymous with violence. From psychotic serial killers to deranged ex-wives, the mentally ill are often depicted as unpredictable and dangerous. But the truth is much more complicated.

People with mental illnesses are much more likely to be the victims of violence than its perpetrators. One study found that men with mental illness were more than twice as likely to be subjected to violent crime than their non-mentally ill counterparts; for women, their risk was tripled.[6] And victims of violent crimes are more likely to become perpetrators themselves.[7]

Some studies have shown a slightly elevated risk of violence in psychiatric patients, particularly if they are acutely and seriously ill. But the elevated risk of violence in people with serious mental illness is minimal: 2.9% vs. 0.8% of the general population.[8] Most people with serious mental illness will never commit violence. The overwhelming majority of violence in the population—about 96%—is not attributable to mental illness.[9]

It's also important to note that violence among the mentally ill occurs primarily in people with personality and substance use disorders, such as drug and alcohol addiction.[7] Violence amongst people with other serious mental illnesses, such as schizophrenia, depression, and bipolar disorder, occurs at much lower rates.[9]

Often, aggression amongst the mentally ill is inextricably tied to confounding factors, such as poverty or a history of abuse; one study even found that psychiatric patients had the same likelihood of committing violence as their non-mentally ill counterparts, once their neighborhood was accounted for.[9] And the biggest risk factors for violence are the same in the mentally ill as they are for the general population: being young, male, single, and poor.[10]

The trope of the violent psychiatric patient is both inaccurate and dangerous. It contributes to the stigmatization of mental illness and may justify the victimization of the mentally ill. The vast majority of people with mental illness will never become violent, and those that do become violent often do so because of the same environmental factors that inspire violence in everyone else.

OCD GIVES YOU SUPERPOWERS

"I'm telling you, I'm right. I checked the oven seventeen times; the dial has been replaced with one that is slightly less black."

Long pause* *Checks the oven dial again

"By George, I think you're right. How'd you know that?"

Obsessive-compulsive disorder is often mispresented as the anal-retentive need for order, a disease of inflexible rituals that gives the character an almost inhuman ability to notice details. In reality, OCD is an anxiety disorder that is characterized by the presence of (surprise!) obsessions and compulsions. Rather than a superpower, OCD can be disabling.

Obsessions are recurrent and persistent unwanted thoughts or urges. Obsessions can range from thinking they left the door unlocked to fearing that they're going to kill someone. Oftentimes, your character will *know* their thoughts are illogical and will try to ignore or suppress them or get rid of them by performing the compulsion.

Compulsions are the actions your character has to take to get rid of those obsessions. For instance, if they can't stop thinking they left the stove on, they might go back and check the stove. If they feel dirty or contaminated, they might wash their hands.

We all have obsessive thoughts and compulsions to some degree. For example, you're standing in line at airport security and keep thinking that you've forgotten your passport. You know you haven't, because you used it to check-in, but you can't stop worrying that you've somehow lost it. So, you keep touching the passport inside your purse/wallet, just to make sure it's there. Obsession = worry that you've forgotten your passport. Compulsion = touching the passport to reassure yourself that it's still there.

The difference for someone with OCD is that these unwanted, obsessive thoughts are distressing, distracting, and can take up a lot of their timethoughts are distressing, distracting, and can take up a lot of their time

   NATALIE DALE, MD

24. CANCER

Xavier's mom died of colon cancer his freshman year of high school; she was only 43 at the time. Ever since he's been terrified of developing cancer himself, so he checks his stool regularly, looking for changes in size, shape, or color. His friends made fun of him, once they discovered his "log-log," where he's tracked every bowel movement since his mom was diagnosed. It's been more than ten years since her death, but he can't help but feel a twinge of anxiety every time he uses the toilet.

BACKGROUND

ONE OF MY BIGGEST PET peeves is when people talk about "cancer" like it's one disease. News flash; it's not! There are more than a hundred different types of cancer that all affect different organs in different people in different ways. Some cancers target babies and some that target the elderly. There are cancers that are inevitably fatal, cancers that make little-to-no impact, and cancers that can be cured with a small procedure. I could write an entire book titled "The Writer's Guide to Cancer," and still not cover everything.

All this means is that if you're going to give one of your characters cancer, you're going to have to be specific. And no, "breast cancer" doesn't cut it. To understand why let's start with some definitions.

WHAT IS CANCER?

Cancer, at its most basic, is an overgrowth of cells. Normally, cells have a lifecycle; they're born, they live, they replicate, and they die. Cancer cells are really good at the replicating part and not so good at the dying part. As they multiply and multiply, they form ginormous globs of cells called tumors. As the tumors grow, they begin to spread into nearby tissue, then further out into the body in a process called *metastasis*.

> Not all tumors are cancerous. A benign tumor doesn't invade into neighboring tissue and doesn't grow back after being removed

Not all cancers follow this exact formula, of course. Some cancers, like leukemia, don't form tumors at all, instead of proliferating within the bloodstream. Some are so slow to invade neighboring tissue that they aren't even considered cancer, though they can develop into cancer if given enough time.

SCREENING

Because his mother was diagnosed with cancer at age 38, Xavier is told he'll need to start getting screening colonoscopies starting at age 28. Preparing for the procedure is torturous; he can't eat, can't drink anything but PEG and water until he's pooping so frequently it feels more like he's peeing out of his a$$. By the time the doctor arrives and gives him the sedative before the procedure, Xavier is more than ready to go to sleep.

Polyethylene Glycol (PEG) is a potent laxative.

Cancer screening is a good way to catch (and treat) cancer early. However, not all cancers can be screened for. And not everyone needs screenings. Here are some basics on the most common types of cancer screening:

- **Breast Cancer:** Screening with mammograms starting around age 40*

- **Cervical Cancer:** Screened with pap smear starting at age 21

*Or younger if your character has certain inherited conditions.

- **Colorectal Cancer:** Screened with colonoscopy starting around age 45*

- **Lung Cancer:** Heavy smokers between the ages 50 & 80 are given a one-time, low-dose chest CT

- **Skin Cancer:** Annual visual examination

Most other cancers have not shown any advantage to screening.

When Xavier wakes up, the doctor tells him that they found—and removed several polyps from his colon. She tells him that the polyps looked benign, but they won't know for sure until the pathology results come in.

Doctors avoid giving cancer diagnoses over the phone. But COVID-19 is changing the landscape of doctor-patient interaction.

NAMING CANCERS

CELLULAR ORIGIN

After what feels like the longest 72 hours of his life, Xavier's doctor calls and tells him to come into the office for results. Xavier is shaking with nerves by the time the doctor walks into the sterile room. She gets straight to the point. Two of the polyps were benign, but the third was cancerous. He has colorectal carcinoma, just like his mom.

Cancer is named based on the type of cell that is growing out of control; breast cancer is caused by an overgrowth of breast cells, gastric (stomach) cancer is caused by the overgrowth of stomach cells, etc. But it gets even more specific, depending on the exact type of cell that is cancerous. Take breast cancer, for example. Your character could have *ductal carcinoma in situ (DCIS)*, a non-invasive cancer* of the milk ducts, which is highly treatable and rarely fatal. Or they could be *inflammatory breast cancer (IBC)*, a highly aggressive disease that targets the skin and lymphatic system. Both are breast cancer, but with very different treatment and prognosis.

*DCIS is actually classified as pre-cancerous, if you want to be technical about it.

STAGING CANCER

The doctor lets Xavier cry. When he's no longer hiccupping, she gently tells him that there's more. The polyp that was removed didn't have clear margins—they weren't able to remove all the cancer in the colonoscopy. He's going to need surgery to remove part of his colon.

Once you know what type of cancer your character has, you need to figure out what stage the cancer is. You've probably heard the phrase "Stage 4 cancer," but what does that mean? While the exact definitions vary by the type of cancer, most cancers can be staged using the TNM system: Tumor, Node, Metastasis.

Tumor refers to a primary tumor; how big it is and how deeply it's embedded itself in the surrounding tissue. **Node** refers to the lymph nodes; how many of the surrounding lymph nodes have detectable cancer cells. **Metastasis** is whether the cancer has spread to other parts of the body. The TNM system is used after surgical resection of the tumor and surrounding lymph nodes; if your character hasn't had surgery, they can't know the TNM score. If the cancer has spread to multiple organs, the exact TNM score might not matter.

After the surgery, Xavier can barely sit still, despite the pain meds and the large scar across his stomach. He's scared of what the results might show, petrified that he's going to follow in his mother's footsteps. He's so anxious, that he barely sleeps. When the doctor arrives to tell him the results, his hands are shaking so hard that he drops the remote while trying to turn off the television. His doctor tells him that the surgery was successful; the margins were clear, the cancerous cells were a moderately aggressive grade, and they didn't find any cancerous cells in his lymph nodes, nor evidence for metastasis. All this put together means he has stage I colorectal carcinoma.

The TNM score isn't the only factor considered when determining a cancer's stage. Imaging, such as CT scans or a PET scan can help show the size of an unresected tumor and can show "hot spots" of tumor activity. Microscope evaluation of cells taken from the tumor can be graded based on the cell's morphology. Blood tests looking for cellular markers can further narrow down the exact type of cancer your character has been struck with. Once the doctor has all the information they can get, they'll determine the cancer's stage.

Most cancer stages range from Stage I to Stage IV, though some cancers (including breast cancer) have a Stage 0.

- **Stage 0** (*In situ*): The cancer is *in situ*, meaning that it hasn't spread at all into the surrounding tissue. It is very easy to treat— once surgically removed, it won't grow back. Stage 0 is considered a precursor to cancer, rather than cancer itself.

  > **Ductal carcinoma in situ** (DCIS) is a form of Stage 0 breast cancer.

- **Stage 1** (*Localized*): The tumor is still very small and has not penetrated deeply into the surrounding tissue. It has not spread to any lymph nodes or to the rest of the body.

- **Stage 2** (*Regional*): The tumor is larger, has penetrated more deeply through the surrounding layers of tissue, and/or has spread to nearby lymph nodes.

- **Stage 3** (*Advance Regional*): Cancer cells have spread into more lymph nodes or have penetrated through more layers of tissue.

- **Stage 4** (*Metastatic*): The cancer has spread to faraway parts of the body.

When the doctor tells him that she doesn't recommend chemotherapy at this time, he jumps up and pulls her into a hug. Unlike his mom, they caught his cancer early. He's going to be OK!

Only once you know the specific type of cancer your character has AND its stage, are you ready to start delving into their symptoms and treatment. So, let's take a look at what kinds of cancers are out there.

TYPES OF CANCER

Another pet peeve of mine is that all women in fiction seem to get breast cancer. And nothing else. What do Samantha (<u>Sex & the City</u>), Xiomara (<u>Jane the Virgin</u>), and Kate (<u>Firefly Lane</u>) have in common? Yup, breast cancer. Can you think of a single female character with colon cancer? Lung cancer? Me neither.

Hazel (<u>The Fault in Our Stars</u>) has thyroid cancer.

MOST COMMON CANCERS

Breast cancer *is* the most common cause of cancer—both in women and in general. Worldwide, it accounted for 2.26 million new cases in 2020. However, lung cancer (2.21 million cases) and colorectal cancer (1.93 million cases) aren't far behind.[1] Let's take a look at a bunch of different causes of cancer in the US:[2]

Men can get breast cancer too! It's rare (less than 1% of all breast cancer is diagnosed in men), but since there's no screening, it's usually caught later and has a lower survival rate.[3]

	Cancer Site[2]	New Cases in US	Deaths	5-year Survival
1	Breast	281550	43600	90.30%
2	Prostate	248530	34130	97.50%
3	Lung	325760	131880	21.70%
4	Colorectal	149500	52980	64.70%
5	Melanoma (Skin)*	106110	7180	93.30%
6	Bladder	83730	17200	77.10%
7	Lymphoma (Blood)	81560	20720	73.20%
8	Kidney	76080	13780	75.60%
9	Uterus	66570	12940	81.10%
10	Leukemia (Bone Marrow)	61090	23660	65.00%
11	Pancreas	60,430	48220	10.80%

	Cancer Site[2]	New Cases in US	Deaths	5-year Survival
12	Thyroid	44280	2200	98.30%
13	Liver	42230	30230	20.30%
14	Stomach	26560	11180	32.40%
15	Brain	24530	18600	32.60%
16	Ovary	21410	13770	49.10%
17	Esophagus	19260	15530	19.90%
18	Cervix	14480	4290	66.30%
19	Testis	9470	440	94.90%
20	Bone	3610	2060	66.80%

I want you to take a look at that last column, the 5-year survival rate. It's the percentage of people who are still alive five years after their initial diagnosis. The higher the number, the better the chances that your character will survive. Breast cancer's 5-year survival rate is over 90%, while lung cancer barely tops 20%. Scroll down a bit further, and you'll see that less than 11% of people with pancreatic cancer are alive five years later.

Of course, these are just vague numbers based on the cancer site, rather than the specific form of cancer. Take brain cancer, for example. If your middle-aged character is diagnosed with an *astrocytoma* (the most common form of brain cancer) their 5-year survival rate is 46%.[5] But if they're diagnosed with a *glioblastoma*, their 5-year survival rate drops to 9%.[5] If they're older, say, over fifty-five, survival rates drop even further.

> *The most common cancer in the US is skin cancer.[4] However, since most skin cancer is slow growing and easy to treat, it's often excluded from prevalence statistics. The exception is melanoma, which can be deadly.

What this means for your writing is that you have to think good and hard about what you want your character's diagnosis to mean. Is it a death sentence that will hang over their head, or a scary period of their life that they will pull through? Do they have a common diagnosis with lots of access to services and support, or do they have a stigmatized diagnosis (more on this later) that they hide from their friends? In other words, let your story dictate the diagnosis you give to your character.

The older your character is, the more likely they are to develop cancer. However, that isn't to say that younger characters can't develop cancer. Some cancers are more likely to be diagnosed at a younger age. Different cancers are more likely to appear at different periods in a person's life. Of course, these aren't hard and fast rules, just general guidelines.

Infancy (<2): No one likes to think about cancer in babies, but it happens. Most of the time, it's due to genetic mutations, whether inherited (passed on from parents) or sporadic (occurring during fetal development). The most common cancers seen in infants are:

- Neuroblastoma

    o Most common cancer in infants; rare in kids older than 10.[6]

- Retinoblastoma

- Brain tumors

CHILDHOOD (2-14):

- Leukemia

    o Most commonly Acute Lymphocytic Leukemia (ALL)

> ALL is strongly associated with Down syndrome.

- Brain & Spinal cord tumors:

    o Tend to affect the *cerebellum,* the part of the brain that coordinates movement

- Wilm's Tumor (kidney tumor)

- Lymphoma:

    o Non-Hodgkin Lymphoma most common

- Embryonal Rhabdomyosarcoma

ADOLESCENTS & YOUNGER ADULTS (15-35):

- Brain cancers:

    o Astrocytomas and oligodendrogliomas are most common.[7]

- Leukemia:

    o Most commonly Acute Myeloid Leukemia (AML)[8]

- Bone cancers

    o Ewing sarcoma (younger teens and tweens)

    o Osteosarcoma (older teens and young adults)

- Germ cell tumors:

    o Teratoma (male or female)

    o Seminoma (male only)

- Lymphoma (Hodgkin Lymphoma)

- Thyroid cancer (teens and young women)

- Rhabdomyosarcoma (teens and young adults)

- Testicular cancer (ages 20-34)

The 5-year survival of people with AML is only 26% (68% if they're younger than 20).[8]

ADULTS (30-64):

- Breast Cancer

- Colorectal cancer

- Cervical cancer

- Melanoma

- Brain tumors (>40 years)

    o Benign: Meningiomas

    o Malignant: Gliomas

Nearly half of all cancer in women under 65 is due to breast cancer.[1]

Breast and colorectal cancer in adults under 40 are almost always due to an inherited genetic syndrome, such as BRCA1/2 or Lynch syndrome.[9]

A few years later, Xavier gets the call that his Aunt Veda, his mother's little sister, has a brain tumor. It's a glioblastoma and it's highly aggressive. He flies out to see her several times, but she's changed, his previously vibrant auntie is somber and bleak. She dies less than a year after her diagnosis. At the funeral, he overhears his rabbi talking with some relatives about his maternal uncle, who had cut ties with the family long ago. Apparently, he had also died recently, of colon cancer, just like his sister. And Xavier's grandmother had died young

OLDER ADULTS (65+):

- Skin cancer: basal cell carcinoma and squamous cell carcinoma

- Breast cancer

- Prostate cancer

- Lung cancer

- Colorectal cancer

- Pancreatic

- Ovarian cancer

- Leukemia: Chronic Myelogenous Leukemia (CML)

- Multiple Myeloma

> Elderly men are more likely to get cancer than elderly women.

CANCER SYMPTOMS

Xavier returned to his doctor and told her what he'd learned at the funeral. His doctor ordered a genetic test, which was positive for Lynch Syndrome, a genetic mutation that increases your risk of cancer, particularly colon cancer.

Every cancer presents differently. Even the same type of cancer (i.e., breast cancer) can result in very different symptoms depending on the exact type of cancer (i.e., DCIS vs. IBC), the age and gender of your character, and how far the cancer has spread. Cancers can sometimes present with vague, non-specific signs, like fatigue and a general feeling of unwellness (*malaise*). Often, people are diagnosed based on screening tests, such as a mammogram or colonoscopy, and feel completely fine.

> People of Ashkenazi Jewish descent are at higher risk of genetic diseases, including Lynch Syndrome.

Once you've decided what type of cancer you want to foist upon your character, you'll need to do your research to figure out what exactly their symptoms will be—if they have any symptoms at all. But don't worry, I won't leave you hanging. Here's a list of some of the most common cancers, and their presentation.

BONE CANCER

- Bone pain and swelling that's worse at night or with activity

- Older teenagers with pain in extremities = *Osteosarcoma*

- Younger teenagers with pain in pelvis, ribs & shoulder = *Ewing's Sarcoma*

BRAIN CANCER

- Changes in personality or behavior

- Nausea & vomiting

- New or worsening daily headaches, particularly in the morning

- Poor coordination or trouble balancing

- Seizures

- Vision changes: blurry vision, double vision, or loss of vision in one eye

> Poor coordination may show up as recurrent falls.

BREAST CANCER

- Often asymptomatic and found during routine screening mammograms

- Breast pain

- Changes in nipple: discharge (other than milk), nipple pulling inwards or inverting

- Lump in breast or armpit, or change in breast shape

- Redness, swelling of breast with thickening and pitting of skin = *inflammatory breast cancer* (IBC)

> Breast skin changes in IBC are called "Peau d'orange"—French for orange peel.

COLORECTAL CANCER

Shortly after finding out about his diagnosis of Lynch Syndrome, Xavier loses his job as an HVAC technician. He gets by on odd jobs, but he can't afford health insurance anymore. Two years go by, then three. He still keeps his "log-log", and he notices that his stools are getting thin and stringy, and harder to push out. They're also darker in color, and sticky, like tar. He stops pooping regularly, becoming more and more constipated. Finally, he stops pooping altogether. His belly bloats up until it hurts so much that he can't walk. Finally, he goes into the ED, where he's diagnosed with a bowel obstruction and taken straight to surgery.

- Asymptomatic early in the disease

    o Diagnosed on routine screening colonoscopy

    o Polyps found on colonoscopy can be cancerous, precancerous, or benign

- Abdominal pain

    o May be caused by a bowel obstruction

> Colorectal cancer is the #1 cause of large bowel obstructions.[9]

- Changes in bowel habits (constipation, diarrhea, 'pencil-thin' stool)

- Blood in stool

    o Bright red = rectum or descending colon

    o Dark, tarry = ascending colon

    o May not be able to see blood; instead, your character may become anemic from blood loss, and will need a test to determine if there's blood in the stool.

- Weight loss

LEUKEMIA

<u>Acute Leukemias (primarily children and young adults)</u>

- Bone pain, particularly in the legs and lower back

    o Children who can't talk sometimes develop a limp due the pain

- Fatigue

- Frequent infections that don't get better with treatment

- Painless, swollen lymph nodes

    o Particularly in armpit, above collarbone, along neck, and in groin

    o Can cause trouble breathing, due swelling of *thymus*, an organ in the chest where white blood cells congregate

- Pale skin, easy bleeding, and bruising

    o Due to *anemia* (low red blood cells)

    o Lots of nosebleeds

- Stomachache, decreased appetite, and weight loss

- Unexplained fevers

Chronic Leukemias (Primarily older adults)

- Often no symptoms; found on routine blood tests

- Painless lymph node swelling and an enlarged spleen

- Recurrent infections

- Fatigue, weight loss, and pale skin that bruises easily are all signs that the disease is advanced

> Chronic leukemia may sound benign but it's a ticking clock. Eventually, it'll cause a **blast crisis:** a life-threatening increase in immature blood cells that don't function properly. A character with a blast crisis will likely die of infection or hemorrhage—author's choice.

LUNG CANCER

- *Clubbing* = widening of the tips of the fingers due to chronic under-oxygenation

- Cough (including coughing up blood), and trouble breathing or wheezing

- Recurrent pneumonia

- Decreased appetite, weakness, and weight loss are signs that the disease is late stage

> Coughing up blood = **hemoptysis**

- Has some crazy complications called *paraneoplastic syndromes* that can do anything from cause extreme bone pain to muscle weakness.

    o If you're going to give your character lung cancer, particularly Small Cell Lung Cancer (SCLC), make sure to look up the appropriate paraneoplastic syndromes if you want to give your character a really hard time.

LYMPHOMA

Hodgkin's Lymphoma (Young Adults (15-30)) and Older Adults (>50))

- Dry cough

- Fever, weight loss, and night sweats = B symptoms

    o Presence of B symptoms is a bad sign (indicates worse prognosis)

- Itchy, dry skin and/or rash

- Painless lymph node swelling is the most common sign

    o Nodes in neck, above collarbone, armpit, and in chest are the most commonly involved.

    o Swollen lymph nodes in chest can be seen on CT scan, used to stage progress

Non-Hodgkin's Lymphoma (Children and Older Adults)

- Belly pain or fullness (due liver swelling)

- Painless lymph node swelling in neck, above collarbone, and in armpit

    o Enlargement happens quickly

- Recurrent infections

- B symptoms rare

OVARIAN CANCER (PRIMARILY OLDER WOMEN)

- Early stages almost always show no symptoms.

- Late-stage symptoms include pelvic pain or discomfort, weight loss, constipation, frequent urination, and swelling or bloating of the belly.

PANCREATIC CANCER

- Usually starts with vague, dull abdominal pain.

- Depression

- Mild diabetes-like symptoms (high blood sugars)

- Tiredness and weakness

- Weight loss, due to both decreased appetite and decreased intestinal absorption of food.

> Early symptoms of pancreatic cancer are vague and hard to diagnose. Once the diagnosis is clear, the cancer has usually progressed too far to be cured.

- Yellowing of the skin and whites of the eyes (*Jaundice*).

PROSTATE CANCER

The early stages of prostate cancer usually don't have any symptoms. That's why doctors perform a *digital rectum exam* (DRE)—put their fingers up their patient's rectum—they're looking for signs of prostate enlargement, hardening, or asymmetry. Believe me, it isn't because they enjoy it.

- Late symptoms occur due to the enlarging prostate blocking the urethra, causing difficulty or pain with urination, as well as needing to go more often (*urinary frequency*).

> Prostate cancer is rarely fatal. The saying is that prostate cancer is a cancer you die with, not a cancer you die from.

- Women cannot get prostate cancer

  o Unless your character is a transgender woman. Then, even if she's had gender-affirming surgery, she'll retain her prostate, and thus can develop prostate cancer, though her risk is lower than that of cis men.[10]

SKIN CANCERS
Melanoma

- A new (or growing) dark spot on the skin that is asymmetric, has irregular borders and shading, and large.

- No systemic effects.

- Can metastasize anywhere including the brain, even after successful removal.[4]

Nonmelanoma Skin Cancers

- *Basal Cell Carcinoma*

  o Most common type of skin cancer: 36 million people are diagnosed in the US every year.[4]

  o Pink, shiny bump, or patch of skin. May have flat scar-like tissue (yellowy-white) around it or an ulcer-like sore at the center.

  o Very rarely fatal.

- *Squamous Cell Carcinoma*

  o Scaly or crusty patch that bleeds occasionally.

  o Also rarely fatal.

TREATMENT

Treatment for cancer usually involves some combination of surgery, chemotherapy, and radiation therapy. Not all cancers require all three modalities—your character's treatment will be decided based on the specific type of cancer, (i.e., small cell lung cancer, or HER2 positive breast cancer), the stage of cancer, and its histological grade, as well as your character's general health and life expectancy. Some will have only chemotherapy, while others will require only surgical resection. Still others may require all three modalities.

SURGERY

When Xavier wakes up, the surgeon tells him that he had a large tumor obstructing his ascending colon, which they removed. But the tumor had spread, and there were several other tumorous lesions; they had to remove the whole colon. Xavier looks down and sees a clear plastic bag filled with brown liquid lying against his belly. He's had a total colectomy; he's going to be pooping in a bag for the rest of his life.

The first step in many cancer treatments is to get a biopsy of the tumor. This procedure helps the oncologist know exactly what type of cancer they're dealing with, and how aggressive it is. Biopsies can be as simple as a "hole-punch" biopsy (used for melanoma) to complicated procedures requiring big a$$ needles, such as those used for transthoracic lung biopsies. Scoping technology, like a colonoscopy or fiberoptic bronchoscopy, can also be used. Some biopsies even require surgery.

Cancer surgery isn't just about cutting out the tumor. When surgeons resect a tumor, they cut a wide swath around the tissue surrounding the tumor. These are called the tumor's margins. "Clear margins" means the cancerous cells are completely contained in the sample that was removed. Sometimes, surgeons will cut out a sample mid-surgery and have it sent to the pathology lab for analysis so that they know they have clear margins before they do anything else.

The other important aspect of cancer surgeries is to remove all lymph nodes that the cancer could have infiltrated. Since doctors can't tell if the cancer has invaded a lymph node just by looking at it, they usually just go through and remove all the ones in the immediate area.

The doctors also had to remove nearly twenty lymph nodes. The pathology report isn't back yet, but the surgeon is pretty sure at least a few lymph nodes were involved. On the bright side, they didn't see any signs of metastasis, but they'll need to do more tests to be sure.

After surgery, all the tissue (the tumor, the margins, and the lymph nodes) are analyzed by a pathologist. The pathology results will detail the exact type of cancerous cell, any tumor markers that may help for treatment, the aggressiveness of the tumor, and how far throughout the body it has spread. But this analysis takes time—somewhere between a few days and a week—and those may be the hardest days of your character's life.

CHEMOTHERAPY

The doctor tells Xavier he is going to need adjuvant chemotherapy once he's recovered from surgery. A few weeks later, Xavier is admitted directly to the hospital for chemotherapy with a drug regimen. The full name is long, Xavier can't remember it all, but the doctors just call it Folfox. He's given an IV infusion of the drug. Within hours, he feels awful; nauseated, and tired, with a pounding headache. He develops a rash on the palms of his hands and sores on the inside of his mouth. The nurse keeps telling him he's doing great, but Xavier secretly wonders if dying might be easier.

Chemotherapy is a drug treatment that targets (and kills) fast-growing cells, such as cancer cells. Unfortunately, hair, skin, blood cells, and the cells lining your airways and gastrointestinal tract (mouth, esophagus, stomach, intestines) are also fast-growing and can be inadvertently targeted. This can lead to a host of side effects, including hair loss, mouth sores, nausea/vomiting, bleeding/easy bruising, light sensitivity, and constipation or diarrhea. Whole-body symptoms, such as fatigue, weight loss, and pain, are also common. If the chemotherapy affects the bone marrow (*myelosuppression*), your character won't have the blood cells needed to clot or fight off infection, so they'll have easy bruising, breathlessness, and an increased risk of infection.

Your character's chemotherapy regimen will be specific to them and their disease, and the side effects they experience will vary as well. Some people will lose their hair and vomit their guts up, while others may have very few side effects of the chemo.

As he nears the end of his chemo, Xavier is exhausted. His mouth is full of sores so that it hurts to eat; not that he's wanted to eat much, since he's always nauseated. He's lost almost twenty pounds and spends most of his days napping. His gums bleed, his nose bleeds, and if he so much as brushes an arm against a table, he'll develop a bruise the size of Texas. He's had pneumonia twice, and once got a skin infection after a blister on his heel failed to heel. When the treatment started, he felt painful pins and needles in his fingers and toes; now, he can barely feel his hands and feet at all.

RADIATION

Radiation kills cells by damaging their DNA, making it impossible for them to continue dividing. Like with chemotherapy, rapidly dividing cells—such as cancer cells—are the most heavily affected. But since all cells need their DNA, all cells can be affected.

For that reason, radiation therapy is both absurdly high dose and extremely targeted. The dose of radiation given over a course of treatment for breast cancer is the equivalent radiation of 600,000 chest x-rays.[11] In order to avoid killing every cell in your character's body, that radiation needs to be targeted specifically at the cancer cells. This means that when your character shows up for their radiation treatment, most of the time will be spent properly positioning them, using boosters and blocks, and rolled up blankets to make sure that they're in the exact position that will allow the radiation to hit the cancerous cells and little else. They also won't get all 600,000 x-rays all at once—the radiation will be dosed out in weekly or biweekly treatments lasting over several months.[11]

External beam radiation uses a machine to direct the radiation.[12]

Internal beam radiation uses radiation placed in the body, such as a surgically- implanted radioactive capsule.[12]

Not every cancer is treated with radiation; in fact, colon cancer is rarely treated with radiation, because it usually responds well to chemotherapy and surgery alone. In contrast, larynx and prostate cancer are often treated with radiation alone—no chemotherapy, no surgery. However, many other cancers, like breast, lung, and rectal cancer, use a combination of chemotherapy, surgery, and radiation therapy. If radiation is used in conjunction with other treatment modalities, it is called "adjuvant radiation."

REAL TALK: STIGMA & CANCER

*After six months on the FOLFOX, Xavier undergoes a series of tests; blood tests, CT scans, and even a PET scan to look for hyperactive cells. Everything looks normal. They tell him he's in remission. Xavier is grateful, but also scared. He's survived this long off social security disability and state Medicaid, but now that he's in remission, he'll be expected to go back to work. But he can't imagine having enough energy to go back to his old job. Plus, how could he get through crawlspaces with a colostomy bag? What would his coworkers think of him walking around with a bag full of literal sh*t?*

Having cancer, any cancer, can be a stigmatizing and isolating experience. Many people with cancer avoid telling their families about their diagnosis because they don't want them to worry. Alternatively, they may avoid telling others because they don't want to be pitied.

Certain cancers, however, tend to have more (or just different) types of stigmas. If your character has testicular or prostate cancer, he may feel like less of a man, while a woman who had a mastectomy may feel as if she has lost her femininity. A trans woman diagnosed with prostate cancer may feel as if her very identity has been compromised.

And then, there are the "lifestyle" cancers, with risk factors associated with lifestyle choices. People with these types of cancers often face a higher level of stigmatization and judgment. This is particularly true for lung cancer, which is strongly associated with cigarette smoking. How would your character feel if they told a friend they'd just been diagnosed with lung cancer, and the friend's first response was, "well, did you smoke?" Unfortunately, it's all too common.

> Anal cancer is also highly stigmatized, particularly for its association with gay men.

BREAKING DOWN THE CLICHÉ: CANCERSPLOITATION

"I'm sorry Bob, but your work has been abysmal lately. Coming in late, missing deadlines…"

"I know, Boss, but you see, my—my niece, Penny. She's been diagnosed with cancer."

"Oh. I'm sorry to hear that, Bob. I didn't know."

"Well, you didn't ask, did you?"

"No, I suppose I didn't."

"So, you'll give me an extension on that project, then?"

"Sure, Bob."

"And, uh, I'm gonna have to leave work early today. Jenny's got her first round of chemo, so I want to be there for her."

"…I thought her name was Penny."

Cancersploitation is when a writer uses cancer as a plot point, intended to pull at the reader's emotions. It may make an unsympathetic character more sympathetic

     NATALIE DALE, MD

or explain away some questionable choices. What it *doesn't* do is delve into the complicated psychosocial or medical aspects of a cancer diagnosis.

There's a whole host of tropes related to cancersploitation. Many are related to impending death causing a character to re-examine their life, whether that means completing their bucket list, mending bridges with loved ones, or deciding not to give a f*ck about what other people think. Falling into one of these tropes isn't necessarily bad—I've talked with cancer survivors who have said they identify with some of these feelings—but be aware that you're doing it.

Other cancer tropes are less savory. The "sick girl" trope, in which a young woman is given a terminal illness (usually cancer) solely to make the protagonist (usually male) sad is old, tired, and ready to be retired.[13] Similarly, the "littlest cancer patient" trope, in which a small child is introduced for the sake of tugging heartstrings and maybe dropping some gems of wisdom along the way, inevitably fails to portray the complexities of a childhood cancer diagnosis. The trouble with these two tropes, in particular, is that the people with cancer are one-dimensional side characters solely defined by their diagnosis. Don't do that.

Your book is not a medical documentary—you don't have to get absolutely every medical detail right to avoid falling into the trap of cancersploitation. But you do need a good reason for why you're giving your character cancer. And you need to show the messy realities of a cancer diagnosis—physical, social, and psychological.

25. DEMENTIA AND DELIRIUM

"Hi Yeye," Yan calls, pushing aside the green hospital curtain, "I brought you..."

She trails off, her words sticking to her throat. Her grandfather looks so small in the white hospital bed, lying on the opposite side of the hip he'd just had surgery on. His thick white hair is shaved on the right side of his head, and she can see the shiny staples holding his scalp in place. She swallows hard; her mother told her that he broke a hip when he fell, but she hadn't said anything about hitting his head.

Yeye seems to notice her discomfort. "Yan," he says with a smile bright as the sunflowers he planted around his porch, "I'm so glad you're here. And you brought a phalaenopsis!"

Smiling, Yan sets the brightly colored orchid on the windowsill and settles into the chair beside him.

BACKGROUND

DEMENTIA IS A PROGRESSIVE AND unrelenting disease characterized by the loss of intellectual function, particularly memory. Often, dementia presents with a loss of autobiographical information—if you need your character to forget their name, or the name of their child, dementia is a better culprit than a head injury (See *Ch. 12: Traumatic Brain Injuries*).

In dementia, the level of consciousness is preserved; your character will maintain their normal levels of energy and activity. Only cognition is impaired.

Delirium, on the other hand, is a sudden decrease in cognitive function accompanied by altered consciousness. It is a form of altered mental status. Most importantly, it is a symptom, not a disease itself, as delirium is almost always caused by an acute medical condition or biological disturbance.

DELIRIUM

The sun has long set before Yan has convinced herself that her grandfather is doing as well as he claims. Stomach growling, she pops down to the cafeteria to grab a late dinner. But when she returns, her grandfather is surrounded by men and women in scrubs, holding him down. He thrashes, hurling insults, pointing repeatedly at garbage, and screaming something about how they shouldn't allow dogs in the hospital. Tina watches in horror as someone injects something into the saggy skin of his upper arm.

"What are you doing?"

"He's insisting he needs to get up," the nurse snaps, "and he really can't do that right now. He just got out of surgery this morning. He's going to pull his stitches out, or worse. I know it's just sundowning, but we had to stop him before he hurts himself."

Yeye sags back in the bed, his eyes dull and glazed over. The nurses hold on for a few more moments, then release him. Yan runs forward.

"Get away from him," she snaps. She hates confrontation, but she's going to have to speak to someone about this unacceptable behavior. And what was he saying about the nurses bringing a dog into his room? Did he think the garbage can was a dog?

> A **hallucination** is seeing something that isn't there.
>
> An **illusion** is incorrectly interpreting a stimulus, such as hearing footsteps and thinking it's gun fire.

Delirium is an acute change in cognition and consciousness. It waxes and wanes, changing by the hour. Your character may be completely cogent one minute and muttering gibberish the next. They may be irritated, anxious, fearful, or even paranoid. Alternately, they could be sleepy and difficult to wake. They may have hallucinations or illusions.

Delirium can happen at any time, but it's more common in hospitalized patients, particularly the elderly. Causes of delirium include infection, drug intoxication or withdrawal, fever, medications (particularly steroids, narcotics, and sedatives), trauma, burns, dehydration, and malnutrition. If your character has recently had surgery, they are at a particularly high risk of developing delirium.

Sundowning is a form of delirium that sets in at night. Your character may be calm and cooperative all day, then run around pulling out their IV and accusing the night nurse of being a Nazi once the sun sets. It's a frustrating and difficult situation for staff, particularly when the family—who isn't there

> Physical restraints are a last resort. Patients hate them, and they're a lot of paperwork.

at night—doesn't believe it's happening. As a writer, you can use sundowning to sow chaos and heighten inter-character tensions.

Delirium is diagnosed clinically with a mental status exam and treated by addressing the underlying cause. If your character is very agitated, they may be given a sedating medication or placed in physical restraints.

DEMENTIA VS. DELIRIUM

	Delirium	Dementia
Consciousness	Altered	Normal
Onset	Acute	Insidious
Course	Fluctuating	Progressive
Hallucinations	Often	Rarely
Reversible	Yes	Rarely

DEMENTIA

After a few days in the hospital, her grandfather is released home. Yan, still finishing her last semester of college, vows to make time to visit every other weekend.

Everyone has heard of Alzheimer's Disease, the insidious disease of the elderly that steals away the memories of our grandparents. Alzheimer's is common and heartbreaking. But it isn't the only form of dementia out there. If you're looking to give a character dementia, take a step back and ask yourself *why* they need this debilitating disease. Are you looking to add strain to an MC trying to care for an elderly parent? Do you need to hide key information inside an inaccessible memory? Or do you need your MC to be slowly losing their grip on reality?

Once you know your answer, take a look at the options below and decide what works best for your story.

Dementia	Age of Onset	Primary Symptoms	Course	Diagnosis	Reversible?
Alzheimer's Disease	Older (65+)	Memory loss, decreased spatial awareness, poor concentration	Progressive	Clinical	No
Chronic Subdural Hematoma	Older (65+)	Memory loss, poor concentration, headache, nausea	Progressive	Brain CT	Yes
Creutzfeldt Jakob Disease	Any	Memory loss, movement changes, muscle spasms	Progressive	Clinical	No
Dementia with Lewy Bodies	Middle-Aged (50+)	Hallucinations, memory loss, movement changes, sleep disorder	Fluctuating	Clinical	No
Frontotemporal Dementia	Middle-Aged (40)	Behavior & Personality Changes. Loss of Language	Progressive	Clinical	No
Normal Pressure Hydrocephalus	Older (65+)	Memory loss, walking difficulty, loss of bladder control	Progressive	Brain MRI	Yes
Pseudodementia	Any	Depression, apathy, memory loss	Progressive	Clinical	Yes
Vascular Dementia	Older (65+)	Memory loss, poor concentration, stroke symptoms	Stepwise	Brain MRI	No

IRREVERSIBLE CAUSES OF DEMENTIA

ALZHEIMER'S DISEASE

We're going to start here because it's both well-known and common. In the US, Alzheimer's is the fourth most common cause of death, and more than 10% of people over the age of 65 are afflicted.[1] The risk of Alzheimer's increases with age, though it can begin as early as age 40.

"What classes are you taking this semester?" her grandfather asks, for the third time this visit.

Yan resists the urge to roll her eyes. "I already told you, Yeye. Aquatic ecology, biostats, and a senior capstone."

His eyes light up. "Aquatic ecology, yes? You know I did my thesis on..." he hesitates, frowning. "On..."

"Macrocystis pyrifera," Yan finishes. "The giant sea kelp, I know."

Symptoms & Progression

Alzheimer's is a disease of memory loss, particularly recent memory. It begins with short-term memory loss, such as having trouble remembering names or forgetting what they just read. They might have difficulty remembering the right word or remembering where they set their keys. They'll complain of trouble concentrating, particularly in loud or social settings. Family members might note poor judgement and subtle changes in personality, like making inappropriate jokes.

As the disease progresses, the memory impairment gets worse. They'll start to forget important events or people from their past, starting with their immediate past and stretching further and further back in time. Your character may seem confused, moody, or withdrawn. To their family's consternation, they'll begin repeating the same questions over and over, and their personality changes becoming more severe. They may wander or get lost in familiar places. During this stage, your character may notice that something is wrong but may be unable to put their concerns into words. Or they might jump straight into denial, refusing to acknowledge their declining memory, even when the evidence is incontrovertible.

> People with intermediate-stage Alzheimer's shouldn't drive; they get easily lost and overwhelmed, creating a dangerous situation for themselves and others. But getting them to relinquish their driver's license is often a nightmare for everyone involved.

Late-stage Alzheimer's occurs once your character can no longer attend to their daily needs, such as cooking or bathing, so they'll need 24-hour care. Mood changes are common, particularly depression and irritability. They may even begin to have hallucinations. At this stage, your character will have trouble remembering the names of family and friends. The further back in their history the relationship extends, the more likely your character is to remember them. I had a patient who couldn't remember her daughter, but she immediately recognized her brother's best friend, whom she'd played with as a child but hadn't seen in nearly fifty years.

In the final stage of Alzheimer's, your character will be completely dependent on others, unable to feed themselves or even use the toilet without assistance. They won't be able to remember their loved ones, and in some cases may even forget their own name. They'll lose awareness of their surroundings and will gradually lose the ability to walk, sit, speak, or swallow. Death comes as a secondary complication of their debilitated state, usually infection.

Diagnosis

Alzheimer's disease is a clinical diagnosis. There are no tests or imaging that can 100% confirm the diagnosis, though a brain CT showing withering of the ridges of the brain (*cortical atrophy*) can provide some evidence. The only confirmatory test comes from a brain autopsy.

From diagnosis to death, the entire process takes somewhere between five and ten years. However, since many people are good at hiding their symptoms, diagnosis is often delayed.

Treatment

There is no cure for Alzheimer's. There are some medications, such as Aricept or Vitamin D, that can help manage symptoms, but no medication or procedure can stop the progression of the disease.

VASCULAR DEMENTIA

Vascular dementia, also called *multi-infarct dementia*, is caused by small, sequential strokes. While the functionality in Alzheimer's presents as a gradual but steady decline, vascular dementia appears stepwise in nature. Your character will suddenly get worse, then plateau. Then, they'll suddenly get worse again.

The symptoms of vascular dementia are very similar to Alzheimer's: confusion, poor concentration, memory loss, trouble making decisions and poor planning. There may also be some signs of stroke, such as unsteady gait or a facial droop.

Vascular dementia is diagnosed clinically, though your character will probably be given a brain MRI and a carotid artery ultrasound to get a better idea of the state of their arteries. They'll also check out your character's blood pressure, cholesterol, and blood sugar.

Once the damage has occurred, it cannot be undone, so the key to treatment of vascular dementia is to prevent further ministrokes. This strategy includes management of blood pressure, cholesterol, and weight.

DEMENTIA WITH LEWY BODIES

After Alzheimer's, dementia with Lewy bodies (DWLB) is the second most common type of progressive dementia. Like Alzheimer's, it is irreversible and progressive. In many ways, DWLB is very similar to Alzheimer's, with confusion, memory loss, trouble concentrating, difficulty naming and the tendency to wander and get lost. Mood changes are common, particularly depression and apathy. However, DWLB has a unique quartet of features that help distinguish it: visual hallucinations, movement changes, and fluctuating mental function.

> Robin Williams famously suffered from dementia with Lewy bodies.[4]

Visual hallucinations are often the first symptom of DWLB. They occur in up to 80% of people with the disorder, and can be highly realistic, detailed, and complex[1]; one patient famously described a little green man who sat beside him and told jokes. Your character may also have hallucinations they can hear, smell, or touch, but the textbook example is a visual hallucination.

Movement changes such as tremors, rigid muscles, slowed movements, and a shuffling, unsteady gait. Your character will also have trouble regulating bodily functions, resulting in sudden drops in blood pressure, constipation, and the inability to control urination.

Fluctuations in mental functioning can be very challenging for your character's loved ones. One moment, they may seem like themselves—the next, they're staring off into space for long periods of time. Similar to delirium, your character can shift back and forth between alert and lethargic with little warning.

REM sleep behavior disorder, in which your character physically acts out their dreams, is the fourth and final hallmark of DWLB. This disorder can lead to some fun (for the writer—not for the people suffering from it) situations; your character could beat up their spouse, break a leg trying to kick down a cement wall, or even jump out a second-story window. If they can dream it, you can make it happen.

Like with Alzheimer's, diagnosis is clinical, and there is no cure. Treatment focuses on mitigating the symptoms, particularly antipsychotics to control hallucinations.

FRONTOTEMPORAL DEMENTIA (PICK'S DISEASE)

Frontotemporal dementias (FTD) are a class of dementias characterized by changes in behavior and language. It is characterized by a steady decline in your character's ability to think and communicate. FTDs are rare in older individuals, but people ages 45-65 are just as likely to have FTD as they are to have Alzheimer's.[2] In general, people with FTD will experience gradual but persistent changes in their behavior, language, and movement. There are two main subtypes of FTD: behavior variant (bvFTD) and primary progressive aphasia (PPA).

Behavioral variant FTD (bvFTD) is characterized by prominent, often disturbing, changes in personality and behavior. If your character has bvFTD, they'll have poor judgment, limited empathy, poor impulse control, and a marked lack of foresight. bvFTD can affect people as young as 20 but is most common in people ages 50-60.[2]

I had a patient with bvFTD who was brought in by his mistress after he struck her. He was irritable, cussed often, and repeatedly sexually harassed me and any other woman who came within groping distance. Only when his mistress found his wife's number in his phone and contacted her did we find out that he was previously a soft-spoken man who never lost his temper and loved to garden. Then, three months prior, he'd left his wife and three kids in the middle of the night, vanishing without a trace.

> bvFTD is a real condition that can substitute for autobiographical amnesia. Your character can take all the actions of an amnestic (leaving their family, not acknowledging loved ones), but instead of forgetting them, they simply no longer care.

Primary progressive aphasia is the second main type of FTD. If your character has PPA, they'll lose language first. It begins subtly; your character may have trouble finding the right words or may not be able to name people or objects. They may have difficulty pronouncing words or speaking in grammatically correct sentences. There are several variants of PPA; in some, your character will retain the ability to understand words, but will not be able to express them, while in others your character might lose the knowledge of the meaning of words.

At first, your character will retain their memory as their ability to speak, read, and write deteriorates. Ultimately, they'll be left unable to utter or understand any form of language.

Because frontotemporal dementias are caused by the loss of neurons to the same area of the brain, there is a lot of overlap between the different variants. If your character has PPA, they may also exhibit personality changes and impulsive behaviors, while a character with the behavioral variant may also develop some language problems. Since the degree of severity and overlap is widely variable, you—the author—have a lot of leeway when it comes to the specific details of your character's illness.

CREUTZFELDT JAKOB DISEASE (CJD)

If you need a young character to develop a fatal disease that changes their personality, CJD is the answer to your prayers. More commonly, though inaccurately, known as "mad cow disease", CJD is caused by an infectious protein called a prion. Rarely, does that prion come from eating the brain of an infected cow, but most of the time, it's a sporadic mutation that happens for no apparent reason.[3]

CJD begins suddenly with a mix of severe neurologic and psychiatric symptoms. Your character may have difficulty walking and speaking, dizziness, numbness or pins and needles (*paresthesia*). They'll experience blurry or double vision and insomnia. Psychiatric symptoms include depression, anxiety, irritability, memory loss, withdrawal from loved ones, and even hallucinations.

As the disease progresses, your character's coordination will worsen, making walking, talking, and even swallowing difficult. Their muscles will twitch and spasm, and they'll lose control of their bowel and bladder. The memory loss will become severe, and your character will become agitated and confused. Eventually, they'll lose the ability to speak or move voluntarily.

CJD is inevitably fatal within one year, though most people die within a few months from infection.[3] There is no cure.

REVERSIBLE DEMENTIAS

Not all dementia is doom and gloom; some dementias can actually be treated. Some of them can even restore your character's mind to what it was. Not all plot twists have to be negative, right?

CHRONIC SUBDURAL HEMATOMA

"Yeye, are you OK?"

It's Yan's third visit; more than six weeks since her grandfather was hospitalized. He's been cleared by his physical therapist to go back to his daily life, but as far as Yan can tell, he's mostly just sitting in his living room watching television. He hasn't gone back to church or his volunteer job at the aquarium.

Yeye rubs at his temples. "I just have a headache, Yingtai. Can you come back tomorrow?"

Yan's frown deepens. "It's me, Yeye. Not Mom."

"Oh, yes, of course," he mutters distractedly. He starts to stand, then turns and vomits onto the floor.

Caused by the breaking of the small veins on the brain's surface, chronic subdural hematomas can be caused by relatively minor trauma, particularly if your character is elderly or an alcoholic. Your character may not even realize they've hurt themselves, and don't tell anyone about the incident, while, unbeknownst to them, blood is leaking into the area surrounding the surface of the brain.

Your character may not feel any symptoms for days or even weeks after the injury. Symptoms will begin slowly and insidiously, with memory loss and mild confusion that is easy to mistake for dementia. However, there's more to it than just the memory loss; your character should also be having headaches, nausea, and vomiting. These extra symptoms should be a red flag to your readers that something more is going on.

> *Over her grandfather's protestations, Yan drives him to urgent care. The doctor orders a brain CT, which shows a large pool of blood that has collected between his brain and the tensile covering called the dura. He's admitted to the hospital for brain surgery to stop the bleeding.*

Diagnosis is with a head CT showing the brain bleed. Treatment is surgery to stop the bleeding.

DEPRESSION (PSEUDODEMENTIA)

Depression causes a decline in cognitive function, particularly in memory and problem-solving. Severe depression can cause such severe cognitive decline that it can mimic Alzheimer's. So, how do you tell them apart? First, your character will have other signs of depression, such as tearfulness, hopelessness, changes in sleeping and eating patterns, and slowed movement. Second, the dementia-like symptoms will improve with antidepressants or electroconvulsive therapy (ECT). As the depression is treated, the signs of dementia will lift.

Pseudodementia can be really hard to diagnose, as Alzheimer's can mimic depression!

NORMAL PRESSURE HYDROCEPHALUS (NPH)

NPH is a reversible cause of dementia that, to the untrained eye, can look just like Alzheimer's Disease. In fact, some studies estimate that as many as 10% of people with other forms of dementia actually have NPH instead.[5] That's a crazy statistic, considering that NPH is totally treatable.

NPH exhibits three classic symptoms: dementia, trouble walking, and trouble controlling the bladder. It's diagnosed by assessing your character's gait and brain function, as well as a brain CT or MRI. A lumbar puncture (a needle inserted into the vertebral column to pull out cerebrospinal fluid (CSF)) is both diagnostic and therapeutic. Treatment is the surgical placement of a shunt; a drain that allows excess CSF to leak out.

SECONDARY DEMENTIAS

Some diseases cause dementia as part of the disease progression. If this happens, your character will experience the symptoms of the disease itself first; the dementia symptoms will come later. These diseases include:

- Brain mass or tumor

- HIV

- Huntington's disease

- Parkinson's disease

- Progressive multifocal leukoencephalopathy

- Syphilis (neurosyphilis)

REAL TALK: DEATH & DEMENTIA

Because death is usually due to secondary complications, it is remarkably easy to extend the life of someone in the final stages of dementia by treating the complication, whether that be pneumonia, a urinary tract infection, or a bowel obstruction. The question, then, is when does your character tell the doctors to *stop* treating those complications. After all, someone with dementia doesn't have the capacity to make these decisions, so your characters must do it for them. Do they withhold lifesaving antibiotics? Send them for a painful and confusing surgery, or allow them to die from a treatable bowel obstruction? The decisions surrounding the death of a dementia patient is a trove of interpersonal and inner conflict.

NATALIE DALE, MD

BREAKING DOWN THE CLICHÉ: ALL OLD PEOPLE HAVE MEMORY LOSS

*"Honey? Where're my glasses?" *Opens the refrigerator* "Never mind. Found them!"*

As your character ages, it's normal for them to forget things—everyone does. But that forgetfulness shouldn't be enough to impact their day-to-day life. If your character is routinely asking the same questions over and over, and having trouble following directions, you might be inadvertently giving them dementia. And dementia is never normal.

	Normal Aging	Dementia
Forgetfulness	Occasionally misplacing items	Losing things and not being able to find them
	Missing a bill payment	Inability to consistently pay bills
Language	Sometimes forgetting a word (on the tip of their tongue)	Forgetting so many words it's hard to hold a conversation
	Needing to be reminded of an acquaintance's name	Forgetting a loved one's name
Orientation	Briefly forgetting the date or day of the week	Not knowing what day or time of year it is
	Forgetting what floor of the hospital they're on	Not realizing they're in the hospital
Poor Decision-making	Falling for a scam	Repeatedly being taken advantage of
	Refusing to dress up for a special occasion	Forgetting to bathe or shower
Spatial Awareness	Getting lost in a new place	Getting lost in a familiar place
	Driving very slowly and overly cautious	Blowing through stop signs or turning in front of traffic
Sleep	Trouble falling asleep, waking up earlier	Awake and wandering (or yelling) at night, drowsy during the day

PART IV: FAQ & FINAL THOUGHTS

26. TOP 10 FREQUENTLY ASKED QUESTIONS

1. HOW DO I GIVE MY CHARACTER AMNESIA? ARE THERE DIFFERENT TYPES OF AMNESIA?

Amnesia is the loss of memory. It is usually acute, meaning it comes on quickly, and self-limited, meaning that it usually improves. Amnesia is differentiated from dementias, like Alzheimer's, in that it does not encompass other cognitive changes, such as getting lost, trouble problem solving, or difficulty finding words. In other words, amnesia is the loss of memory without any other loss of function.

There are lots of different types of amnesia. Some types of amnesia are completely normal. **Infantile amnesia**, for example, is the inability to remember childhood memories beyond the age of three or so. Everyone has this type of amnesia, though some can form memories at an earlier age than others. There are two main types of amnesia: anterograde and retrograde.

Anterograde amnesia is the inability to form new memories. It can be temporary, as in the case of alcohol-induced amnesia, or blackouts; or permanent if certain parts of the brain are damaged. Anterograde amnesia is often seen after concussions or other traumatic brain injuries. Chronic alcoholism, strokes, electroconvulsive therapy (ECT), brain inflammation, and certain brain surgeries can also cause anterograde amnesia.

Retrograde amnesia is the loss of previously formed memories. Usually, most recent memories are lost first while older memories are retained. Retrograde amnesia is the type of amnesia commonly found in Alzheimer's disease and other dementias. Other causes of retrograde amnesia include concussions and other traumatic brain injuries, stroke, chronic alcoholism, seizures, brain inflammation, and anoxic brain injury.

> Anterograde amnesia is caused by damage to the **hippocampus**—a part of the brain that consolidates memory.

Notice how there's a lot of overlap in the causes of these two types of amnesia? That's because a single insult to the brain—such as a traumatic brain injury—can cause both anterograde and retrograde memory loss. There are also other types of amnesia, which occur under specific conditions. They include:

Autobiographical amnesia is the loss of memory about ones-self. It ranges from loss of memory of specific personal events (usually traumatic) to loss of general autobiographical information (name, likes/dislikes, family members, etc.). It is very rare. There are two causes of autobiographical amnesia: diffuse brain damage (meaning your character will have other signs of major brain damage as well) or dissociative amnesia.

Dissociative amnesia is a poorly understood psychiatric disorder, brought on by trauma or stress, that causes autobiographical amnesia. It is surprisingly common, affecting ~1.8% of the population.[1] Most of the time, the autobiographical amnesia is localized, meaning that your character has lost memories of a traumatic event, or for certain periods of time (though this period can be months, or even years). Generalized autobiographical amnesia, in which your character completely forgets their entire life history and/or their personal identity, is extremely rare. When it does happen, generalized amnesia usually occurs in victims of sexual assault and in combat veterans.

If you need your character to forget who they are and wander into a new place, dissociative amnesia is probably the type of amnesia you're looking for. They don't need to be physically injured, but they do need some sort of traumatic event that can spark this condition.

Drug-induced amnesia is caused by a class of drugs called sedatives. It is a temporary effect that can cause your character to "blackout" for a certain period. How long the blackout lasts—and how your character feels afterward—depends on both the drug and the dose given. Drugs that cause amnesia include:

- **Benzodiazepines** like Xanax and Ativan.
- **Barbiturates** are used for general anesthesia, like phenobarbital and pentobarbital.
- **Date rape drugs** like "Roofies" (*Rohypnol*), GHB, and Ketamine.
- **Sleep aids** like Ambien and Lunesta.

If you want to give your character amnesia for a limited amount of time, drug-induced amnesia is probably your best bet. They'll lose memory of what they did during a period of time, but they won't have long-term cognitive effects that could hinder your story.

Post-traumatic amnesia (PTA) is a specific type of amnesia that occurs after brain injury; particularly traumatic brain injuries big enough to cause your character to lose consciousness (see *Ch. 10*). It is a form of anterograde amnesia (your character can't make new memories) that also impacts personality and executive function. Your

character will be confused and possibly distressed and anxious, or they may not be able to acknowledge that they're injured and in the hospital at all. They may not be able to recognize friends and family, and they might act out of character—suddenly becoming aggressive, violent, or unusually docile. PTA is a self-limited condition; it can last for only a few minutes, or up to hours. Very rarely, it can last months. There is no way to know for sure how long it will last.

If you're looking for a type of amnesia that is short-lived and causes your character to act unlike themselves and/or be unable to recognize their loved ones, PTA might be the best option. And if your character is emerging from a coma, they will very likely have PTA as well.

Transient global amnesia (TGA) is one of my personal favorite types of amnesia, because it can happen to anyone, lasts for 24-hours or less, and has no long-term sequelae. TGA causes a single episode of sudden memory loss. It causes both anterograde and retrograde amnesia, though autobiographical memories, and the ability to perform complex tasks are retained. If your character has TGA, they will be disoriented, confused, and possibly anxious. They'll ask the same question over and over, such as where they are or what day it is. They'll remember things that happened a long time ago but will lose the memory of recent events. TGA only occurs once in a lifetime and is more common in middle age. The exact cause of TGA is unknown; some theories believe it is a type of seizure, and others believe it is more likely to be due to low oxygen flow to the brain. However, if the symptoms occur more than once (twice at most), the memory loss is probably due to a more common neurologic disease, such as a transient ischemic attack, or mini stroke (See *Ch. 7: Stroke*).

2. HOW ARE MEDICATIONS ADMINISTERED? WHY CAN'T I JUST INJECT EVERYTHING INTO THEIR NECK?

There are lots of ways to administer a drug or medication. Some, like pills, are straightforward, but there are other fun and unique routes of administration that you might want to use on your characters. Let's start with the obvious:

ORAL
Taking medications by mouth is probably the most common route of administration.

The main advantage is that it's easy and painless. The medication passes through the stomach and into the small intestine where it is absorbed by the body. Advantages are that it's easy and painless. Disadvantages are that the drug needs to withstand the acidic environment of the stomach and that your character needs to be able (and willing) to swallow. But the biggest disadvantage of oral meds is that they take time to work. After all, they have to pass through the stomach and into the small intestine before they can be absorbed and start working. So, if your character needs the drug to begin to take effect sooner than 20-30 minutes, the oral route probably won't work.

Drugs given by the oral route don't have to be pills. They can be capsules, tinctures, teas, gummies, chocolate, baked goods; if you can imagine your character ingesting it, it can be given as an oral drug. Examples of oral drugs include many over-the-counter medications, like ibuprofen or cough syrup, as well as prescription medications. Illicit drugs that are most commonly taken orally include ecstasy, amphetamines, LSD, psilocybin ("magic mushrooms"), and date rape drugs, like Rohypnol ("roofies"), ketamine, and GHB.

For more on the effects of illicit drugs, see Volume 1: Setting & Character, Ch. 17: Drugs & Addiction.

INTRAVENOUS (IV)

Intravenous medications are given straight into your character's veins. Legally, only a few medical professionals—doctors, nurses, PAs, and paramedics—can give IV medications, though many illicit drug users are adept at doing so as well. There are two types of IV medication administration: bolus and infusion. An IV bolus, or "push," is a rapid, one-time injection of the medication. An infusion is the controlled administration of the medication over time. To receive an infusion, your character will need an IV catheter; an indwelling piece of plastic, usually in the veins of the hand, which allows medical professionals to administer medications easily without having to puncture the vein multiple times.

To administer an IV medication, your character must find a vein, clean the area, puncture the vein using a needle, then "push" the medication into the vein. If there's an IV catheter in place, they'd use that instead. The veins used are almost always the veins in the arm, hand, or foot. Medications are only injected into a vein in the neck in very specific circumstances, and even then, they need a minor surgical procedure to insert the catheter first.

For more on why you shouldn't inject in the neck, see Ch. 11: Head Neck & Throat Injuries.

There's no advantage to injecting most medications into the neck—the medication won't get to the brain any faster than through a vein anywhere else in the body—and it is extremely dangerous. So please, stop injecting your characters in the neck.

Since IV meds are delivered directly into the bloodstream, they work fast—often in less than a minute. However, it takes skill to find a vein and inject into it; this isn't something your character can do in the middle of a fight.

Medications given by IV tend to have strong effects and are often used in life-or-death situations. Some examples include strong pain relievers, like morphine, drugs to induce general anesthesia (propofol), blood pressure stabilizers (epinephrine, adrenaline), and potent antibiotics (vancomycin). Illicit drugs that are taken IV ("injection drugs") include heroin, amphetamines, and cocaine.

INTRAMUSCULAR (IM)

In my opinion, intramuscular administration of drugs is where it's at for writers. It has a relatively fast absorption—several minutes to full effect—and is easy enough that anyone can do it. All your character has to do is stick a needle in a large muscle and inject the medication. The upper, outer edge of the butt-cheek is the preferred site (*dorsogluteal site*), but any large muscle—the thigh, the upper arms—will work. Intramuscular medications can also be used in violent or agitated patients that won't sit still long enough for an IV to be placed.

Medications given intramuscularly include vaccines, some antibiotics, and contraceptive shots. Some sedatives and antipsychotics can also be given intramuscularly. If you're looking to use a medication to subdue a violent character, IM sedatives might be your option (See FAQ #4 for more).

INHALATION

Drugs given by inhalation are another excellent choice for writers. Inhalation works fast, usually within 5-10 minutes. There are a few different ways to deliver aerosolized medications. A nebulizer aerosolizes liquid medication into a mist that is inhaled while your character wears a face mask. Inhalers, on the other hand are handheld devices that your character sprays into their mouth as they breathe in. Nebulizers are easier to use, especially for children.

The most commonly used inhaled medications target the lungs, such as the inhaled steroids (Fluticasone) and rescue inhalers (Albuterol) that treat asthma and COPD. However, inhaled medications can also be used to induce anesthesia. Ether and chloroform are the two most famous (among writers) inhaled anesthetics, though they are rarely used in contemporary medical practice (See FAQ#4). Illicit drugs delivered through inhalation include marijuana, cocaine, heroin, amphetamines, PCP, salvia, and opium.

TRANSMUCOSAL

This is a weird one. Mucosal surfaces are the moist inner lining of your body cavity. Pretty much your entire gastrointestinal tract, from your mouth to your rectum, is lined with mucosa. The mucosa is filled with blood vessels; if your character dissolves a drug close to a mucosal surface, it will get absorbed straight into the bloodstream.

Since the drug goes straight into the bloodstream, they work pretty quickly—usually less than a few minutes. There are several different mucosal surfaces:

- Buccal = tucked in the cheek

- Intranasal = inside the nose

- Rectal = inside the rectum

- Sublingual = beneath the tongue

- Transvaginal = inside the vagina

> Technically, snorting is a form of transmucosal administration.

Transmucosal drugs are not super common—people generally don't like stuffing medications up their bums. However, they're great for self-administered medications, or to administer medication to an unconscious person without IV access. If your character needs the medication to start working quickly, or if they can't swallow, transmucosal administration is often used. Examples include drugs used for migraines, heart attacks, severe nausea, fever, pain, and seizures.

Illicit drugs that are snorted, including cocaine, heroin, and ecstasy, utilize transmucosal (intranasal) administration. Some legal drugs, like bath salts, certain opioids, and benzodiazepines, can also be snorted if your character is abusing them.

TRANSDERMAL

Medications delivered through a patch on the skin are considered transdermal. The drug penetrates through healthy skin and is absorbed into the tiny blood vessels running just underneath. Drugs delivered in this manner tend to work slowly but steadily, providing a constant and continuous source of the drug. Common medications delivered transdermally include nicotine ("the patch"), fentanyl (a strong opioid), and scopolamine (anti-nausea).

Because transdermal patches deliver drugs at a set rate, it is not a commonly abused route of administration. However, fentanyl is an extremely strong opioid (much stronger than heroin) that comes in patches. Fentanyl patches may cause addiction, especially when used for a long period of time. If your character is already

> For more on the misuse of opioids and the opioid crisis, see Volume 1: Setting & Character, Ch. 17: Drugs & Addiction.

addicted, they may misuse the fentanyl patches by using more than one at once or finding more efficient ways to administer the drug, such as ingesting the patches orally. This is an incredibly dangerous practice, as fentanyl is 50-100 times stronger than morphine.[2]

3.   WHAT HAPPENS TO MY CHARACTER'S BRAIN WHEN I KNOCK THEM UNCONSCIOUS?

OK, so writers don't actually ask me this question. But with how often they write about characters getting knocked unconscious, they really should.

Hitting a character over the head to knock them unconscious is a trope—particularly if the hero is knocking someone unconscious rather than "hurting them"—and an overused one at that. As a former neurologist, this is one of my pet peeves. Hitting someone over the head IS hurting them; it's called a traumatic brain injury (TBI). And while TBIs vary in severity, even a hit that isn't strong enough to knock them out can cause a concussion. And concussions can be debilitating. So, let's go over the severity (and prognosis) of head injuries based on how long your character is unconscious.

No loss of consciousness: Even without a loss of consciousness, your character may still have a concussion after a knock to the head. In fact, most people with concussions never pass out at all. Concussion severity has three grades; grades 1 & 2 do not involve any loss of consciousness. Only the most severe—grade 3—involves any loss of consciousness, even if it is only for a few seconds.

See Ch. 12: *Traumatic Brain Injuries* for more on concussions.

Symptoms of concussion include headache, nausea/vomiting, ringing in the ears, blurry vision, numbness and tingling in their extremities, dizziness, sensitivity to light or sound, confusion, trouble concentrating, memory problems, depression, moodiness, or inability to control their temper. Someone observing your character with a concussion might notice that they are clumsy, speaking slowly, asking the same questions over and over, and appearing confused or dazed. The severity of these symptoms ranges from mild to completely debilitating. Usually, the higher the grade of the concussion, the worse the symptoms, though this is not always the case.

Most people with concussions, particularly those with grade 1 & grade 2 concussions, tend to recover fully within a few days to weeks. However, your character could still develop persistent post-concussive syndrome, in which symptoms last up to a year. It's also important to note that multiple head injuries, especially ones that cause them to pass out, can lead to long-term brain

If you have a character who is too powerful and you need to hobble them without killing them, persistent post-concussive syndrome might do the trick!

damage, specifically a nasty condition called *chronic traumatic encephalopathy* (See *Ch. 12: Traumatic Brain Injury*).

Brief unconsciousness (Seconds-30 minutes) is considered a mild head injury. There are two main reasons your character might briefly lose consciousness: severe concussion and epidural hematoma.

If your character loses consciousness—even just for a few seconds—their concussion is considered Grade 3. Recovery from a Grade 3 concussion will take at least a few weeks.

> **Thirty minutes** is the maximum amount of time you can get away with your character being unconscious if you don't want them to have permanent brain damage. Even so, the less time they're unconscious, the better.

If your character wakes up with a Grade 3 concussion, they will be very confused, and will likely not know where they are or what happened recently. They'll be clumsy and in pain. If you're going for comedy, they might drive their interrogator crazy by repeating the same d*mn question over and over. But if you need them to fight off your bad guy or figure out a brilliant escape plan, then they're going to fail.

The other reason your character might briefly lose consciousness is a much more dangerous condition called an *epidural hematoma*, a type of potentially fatal brain bleed. Your character will briefly lose consciousness right after the incident, then wake up insisting they're ok. But don't be fooled; they'll continue to bleed into their brain, develop a nasty headache, and then, after a few hours—days at the most—will fall back into unconsciousness. Once this happens, they won't wake up again; their brain has herniated, and they are dead. To prevent death, your character will need neurosurgery to stop the bleeding and decrease the pressure on the brain. If you're looking to kill off a relatively young, healthy character who refuses to go to the hospital, an epidural hematoma will work well.

> See Ch. 12: *Traumatic Brain Injuries* for more on brain bleeds.

Less than 6 hours of unconsciousness is considered a moderate head injury. But don't be fooled by the word "moderate"—these types of injuries have major consequences. One study found that 71% of patients with moderate TBI required admission to the ICU, 6% died of their injuries, and nearly 50% were permanently disabled.[3] Another study found that five years after their injury, more than 50% of moderate-severe to severe TBI patients were dead or worse off than

> Surviving a moderate-severe TBI cuts 9 years off a person's life expectancy.[5]

when they were first injured.[4] And remember, these are the numbers for recovery *with treatment*. Without treatment, fatality will skyrocket.

If your character is unconscious for more than thirty minutes, don't expect them to do much of anything when they wake up. They'll be groggy, confused, and weak, and will probably have posttraumatic amnesia to boot. Plus, once you're at this level of a head injury, your character will need to be hospitalized and in the ICU. If that isn't possible for your story, don't keep them unconscious for longer than 30 minutes.

More than 6 hours of unconsciousness is considered a severe brain injury, and the prognosis is terrible. One study found that over 20% of people with severe TBI die of their injuries, while another nearly 60% live with moderate to severe disability.[4] About 3% will have a good recovery, and the remainder will remain in a persistent vegetative state.

Severe traumatic brain injuries are managed in the ICU. Your character may need neurosurgery, blood pressure monitoring, and monitoring of the pressures in the brain, among about a million other things. If your character has a severe traumatic brain injury and isn't in the hospital, they're as good as dead.

These numbers are for closed injuries, like a sword hilt to the head. Penetrating brain injuries—like gunshot wounds—have even higher fatality rates.

4. SO, IF I CAN'T HIT THEM ON THE HEAD, HOW DO I MAKE A CHARACTER FALL UNCONSCIOUS?

In short, drugs. There are tons of drugs—both legal and illegal—you can use to incapacitate a character. The method of administration and the drugs you use are going to depend on your specific situation: how sedated the character wants the victim to be and how long they want the victim to remain sedated.

Notice how I keep saying "sedated" instead of unconscious. Unconscious isn't a medical term, it's too vague. Instead, I'm going to use the term sedated, meaning that the victim is sleepy, calm, or relaxed. Depending on your story needs, your character can be minimally sedated (relaxed and calm, sleepy or lightly asleep), moderately sedated (similar to being fast asleep), or deeply sedated (can't be woken, but will move away from pain). If your character becomes so deeply sedated that they don't respond at all to pain, then they are in the deepest level of sedation—general anesthesia—and they will likely stop breathing on their own. Don't let the victim become this sedated unless you're killing them off.

ORAL MEDICATIONS

Administering a drug orally is going to give your character the most options in terms of which drug they want to use. However, the victim will first have to ingest the drug, then wait at least half an hour (usually longer) for it to take effect. There are a lot of prescription (and non-prescription) medications out there that can cause sedation.

- **Benzodiazepines** (called "benzos") are notorious sedating medications. Diazepam (brand name Valium) and Alprazolam (brand name Xanax) are two famous examples. Of the legal benzos, Diazepam has the fastest onset (15-60 minutes), and effects last around 5 hours.[5] However, Flunitrazepam, commonly known by the brand name Rohypnol—or by the nickname "roofies"—starts acting even faster, within 15-20 minutes.[6] Rohypnol is illegal in the US and, when sold legally in countries like Mexico, comes with a blue dot in the center so that it will discolor a drink if it is put into it.

- **Barbiturates** also cause significant sedation; so much so that they're given IV to induce anesthesia. When taken orally, short-acting barbiturates like pentobarbital and amobarbital can take effect in as little as twenty minutes.[7]

- **Opioids** cause significant sedation, but only when taken at dangerous levels. If your character is deeply sedated from opioids, they are in danger of stopping breathing.

- **Date rape drugs** like ketamine and GHB cause both sedation and amnesia. (See Volume 1: Setting & Character, *Ch. 17: Drugs & Addiction*).

If your story needs fast onset, deep sedation that the victim takes orally, benzos or barbiturates are probably your best bet. But benzos, barbiturates, and opioids are all Schedule 2 drugs, meaning that they are tightly controlled and illegal to use outside of a controlled setting. If your story is set in the contemporary USA, your character is going to have to jump through some serious hoops to get their hands on these drugs. However, there are still a few sedating medications your character might be able to access more easily.

- **Atypical antipsychotics,** like Olanzapine and Quetiapine, are notoriously sedating. So much so that doctors often give a low dose to patients in the hospital who can't sleep. At higher doses, the need to sleep becomes irresistible. Antipsychotics won't cause your character to become deeply sedated, as benzos or barbiturates can, but they will make your character fall fast asleep.

- **Sleep aids**, like Lunesta and Ambien, can be given to entice a character to sleep. But their sedating effect is not as strong as the other medications; they'll probably just make your character feel sleepy.

INTRAMUSCULAR INJECTION (IM)

If you need a character to be rapidly sedated, intramuscular injection is a good choice. The drug can be injected into a large muscle, like the buttocks, thigh, or upper arm, in seconds. There are three main types of injectable sedatives.

Ketamine is a sedating drug that causes a trance-like state, sometimes called *twilight sedation*. The victim will be awake and responding to questions, but they won't feel pain or remember anything that happened while they were under the influence. Ketamine is a derivative of the dissociative/psychedelic drug PCP; if you're writing from the POV of the character under the influence, they will feel detached from the world or in a dreamlike state. They may have hallucinations, distorted perceptions, feelings of bliss, or an out-of-body experience. However, since ketamine is also a powerful amnestic, they won't remember any of it once the drug is out of their system.

IM ketamine is often used by paramedics in the field when they need to sedate a violent or aggressive patient. It is also used on children, or anyone who needs to be quickly sedated but, for one reason or another, doesn't have IV access. Ketamine takes effect quickly—usually in about 4 minutes—and lasts somewhere between 15-30 minutes.[8] Four minutes might seem like forever during a fight, but if your character needs to subdue an opponent with medication during a fight, IM ketamine is probably your best bet.

> Ketamine and Midazolam are highly controlled Schedule 2 drugs. Your character is going to have to get creative to get their hands on some.

Midazolam is a benzodiazepine medication that can be given IM. It works fast, taking effect in as little as five minutes.[9] The sedating effects can last for an hour or two.

Haloperidol is another sedating medication that can be given IM. It's an older antipsychotic medication that has traditionally been used to calm aggressive or agitated psychiatric patients. It takes a while to take effect—around 17 minutes—and causes mild sedation.

INHALED ANESTHETICS

Inhaled anesthetic medications, like ether and chloroform, are beloved techniques used by writers to knock out their characters. But they don't work the way you see on TV.

Diethyl Ether was the original anesthetic, first described in 1729.[10] It has a strong, sweet smell and boils at a low temperature, so will vaporize on its own when held up to the victim's mouth. A beloved tool of writers, ether is not as useful as you might think. First, it takes a long time to work—somewhere between 15-25 minutes of constant administration, depending on the dose given and the depth of sedation required.[11] Second, it causes a whole mess of side effects, including coughing fits, nausea/vomiting, rash, and even convulsions. Finally, it's highly flammable. The main advantage of ether is that it is easily available; it's a common lab solvent. Your character could buy it online and have it shipped to their house.

Chloroform, like ether, is a colorless liquid that smells and tastes very sweet. Originally used to induce anesthesia, it is no longer used in the medical setting due to its propensity for causing liver damage and heart problems.[12] Unlike what you've probably seen, chloroform also takes a long time to take effect. The higher the dose, the faster the sedation will take effect, but it will still take several minutes at the least, giving the victim plenty of time to fight back.

Modern anesthetic gases, like desflurane, halothane, or sevoflurane, work much faster, usually in less than a minute. However, they induce sedation so deep that the victim won't be able to breathe on their own. They're also quite difficult to acquire, as they require significant equipment (gas canisters, anesthesia gas machine, face mask) to administer.

Nitrous oxide, also called "laughing gas," will not knock your character out on its own. They might feel dizzy and disoriented, though, which could work, depending on the needs of your story. Nitrous oxide works fast, it usually takes just a few minutes.

Because ether and chloroform take so long to take effect, and because the victim needs to constantly be breathing the substance during that time, they are terrible options for sedating an unwilling victim. Real-life criminals who have tried to utilize ether and chloroform to subdue their victims have been notoriously unsuccessful, mainly because the victim can—and will—fight back.[13]

5. WHERE SHOULD I STAB MY CHARACTER IN ORDER TO KILL THEM? WHAT IF I WANT THEM TO BE INJURED BUT NOT MORTALLY WOUNDED?

Trauma—especially penetrating trauma—is often about luck. A knife could nick an artery and kill your character in seconds, or it could miss the artery by a millimeter and your character is fine. People have survived being shot over and over at point-blank range, while others have been killed by a single accidental knife thrust. Minute variations in anatomy (the thickness of fat layers or an artery that diverts slightly from the usual course) certainly contribute. But, particularly with gunshots, survival often comes down to sheer, dumb luck.

As a writer, this is great news. It means you can feel free to stab, shoot, or hit your character pretty much anywhere, and it won't be unbelievable if they don't die of their wounds. That said, you probably don't want to stretch your story's plausibility too far. Some locations are more likely to result in fatal wounds than others. To help your character's injuries seem more realistic, here's a quick overview of areas that are likely to be more or less lethal.

AREAS LIKELY TO BE MORE LETHAL

Back of the head, where the skull meets the spinal cord. A good hit here will severe the spinal cord where it meets the brainstem, leading to instant death. But remember, this is a hard target to hit. The knife would have to slip perfectly between the skull and C1. Unless your character is very skilled, the knife is more likely to glance off the bone and cause nothing but a flesh wound. If they're using a gun, however, a bullet to the back of the head is highly likely to be lethal.

Front of the neck, where the carotid artery runs. Feel your Adam's apple, then slowly move your fingers sideways until you can feel your pulse beneath your fingers; that's your carotid artery. A cut there will make your character bleed out in seconds. It could also cut through the trachea (the windpipe) making it difficult for your character to breathe.

Above the collarbone: The space between the collarbone and the neck (called the "root of the neck") carries several large blood vessels, including the brachiocephalic trunk, a giant branch of the aorta that splits to become the carotid artery and the subclavian artery. There are a bunch of nerves that run

through this area. It is also relatively unprotected by bone, though the structures run somewhat deeper. A stab injury here could have devastating consequences.

Left chest: Really, anywhere in the chest could be bad-news-bears. Penetrating injury to the lung can cause the lung to fill with blood, or it could cause a sucking chest wound, or it could cause the lung to collapse. Injury to the great vessels could cause massive hemorrhage. But if you really want your character to kill their victim quickly, have them aim for the heart.

The heart sits in the left-middle of the chest. Much of it is protected by the breastbone, so a blade would have trouble penetrating it. However, the left ventricle—the workhorse of the heart—extends down and to the left, all the way to the *midclavicular line*, an imaginary line drawn straight down from the middle of the collarbone. In men, the nipple sits just to the right of the mid-clavicular line, at the fourth rib. If your character aims just the right of the nipple, between the nipple and the breastbone, they have the best chance of hitting the ventricle.

Even a direct hit to the heart won't kill your character instantly. They'll still die of hemorrhage, which can take up to a few minutes.

Armpit: The axillary artery (a large artery that supplies blood to the arm) runs through the armpit, alongside a complex bundle of nerves called the *brachial plexus*. A penetrating injury here will not only cause massive hemorrhage but could also cause significant damage to all of the nerves supplying the arm. The radial artery (the artery in the wrist that is cut when slitting a wrist) will still cause your character's victim to bleed out, but since it is a smaller artery, it will take longer. It's also going to be harder to hit in a fight.

Upper right abdomen: The liver is a highly vascularized structure. A large organ located on the right side of the abdomen, just below the ribcage, the liver is an easy target to hit. A strike here will cause a massive hemorrhage.

Lower back/Flank: The kidneys are another highly vascularized organ. Located on either side of the spinal cord, the kidneys sit just below the ribcage. A penetrating injury here can cause significant internal bleeding. However, most traumatic kidney injuries are due to blunt trauma.[1]

Groin: The femoral artery is a huge artery that runs close to the surface in the groin. Injury here could cause your character to bleed out in minutes. You can feel your own femoral pulse to get an idea of how big it is: press your finger into the crease of your thigh, right in the middle between your hip bone and your pubic bone.

AREAS LIKELY TO BE LESS LETHAL

Head: The skull is really thick. If your character is being attacked with a small blade, it's unlikely to be able to penetrate through the skull. The scalp and face wounds will bleed like h*ll, but they probably won't be lethal. All bets are off if your character is being attacked by a sword, or worse, a gun.

If your character is being attacked with a weapon that can penetrate the skull, they will probably have some pretty serious injuries. Penetrating injuries to the front of the head are less likely to cause death than penetrating injuries to the back. But these injuries still cause lasting damage. Gunshots are particularly bad, as the shock wave created by the high velocity of the bullet can damage the tissue that was not in the direct path of the bullet. If you want your character to walk away from a fight, I highly recommend you do not shoot them in the head.

As discussed in *Ch. 12: Traumatic Brain Injury,* non-penetrating injuries to the head can also be deadly. They can cause brain bleeds and other traumatic brain injuries which, even when not lethal, have the potential to cause lifelong disability. So, if you're looking to avoid long-term rehabilitation and potential disability, not to mention death, I'd stay away from major trauma involving the head.

Chest: Really, there isn't a great place to be stabbed in the chest. But if you're looking for a chest wound that might not kill your character, try stabbing them on the right side, near the collarbone. The upper parts of the lung often aren't as important for gas exchange and, as long as you don't hit above the collarbone, you'll probably miss any nerves and big blood vessels as well

Back: The shoulder blades protect smaller blades and even low-velocity bullets.

Abdomen: Most gut wounds take a long time to kill. There are certainly blood vessels in the abdomen that could kill your character quickly, but it's very believable that the penetrating tool could miss anything major.

Extremities: If you want to avoid lethal damage to your character, injuring the extremities is your safest bet. There are a lot of muscles and bones there. Your character would have to have an unlucky strike to hit a good artery, and since you're the one writing this scene, that's pretty easy to avoid.

6. WHAT DOES A PSYCHIATRIST DO? HOW IS THAT DIFFERENT THAN A PSYCHOLOGIST?

The short answer is that **psychiatrists** treat people with mental disorders using medications, while **psychologists** treat people using psychotherapy. This is a gross overgeneralization, but I wanted to get it out there. For the full story, keep reading.

PSYCHIATRIST

A psychiatrist is a medical doctor. They go to medical school and complete residency like any other physician. A psychiatrist's specialty is mental disorders, ranging from mood disorders like depression to substance abuse disorders like alcoholism. Their job is to diagnose and treat psychiatric diseases, and they usually do so by providing prescription medications and following up on their patients'.

Your character's first appointment with a psychiatrist will probably be a long one. The psychiatrist will go over your character's symptoms, as well as all their medications, medical history, and family history. During this evaluation, the psychiatrist will also perform a detailed physical exam, though your character might not notice. A psychiatrist's physical exam is close observation, watching the way your character moves, dresses, thinks, and talks. Once the exam is completed, they'll explain your character's diagnosis and, if the condition warrants it, prescribe medications and/or therapy. Subsequent appointments will be shorter, often as short as 15 minutes, and occur less and less frequently as your character improves. During these appointments, the psychiatrist will evaluate your character's response to treatment. They'll ask about the side effects and efficacy of the medications and will adjust dosages or change medications as necessary.

While psychiatrists can technically perform therapy, they generally don't, simply because they can't bill for it. Instead, most psychiatrists will recommend that your character see a psychologist or therapist.

PSYCHOLOGIST

A psychologist is not a medical doctor, though most clinical psychologists have doctoral degrees, such as a Ph.D. in Psychology or a Doctor of Psychology (PsyD). A clinical psychologist's job is to assess and treat mental, psychosocial, emotional, and behavioral issues. Many, though not all, provide psychotherapy. Psychotherapy comes in many forms, from Freudian psychoanalysis to cognitive behavioral therapy.

Psychologists use interviewing and psychotherapy techniques to help your character work through their mental illness and/or emotional struggles. They cannot prescribe medications, but they can give your character homework—exercises to practice or a journal to maintain. Therapy sessions usually last 30-60 minutes and are conducted regularly; weekly or even more frequently if your character is in crisis. Psychotherapy is often used in conjugation with medications.

Not all therapy is provided by psychologists. Social workers, clergy, professional counselors, psychiatrists, and licensed therapists can also provide types of therapy.

7.   WHAT IS PSYCHOSIS?

Psychosis is a condition wherein changes in your character's thoughts and perceptions cause them to lose touch with reality. It is less of a diagnosis and more of a symptom, a description of your character's mental state. A period of time in which your character experiences psychosis is called a psychotic episode. These episodes can be caused by a variety of different diseases, including schizophrenia, depression, and bipolar disorder. To be diagnosed with psychosis, your character will need to have either delusions or hallucinations.

Delusions: Fixed, false beliefs. Examples include your character thinking she is Marilyn Monroe or believing that aliens are listening to her thoughts.

Hallucinations: Seeing and hearing things that are not there. Examples include hearing disembodied voices, seeing flashing lights, or feeling bugs crawling over their skin. Complex hallucinations (hallucinations that utilize multiple senses) are rare.

Your character's experience of psychosis may vary with their mood and diagnosis. For instance, if your character is experiencing a manic episode, they are more likely to have delusions of grandeur, such as believing that they are touched by God or the reincarnation of a beloved public figure. If they are depressed, they might hear voices telling them that they are a piece of sh*t. If your character is a paranoid schizophrenic, they might believe that the government is spying on them and might even see special agents stalking them through the grocery store. Psychoses in bipolar disorder and depression tend to be mood-congruent and shorter in duration compared to schizophrenia and its related disorders.

> Hallucinations and delusions that are aligned with your character's mood are called **mood congruent**. If unaligned, they are **mood incongruent**.

8. WHAT CAUSES INFERTILITY? HOW WILL MY CHARACTER KNOW THEY'RE INFERTILE?

Infertility is startlingly common; in the US, 1 in 4 couples struggle to get pregnant, stay pregnant, or both.[14] While infertility is often seen as a female problem, the male partner is a contributing factor at least half of the time. In the US, infertility is diagnosed after a heterosexual couple has been having regular, unprotected sex for at least a year. In general, your character won't know they are infertile until they begin trying to conceive unless they've had a procedure (vasectomy, testicular radiation, tubal ligation, etc.) that impacts fertility. It is also possible that your character's fertility decreased with age; they might have been able to conceive at 20 but can no longer do so at 35.

Infertility comes in three main flavors: problems with the man (*male factor infertility*), problems with the woman (*female factor infertility)*, and unexplained.

Male factor infertility is generally caused by problems with the sperm, the testicles, hormones, structural problems that block the flow of semen, or any combination of the above.

- Sperm problems occur when there aren't enough sperm or the sperm are low quality, poor swimmers, genetically abnormal, or malformed.

> Tobacco, marijuana, alcohol, and steroid use can contribute to male infertility.

- Testicular disorders include infections, medications, trauma, or surgeries that impair the testicles' ability to create sperm. *Varicocele,* a condition of enlarged veins in the testis that overheats the sperm, is one of the most common causes of male infertility.

- Structural disorders include vasectomy, inability to ejaculate, and backward ejaculation.

The first step in the workup of male factor infertility is a *semen analysis*, a test that evaluates the volume, number, concentration, morphology, and quality of the sperm and semen. This is not a test that is normally performed; your male character would not be given a semen analysis as part of a regular checkup. Semen analyses often have to be done through specialized labs; your character may have to pay out-of-pocket for this particular exam. Other tests for male infertility include a physical exam, testicular and/or rectal ultrasound, genetic testing, hormone testing, and an evaluation of the urine after ejaculation.

Treatment of male infertility depends on the cause. Sometimes, the treatment is as simple as wearing boxers instead of briefs and avoiding hot tubs, bicycles, and drugs. However, if the man's infertility is severe, couples may need to utilize assistive reproduction techniques, such as in-vitro *fertilization* (IVF), to conceive.

Female infertility can be caused by problems in the eggs, the ovaries, the fallopian tubes, the uterus, or some combination of all four.

- Problems with the eggs tend to happen in older women. Women are born with a fixed number of eggs; as they age, the number may dwindle, and/or the quality may decrease. If your infertile character is over thirty-five, or if she's experiencing early menopause, egg quantity and quality is likely a contributing factor.

- Problems with ovulation, on the other hand, can occur at any time in a woman's life. If your character has an eating disorder, polycystic ovarian syndrome (PCOS), thyroid or another hormone imbalance, or even is just skinny and athletic, she might not ovulate regularly. Without ovulation, there can be no pregnancy.

- If the problem is in the fallopian tubes, it is usually due to scarring. The most common reason a tube would become scarred is because of a *pelvic inflammatory disease* (PID), caused by infection with gonorrhea or chlamydia. A previous ectopic pregnancy can also cause fallopian tube scarring.

- Uterine problems include scarring, abnormal uterine growths such as polyps or fibroid, or an unusually shaped uterus.

- *Endometriosis*, a hormonal disease that causes uterine tissue to grow outside the uterus, can impact all aspects of female infertility.

Diagnosis of female infertility can be a long and uncomfortable process. Your character will start by getting a pelvic exam and a transvaginal ultrasound to evaluate her uterus and ovaries. She also might need blood tests to monitor her hormones, genetic testing, and invasive imaging tests such as *hysteroscopy* (a camera inserted into the uterus through the vagina), a *sonohysterogram* (an ultrasound of the uterus), and/or a *hysterosalpingogram* (a dye test to evaluate the fallopian tubes).

Treatment of female infertility depends on the cause. Often, the first step is Clomid, a hormonal medication used to induce ovulation.

Unexplained fertility occurs when a couple can't conceive, but the doctors can't find anything wrong. Somewhere between 15-30% of infertile couples will never figure out why they can't conceive.[15]

9. MY HERO/HEROINE HAS TO RETURN TO THE SMALL TOWN WHERE THEY GREW UP IN ORDER TO CARE FOR A LOVED ONE. WHAT SORT OF CHRONIC CONDITION MIGHT NEED FULL-TIME CAREGIVING?

There are a lot of different conditions that could fit this bill, but they tend to fall into one of four categories: mobility difficulty, dementia, mental illness, and generalized weakness/frailty. Of course, many conditions blur the lines between those categories. Here are a few examples of conditions that could require full-time caregiving in order to stay in their own home.

DEMENTIA

- **Alzheimer's disease** (See *Ch. 24: Dementia & Delirium*) is the obvious candidate when you think of a character who will need long-term caregiving. In the early stages, people with Alzheimer's are prone to wandering and getting lost. As the disease progresses, your character will need to help their loved one with all sorts of daily activities, ranging from feeding/dressing/bathing themselves to helping them turn on the TV.

- **Dementia with Lewy Bodies** (See *Ch. 24: Dementia & Delirium*) is a form of dementia that is also associated with hallucinations, Parkinsonian movements, and REM sleep disorder (physically acting out their dreams).

MOBILITY

- **Recent surgery**: If your character had recent large surgery, particularly if they fractured their hip or their pelvis, they're not going to be getting around on their own for at least a few weeks. This is a good option if you need your character to provide caregiving unexpectedly (after all, no one plans a broken hip) or for a short period of time.

- **Multiple sclerosis** (See *Ch. 21: Autoimmune Disease*) is a progressive neurologic disease caused by the immune system attacking the brain and spinal cord. Symptoms range from mild numbness/tingling in one hand to complete paralysis on half the body. If your character's loved one experiences an MS exacerbation that seriously impedes their mobility, your character may need to help them adjust to their new disability. MS symptoms sometimes improve and sometimes don't, so if you're looking for a condition where your character has no idea how long they'll be needed for, MS is a good option.

- **Parkinson's Disease** is a neurodegenerative disease that usually begins with mobility issues (a tremor in the hands and a shuffling gait). As the disease progresses, the character will become stiff and immobile, almost as if they are being frozen inside their body. This is called "Parkinsonian movements." As their mobility worsens, they will also begin to lose their memory.

- **Stroke** (See *Ch. 7: Stroke*): A stroke may leave your character paralyzed on half their body. Even if their symptoms are improving, or if they are able to walk, they may have difficulty feeding, bathing, and dressing themselves. This is a good condition if you're looking for a sudden illness that will likely need long-term caregiving.

- **Advanced diabetes** (See *Ch. 19: Diabetes*) can result in mobility issues due to peripheral neuropathy, diabetic ulcers, and even amputation. It can also cause blindness.

- **Traumatic spine injuries** (See *Ch. 13: Spine & Spinal Cord Injuries*): A character with a traumatic spine injury may be newly paraplegic or tetraplegic. While the goal for these characters is for them to learn to live as independently as possible, the first few months after the incident will require lots of hands-on care ranging from toileting and bathing to feeding.

MENTAL ILLNESS

- If your character has severe **depression** (either unipolar or bipolar)—particularly if they made a suicide attempt—they will need someone to stay with them while they recover. Remember, antidepressants take up to six weeks to start working. During that time, your caregiver character will need to drive their loved one everywhere, stay with them while they're awake, administer medications, and make sure they don't have access to lethal means.

- A character with **schizophrenia**, particularly if it is a new diagnosis or if they have gone off their medications, may need some caregiving as they adjust to their diagnosis and medications.

GENERALIZED WEAKNESS

- **Cancer** (See *Ch. 24: Cancer*): There are three main parts of the cancer journey that are most likely to require caregiving. First, if the character is recovering from a major surgery, such as a mastectomy or a total colectomy. Second, during chemotherapy, particularly if the character is having significant side effects from the chemo. And third, at the end of life, when your character will become too weak/fatigued to do much of anything.

- **Autoimmune deficiency syndrome (AIDS)** (See *Ch. 5: Fever*): As their disease progresses, people with AIDS can become very weak or even bedbound. Alternatively, they may feel totally fine, but their white blood cell count is so low that going out into public spaces (grocery store, restaurants, etc.) could literally endanger their life.

- **Chronic heart/lung disease** (See *Ch. 20: Chronic Breathlessness*): If your character has severe chronic heart or lung disease, such as COPD or CHF, they're going to become very out of breath, even with minimal exertion. They may need help with activities that require exertion, such as shopping, cooking, and cleaning.

If you decide to write a character with a chronic illness, do your research, not only about the specifics of the disease but also about what it's like to have a chronic illness. People with chronic illnesses face significant stigma.

Giving blood vein to vein, like you sometimes see in movies, is generally a terrible idea. But blood transfusions can be legitimately lifesaving. If your character is trying to save someone's life after a massive hemorrhage, being able to give them blood could save their life. But if your character doesn't have access to a hospital or blood bank, how can they do that? Turns out, there is a way to transfuse blood in the absence of a blood bank. But first, let's go over the basics of blood types and blood transfusions.

BLOOD TYPES

Red blood cells have two different types of proteins on them: ABO proteins and Rh proteins. AB proteins can be either A-type or B type. If your character has both, they're AB. If your character has neither A nor B, they are considered type O. Rh proteins are either present (positive) or absent (negative). Clear as mud? The following table should help.

> O+ is the most common blood type.

AB Type	Rh +	Rh -
A	A+	A-
B	B+	B-
Both	AB+	AB-
Neither	O+	O-

If your character has an A protein and an Rh protein, they're A+. If they have both A and B, but no Rh, they're AB-. If they have no proteins at all, they're O-. So, why does this matter?

Because the immune system reacts to these proteins. Your character's body is used to the proteins they were born with, but if you suddenly give your character blood with the wrong type of protein, it will spell disaster.

Blood transfusion with the wrong type of ABO protein causes your character's immune system to attack the red blood cells, leading to a massive breakdown called an *acute hemolytic transfusion reaction.* Even small amounts of the wrong blood type, as little as two teaspoons worth, can cause this potentially

> If the Rh proteins don't match, it's less disastrous. However, if an Rh- woman is exposed to Rh+ blood, then gets pregnant with an Rh+ baby, the baby could die.

fatal condition.[17] Your character will quickly develop fever, chills, trouble breathing, muscle aches, chest pain, nausea and abdominal pain and blood in their urine as their kidneys start to fail. Treatment is with IV fluids and dialysis, but even with treatment, the condition is often fatal.

Luckily, this condition is completely preventable: just give the victim the correct blood type. A-type blood needs A-type blood, and B-type blood needs B-type blood. Since O-type blood has no proteins, the immune system won't react to it. For that reason, it is considered the universal donor, as pretty much anyone can receive O-type blood. Below is a table of compatible blood types.

Victim's Blood Type	Donor Blood Type Compatibility			
	A	B	AB	O
A	Yes	No	No	Yes
B	No	Yes	No	Yes
AB	Yes	Yes	Yes	Yes
O	No	No	NO	Yes

So, if your character knows that they're a universal donor (O-type blood), can they just hook themselves up?

Not so fast. Whole blood transfusions (blood as it comes out of the veins) are extremely rare. Instead, doctors give components of blood, based on the needs of the patient.

WHOLE BLOOD VS. BLOOD COMPONENTS

When blood is donated, it is separated into its components—red blood cells, plasma, and platelets. The red blood cells, which carry oxygen to the tissue, are concentrated and given to patients as *packed red blood cells.* This is the most common type of blood given when the victim has hemorrhaged. The plasma and platelets are used for other conditions.

There are many reasons packed RBCs are preferable to whole blood. For one, it's a lot of extra fluid that can put a strain on your character's heart. Another is that the plasma contains the immune cells, called antibodies, which attack the RBCs. Because all people with type O blood have antibodies against the A and B proteins, whole blood must be a perfect match; type O blood cannot be used as a universal donor. However, there is one instance when whole blood is used for transfusions: the military.

Warm, fresh whole blood transfusions have been used by the military since World War 1 and continue to be used in combat today.[14] Due to difficulty storing blood components in war zones, the military has started using walking blood banks—soldiers with the correct blood type who is "on-call" to give blood whenever necessary. But not just anybody can be a walking blood bank.

Due to the impracticality of matching the blood type perfectly, the military only uses soldiers with an extremely specific blood type: O-type blood with low numbers of antibodies to the A and B proteins.[18] If they don't have super low antibodies, their blood will cause an acute reaction, so they need to be tested for the antibody levels before they become a walking blood bank. They also need to be tested for blood-borne diseases like HIV, hepatitis, and malaria. Walking blood banks can be called in to give blood at any time. They give blood like any donor - into a bag—which has to be regularly rocked to keep the components mixed. Then the blood is infused into the victim from the bag.

DIRECT VS. INDIRECT TRANSFUSIONS

No one in contemporary medicine performs direct, arm-to-arm transfers anymore. Indirect transfers are better for many reasons; they allow for blood typing and screening for blood-borne diseases, and they allow for blood component transfusions and can be given at a set quantity and rate. If your character has access to a healthcare system—any healthcare system—they will get their blood transfusion through an IV connected to a bag on a post.

But if your character is out in the middle of nowhere and the victim is going to bleed out any minute, a direct arm-to-arm transfusion could work. After all, when blood transfusions were first invented, this is how it was done. It certainly isn't an ideal situation, but if your story requires it, you could make it work.

Early transfusions used a syringe to extract blood from the donor and inject into the recipient. Later iterations literally sewed the donor's artery to the recipient's vein. Only in the 1900s did someone figure out how to use IV cannulas and tubing.[19]

FINAL THOUGHTS

WHEN I FIRST STARTED WRITING stories, I thought I had to get every fact exactly right. I would spend hours of my writing time on the Internet, trying to figure out exactly how fast a horse could travel over mountainous terrain, or how quickly packaged food spoils during space travel. Often, the frustrating answer was "it depends," and I'd have to make my best guess. Then my story would change, and that detail would become irrelevant anyway.

Don't be like me.

In the end, you're writing fiction. Readers expect to suspend disbelief, at least to a certain extent. Your story—the needs of your plot and character arcs—should always come first. The medical details can be filled in later.

I've structured this book so that you can do exactly that. Need a character to go to a hospital for chest pain? There's a chapter for that. Your character has been beaten within an inch of her life, but you need her to walk out of the hospital after only a few days? I've detailed how the severity of traumatic injuries can often come down to sheer dumb luck. I've even given you a list of anatomic locations that are less likely to cause lasting damage if your character is injured there. In writing and organizing this book (and its companion, Volume 1: Setting & Character), I have tried to emphasize how realistic medical details can inform and improve your story, rather than hinder it.

There are a few exceptions. If your story relies on a completely unrealistic medical situation—such as a character going into a medically induced coma after a car accident, then waking up two years later with no health problems besides losing all their memories—then I suggest you try to find a way to alter your plot. Not only are such plot points overused and unbelievable, but misrepresentation—particularly of addiction, brain injury, chronic pain, comas, CPR, disability, and mental illness—can be actively harmful. I've done my best to highlight the conditions most harmed by misrepresentation, particularly in the "Real Talk" subsections. What we write matters; real people can be affected by our words. I hope you take these suggestions to heart and don't write a story that perpetuates erroneous representations of already stigmatized or misunderstood medical conditions.

I wanted to end this book by saying something clever. Instead, I'll say something that is true. When I left medicine, I thought I would hang my diploma on a wall and never use that knowledge again. That the tens of thousands of hours—and the hundreds of thousands of dollars—spent on my medical training would go to waste. Instead, this "Writer's Guide to Medicine" series has given me the opportunity to blend my passion for writing with my medical knowledge. Thank you, reader, for helping make this dream come true.

APPENDIX 1: DOCTOR SPECIALTIES

MEDICAL SPECIALTIES

PRIMARY CARE

Primary care providers (PCPs), also called general practitioners (GPs) specialize in routine healthcare and disease prevention: vaccinations, checkups, and common medical concerns. PCPs have a long-term relationship with their patients and are often a patient's first point of contact in the medical world. Two types of doctors can become PCPs: family medicine and internal medicine

- **Family Medicine** doctors take care of the whole family: babies, children, adults, elderly, and even pregnant women.

- **Internal Medicine** doctors specialize in the care of adults.

HOSPITALIST

Hospitalists are doctors who specialize in caring for patients in the hospital. They are the primary provider of care while the patient is hospitalized. Most hospitalists are internal medicine physicians.

INTERNAL MEDICINE SUBSPECIALTIES

If an internal medicine doctor does not want to be a hospitalist or a primary care physician, they may decide to pursue a fellowship to further subspecialize. Potential subspecialties include:

- **Cardiology**: Heart and vascular system

- **Endocrinology**: Hormonal disorders, particularly diabetes

- **Gastroenterology**: Diseases of the GI system, such as the stomach, liver, gallbladder, and intestines

- **Geriatrics:** Elderly patients

- **Hematology/Oncology**: Cancer and diseases of the blood

- **Hospice and Palliative Care:** End-of-life care

- **Infectious disease**: Transmissible diseases, such as HIV

- **Nephrology**: Diseases of the kidney

- **Pulmonology**: Diseases of the lungs

- **Rheumatology**: Diseases of the joints and muscles

NEUROLOGY

Neurologists specialize in diseases of the brain, spinal cord, and nerves. Diseases treated include migraines, stroke, epilepsy, Parkinson's disease, and nerve injury, such as carpal tunnel. A neurologist can see patients in the hospital or the outpatient clinic.

DERMATOLOGY

Dermatologists are doctors who specialized in skin, hair, and nails. They care for conditions ranging from acne to life-threatening rashes. Dermatology is considered both a medical and a surgical specialty. Dermatologists see patients in the clinic and often perform minor surgical procedures, such as skin biopsies and intralesional injections.

SURGICAL SPECIALTIES

Surgery is the treatment of a disease through an operation. Conditions treated through surgery range from appendicitis to cancer. But surgeons don't just operate; they also evaluate the patient prior to the surgery, explain the surgery and its inherent risks, and monitor the patient after the surgery.

GENERAL SURGERY

General surgeons can perform surgery on nearly any organ system. They specialize in in-depth knowledge of human anatomy and can perform a wide variety of procedures, including laparoscopic surgeries. Procedures performed by general surgeons include appendix removal (*appendectomy*), gallbladder removal (*cholecystectomy*), hernia repairs, and wound debridement. They also perform procedures such as colonoscopies and endoscopies.

GENERAL SURGERY SUBSPECIALTIES

Once a surgeon has completed their residency in general surgery, they can go on to further subspecialize. Possible subspecialties include:

- **Cardiothoracic surgery**: Specialists in managing surgical conditions within the chest.

- **Colorectal surgery:** Specialists in the lower GI system, particularly the colon and rectum.

- **Orthopedic surgery:** Specialize in procedures on the joints and bones.

- **Pediatric surgery:** Specializes in surgeries for children.

- **Plastic surgery:** Specializes in cosmetic procedures, including reconstructive surgery for burn victims and mastectomy patients.

- **Surgical oncology:** Performs surgical procedures related to cancer, such as biopsies and lumpectomies.

- **Trauma surgery:** Evaluates the trauma patient and performs surgeries to stabilize patients with acute trauma, such as motor vehicle crashes, gunshot wounds, and severe falls.

- **Vascular surgery**: Evaluates and treats diseases of the blood vessels, such as stroke, aneurysm, and blood clots.

NEUROSURGERY

Neurosurgery specializes in surgeries related to the brain, spinal cord, and nerves. Conditions treated include brain tumors, spinal deformities, herniated discs, head injuries, and nerve injuries, such as carpal tunnel.

OPHTHALMOLOGY

Ophthalmologists care for the eyes. They provide visual aids, such as glasses and contacts, and can also perform surgeries on the eye.

OTOLARYNGOLOGY

Otolaryngologists are also known as Ear, Nose, and Throat doctors (ENT doctors). They perform hearing tests and can perform surgeries on the nose and mouth, such as repairing a deviated septum or cleft lip. Conditions treated include hearing loss, snoring, and sinus problems.

UROLOGY

Urologists specialize in diseases of the urinary system, such as kidney stones (*nephrolithiasis*) and incontinence. They also perform surgical procedures, such as prostate biopsies.

OTHER SPECIALTIES

ANESTHESIOLOGY

Anesthesiologists do more than put patients to sleep. Their job is to keep the patient alive and pain-free during surgery. They evaluate patients before their surgery and talk to the patient about what they can expect from the procedure. In the OR, they induce anesthesia, intubate the patient, and monitor the patient's level of consciousness, vital signs, and pain control during surgery. If there's an emergency during surgery, anesthesiologists are on the front line, maintaining the anesthesia while preventing the patient from dying on the table. After the surgery, they monitor the patient as they recover.

If your character needs surgery, they will meet with the anesthesiologist before the procedure. The anesthesiologist will be the one to roll them back to the OR and the one who helps your character onto the surgical table. The anesthesiologist will be the last face your character sees before they lose consciousness.

EMERGENCY MEDICINE

Emergency medicine physicians work in emergency departments, caring for anyone and everyone who shows up at their door. It is a fast-paced and unpredictable specialty. An EM doc might go from treating a patient with a toe fungus one minute to a major multiorgan trauma the next.

EM doctors are true generalists: anything that walks through their door, they must know how to treat. They perform all sorts of different procedures, from pelvic exams to the famous *resuscitative thoracotomy*—more commonly known as "cracking the chest." They evaluate patients quickly and are skilled in the art of knowing who's about to die and who can wait it out.

A note about trauma: Most major traumas are seen at trauma centers—high-level hospitals with lots of resources. EM doctors work at trauma hospitals and care for the vast majority of patients. But if someone comes through the door with a major multi-organ trauma—think car accidents or multiple gunshot wounds—they will be cared for by a team of doctors led, not by the ED physician, but by the trauma surgeon.

> For more on trauma centers, see <u>Volume 1: Setting & Character</u>, *Ch. 2: Trauma Center.*

OBSTETRICS AND GYNECOLOGY (OB/GYN)

Ob/Gyn physicians provide both medical and surgical care relating to the female reproductive system. They provide routine women's healthcare, such as pap smears, birth control, and STD testing. Ob/Gyn doctors care for women during pregnancy and deliver babies, both vaginally and through cesarean sections. They also care for women with gynecological cancers, such as ovarian cancer.

Ob/Gyn physicians provide both medical and surgical care relating to the female reproductive system. They provide routine women's healthcare, such as pap smears, birth control, and STD testing. Ob/Gyn doctors care for women during pregnancy and deliver babies, both vaginally and through cesarean sections. They also care for women with gynecological cancers, such as ovarian cancer.

PSYCHIATRY

Psychiatrists evaluate and treat patients with mental illness. They can work inpatient, either on the psychiatric ward or as a consultant on the floor, or in outpatient clinics. Diseases treated include depression, anxiety, bipolar disorder, schizophrenia, ADHD, eating disorders, and autism. Subspecialties include forensic psychiatry and child psychiatry.

For more on psychiatrists and how they differ from psychologists, see FAQ#6.

RADIOLOGY

Radiologists are experts in medical imaging. Their job is to diagnose and treat patients based on medical imaging. They are experts at reading X-rays, CT scans, MRIs, ultrasounds, PET scans, and more. Some radiologists, called interventional radiologists, use imaging techniques to guide invasive procedures. Examples include CT-guided biopsies, placement of feeding tubes, and the surgical widening (stenting) of arteries.

GLOSSARY

A

- **A&Ox4:** Alert and oriented to person, place, time, and situation.

- **A1C:** Hemoglobin A1C, marker of blood glucose control.

- **AAA:** Abdominal aortic aneurysm ("triple A")

- **Abdomen:** Anatomic term for the belly area.

- **Abdominal:** Relating to the abdomen.

- **ABG:** Arterial Blood Gas

- **Abortion:** Loss of pregnancy before 20 weeks' gestation. Can be spontaneous, medical, or surgical.

- **Abrasion:** A wound where the skin has been scraped away.

- **ACA:** The Anterior Cerebral Artery

- **ACL:** Anterior cruciate ligament of the knee.

- **ACLS:** Advanced Cardiac Life Support

- **ADLs:** Activities of Daily Living, such as dressing, eating, and bathing.

- **ADD/ADHD:** Attention Deficit Disorder/Attention Deficit Hyperactivity Disorder.

- **AED:** Automated External Defibrillator

- **ALL:** Acute Lymphocytic Leukemia

- **Allergic rhinitis:** Runny nose due to allergies.

- **ALS:** Amyotrophic Lateral Sclerosis. Also called Lou Gehrig's Disease.

- **Alzheimer's disease:** A common type of dementia.

- **Amiodarone:** Medication used to treat potentially fatal heart rhythms.

- **AML:** Acute Myeloid Leukemia

- **Amputation:** Removal of a limb or digit. Can be traumatic (accidental) or surgical.

- **ANA:** Antinuclear Antibody. Test for lupus.

- **Anaerobes:** Bacteria that thrive in low-oxygen environments. Often aggressive, with a pungent smell.

- **Analgesia:** Pain relief.

- **Anaphylaxis:** Dangerous allergic reaction causing hives and throat swelling

- **Aneurysm:** A bulge in a blood vessel (usually an artery).

- **Angina:** Chest pain due to narrowed coronary arteries. Can be stable or unstable.

- **Anosognosia:** A neurologic deficit in which the victim is unaware of their neurologic or psychiatric condition(s).

- **Anoxic:** Due to lack of oxygen

- **Anterograde amnesia:** Inability to form new memories

- **Antivenom:** Treatment for venomous snakebites.

- **Antipyretics:** Antifever medications

- **Aorta:** The thick, muscular artery that carries blood from the heart to the rest of the body.

- **Aortic arch:** The curved, top portion of the aorta.

- **Aortic stenosis:** Narrowing of the aortic valve

- **Aortic valve:** Heart valve located between the left ventricle and the aorta

- **Aphasia:** Difficulty speaking/communicating due to neurologic problems

- **APP:** Advanced Practice Provider

- **Apnea:** Stop breathing.

- **Aprosody:** Lack of normal intonation in speech.

- **Arachnoid mater:** The spidery covering of the brain located between the dura mater and the pia mater.

- **ARDS:** Acute Respiratory Distress Syndrome

- **Arrhythmia:** Irregular heart rhythm

- **Artery:** A large blood vessel leading away from the heart

- **Arteriogram:** Imaging technique used to visualize the arteries.

- **Ascites:** Fluid buildup in the abdomen.

- **Aspirate:** To inhale material into the lungs OR to pull material from the body using suction.

- **Asymptomatic:** No symptoms

- **Astryocytoma:** A common type of brain cancer

- **Asystole:** No electrical activity of the heart (flat lining)

- **Ataxia:** Impaired balance or coordination that often leads to trouble walking.

- **Atelectasis:** Collapse of the alveoli of the lungs.

- **Atherosclerosis:** Plaque buildup in arteries

- **Ativan (Lorazepam):** Benzodiazepine medication used to treat anxiety

- **ATP:** The energy unit of all cells.

- **Atria:** The top two chambers of the heart

- **Atropine:** Medication used to treat slow heart rate

- **Aura:** A constellation of symptoms that occurs right before a migraine or seizure.

- **Autobiographical amnesia:** Loss of memory about oneself. Rare.

- **Avolition:** Lack of motivation.

- **Avulsion:** An injury in which the skin/underlying tissue are ripped off the underlying muscle/bone. Also called **degloving**.

B

- **β-hCG:** Beta-Human Chorionic Gonadotropin. The hormone produced by the developing embryo.

- **B-Symptoms:** Constitutional symptoms, including fever, weight loss, and night sweats.

     NATALIE DALE, MD

- **Backboard:** Rigid plastic board used to transport injured patients.

- **Bag Valve Mask (BVM):** Rigid plastic balloon that attaches to face mask, used to force air into lungs during CPR

- **BD:** Bipolar Disorder

- **BIPOC:** Black, Indigenous, People of Color

- **Blood glucose:** Blood sugar

- **Blood pressure (BP):** The force of blood against the walls of the arteries.

- **Blanching:** Skin that turns white when pressed.

- **BLS:** Basic Life Support

- **BMI:** Body Mass Index

- **Botox:** Paralytic made from the potent neurotoxin *botulinum*. Used in migraine and wrinkle prevention.

- **Bowel rest:** Total abstinence from food intake.

- **Brachial Plexus:** Complex of nerves that innervate the arm.

- **Bradycardia:** A slow heart rate

- **Bradypnea:** A slow breathing rate

- **BRCA1/BRCA2:** Breast cancer gene 1/2. Tumor marker for breast cancer.

- **BSA:** Body Surface Area

- **BvFTD:** Behavioral Variant Frontotemporal Dementia

C

- **C-#:** Cervical vertebra and number. (i.e., C1 = first cervical vertebra, C7 = seventh cervical vertebra)

- **C-section:** Cesarean delivery. Surgical delivery of a baby.

- **CABG:** Coronary Artery Bypass Grafting (open heart surgery).

- **CAD:** Coronary Artery Disease

- **Cadaver:** Dead body

- **CAP:** Community Acquired Pneumonia.

- **Capillaries:** Tiny blood vessels where gas exchange occurs.

- **Cardiac:** Of or relating to the heart

- **Cardiac tamponade:** When the space between the heart and the pericardium fills with blood, impeding the heart's ability to contract.

- **Carotid artery:** The large artery in the neck (where you take your pulse)

- **Catatonia:** Abnormal movement and behavior due to a psychiatric condition characterized by decreased reactivity to the environment.

- **Cauda equina:** The nerve roots at the base of the spinal cord. Named because they look like a horse's tail.

- **Cavitation:** A type of injury caused by a high-energy projectile.

- **CBT:** Cognitive Behavioral Therapy

- **CDC:** Center for Disease Control

- **Census:** How many patients a provider is responsible for caring for at any given time.

- **Cephalopelvic disproportion:** When the baby's head is too big for the woman's pelvis.

- **Cerebellum:** The part of the brain that controls coordination

- **Cervical Collar (C-Collar):** Rigid plastic collar used to immobilize the neck and prevent vertebral fragments from severing the spinal cord.

- **Cervical Spine (C-spine):** The 7 vertebrae in the neck.

- **Cervix:** Latin for *neck*. The lower part of the uterus.

- **Clostridium dificile (C. diff):** Contagious bacteria notorious for causing malodorous diarrhea.

- **CHAD-VASC:** Score used to calculate stroke risk.

- **Chest compressions ("compressions"):** Pressing on the chest during CPR

- **Chest tube:** Thin plastic tube inserted in the chest to remove fluid or air from the thorax.

- **CHF:** Congestive Heart Failure

- **Chronic Bronchitis:** A type of COPD associated with chronic cough and sputum production.

- **Cirrhosis:** Scarring of the liver

- **Circumferential injury:** When injury, usually burn or other scar tissue, goes all the way around a limb.

- **CJD:** Creutzfeldt Jakob Disease. Also called Mad Cow Disease.

- **CK:** Creatinine Kinase, a protein found in muscle

- **Clouded:** A state of mildly impaired consciousness or fogginess.

- **CMV:** Cytomegalovirus.

- **CNA:** Certified Nursing Assistant

- **CNM:** Certified Nurse Midwife

- **CNS:** Central nervous system—the brain and spinal cord.

- **CO:** Carbon Monoxide.

- **Coagulopathy:** Problems with blood clotting.

- **Code blue ("Code"):** Code called on the hospital overhead system if someone's heart stops beating.

- **Code team:** The medical team responsible for responding to Code Blues.

- **Colostomy:** Surgical opening connecting the colon to an external containment device (colostomy bag).

- **Coma:** A state of complete unconsciousness, characterized by lack of responsiveness to any stimuli.

- **Comatose:** The state of being in a coma.

- **Congenital:** A condition that has been present since birth.

- **Conjunctiva:** The clear coating of the eyes.

- **Conjunctivitis:** Red, itchy eyes due to inflammation of the conjunctiva.

- **Constitutional:** Affecting the whole body.

- **Contractures:** Painful tightening of scar tissue.

- **Contusion:** A bruise

- **Convulsions:** Uncontrolled muscle contractions that cause violent shaking of the limbs.

- **COPD:** Chronic Obstructive Pulmonary Disease

- **Cord prolapse:** The umbilical cord being compressed during delivery.

- **Coronary arteries:** The arteries that carry blood to the heart muscle.

- **COVID:** Coronavirus-19

- **COW/WOW:** Computer on Wheels/Workstation on Wheels

- **CPAP:** Continuous Positive Airway Pressure device.

- **CPR:** Cardiopulmonary Resuscitation

- **Crepitus:** The grating sensation of bone rubbing on bone or cartilage. Also, the bubbly feeling of free air under the skin.

- **Cricothyrotomy/Cricothyroidotomy:** Emergency procedure used to establish an airway by cutting through the front of the neck and into the windpipe.

- **CRNA:** Certified Registered Nurse Anesthetist

- **CRP:** C-reactive protein. Blood test for inflammation.

- **CSF:** Cerebrospinal Fluid

- **CTE:** Chronic Traumatic Encephalopathy

- **CT Scan:** Computed Tomography Scan

- **CVA:** Cerebrovascular Accident. The medical term for stroke.

- **Cyanosis:** Blue-tinged skin around the mouth, fingers, and toes due to lack of oxygen.

D

- **D&C:** Dilation & Curettage. A surgical procedure used to remove the contents of the uterus. Used in many situations, ranging from removal of cancerous tissue to surgical abortions.

- **DAI:** Diffuse Axonal Injury

- **DCIS:** Ductal Carcinoma in Situ

- **Defibrillation:** Providing an electric shock to try and return the heart to its normal rhythm

- **Degloving:** An injury in which the skin/underlying tissue are ripped off the underlying muscle/bone. Also called **avulsion injury**.

- **Dehydration:** A negative fluid balance. Can be caused by inadequate water intake or by fluid losses.

- **Delusion:** Fixed, false belief. A sign of psychosis.

- **Dialysis:** Treatment that removes toxins and waste products from the blood. Used for patients with severe kidney disease.

- **Diaphragm:** The muscle that controls breathing.

- **Differential Diagnosis:** A list of possible disorders that could be causing symptoms, ranked from most likely (or most dangerous) to least likely.

- **DIP:** Distal Interphalangeal joint.

- **Diplopia:** Double vision

- **Dissociative amnesia:** A psychiatric disorder that causes autobiographical amnesia. Usually brought on by trauma

- **Dissociative fugue:** Dissociative amnesia plus travel.

- **Distal:** Further from the center of the body.

- **DKA:** Diabetic Ketoacidosis. A high blood sugar crisis.

- **Deep Vein Thrombosis (DVT):** A blood clot in the veins, usually found in the veins of the calf.

- **DM:** Diabetes Mellitus

- **DMSO:** Dimethyl sulfoxide

- **DMT:** Disease Modifying Therapy

- **DNR:** Do Not Resuscitate

- **Drowning:** Death by suffocation due to submersion in liquid.

- **Dura mater:** The thick, cloth-like covering between the skull and the brain.

- **DVT:** Deep vein thrombosis.

- **DWLB:** Dementia with Lewy Bodies

- **Dysarthria:** Difficulty speaking due to mechanical problems.

- **Dyspnea:** Trouble breathing.

- **Eclampsia:** Seizures due to high blood pressure during pregnancy

- **ECT:** Electroconvulsive Therapy

- **ED:** Emergency Department

- **Edema:** Swelling due to excess fluid.

- **Electrocardiogram/Electrokardiogram (ECG/EKG):** Test to look at the electrical rhythms of the heart

- **Electroencephalogram (EEG):** Test to look at the electrical pattern of the brain

- **Electromyography (EMG):** Nerve conduction test.

- **Electrolytes:** Chemicals in the blood, such as sodium and potassium, which are used to maintain many cellular processes.

- **Embryo:** An unborn human prior to 8 weeks gestation

- **EMDR:** Eye Movement Desensitization and Reprocessing

- **Emphysema:** A type of COPD

- **Endometritis:** Inflammation of the uterus.

- **Endotracheal tube (ET tube):** Thin plastic tube used for intubation.

- **EMT:** Emergency Medical Technician

- **Epidermis:** The top layer of skin.

- **Epilepsy:** Seizure disorder characterized by abnormal electrical activity of the brain.

- **Erythema migrans:** A bullseye rash from a tick bite.

- **ESR:** Erythrocyte sedimentation rate. Blood test for inflammation.

- **ESRD:** End Stage Renal Disease

- **Extracorporeal Membrane Oxygenation (ECMO):** Machine that oxygenates blood outside the body, similar to a heart-lung machine.

- **Extubate:** The process of pulling out the endotracheal tube.

- **Fallopian tube:** The tube that connects an ovary to the uterus.

- **Fascia:** The connective tissue deep below the skin.

- **FAST:** Focused Assessment with Sonography for Trauma

- **Febrile:** To be feverish, to have a fever.

- **Femoral artery:** The large artery in the groin.

- **Femur:** The thigh bone. Longest and thickest bone in the body.

- **Fetus:** An unborn human after 8 weeks of development.

- **Fetal malposition:** When the fetus is not positioned properly, such as a breech birth

- **Fever:** Abnormally high body temperature (>100.4°F)

- **Fibula:** The thin, delicate bone of the lower leg.

- **Fluid resuscitation:** Giving fluids to restore blood volume, blood pressure, or increase perfusion to the organs.

- **FOAS:** Focal Onset Aware Seizure

- **Foley:** A plastic tube inserted into the urethra and left in place to drain the bladder.

- **Forceps:** Surgical instrument used for grasping small objects.

- **Fracture:** A broken bone

- **Frostbite:** When water in skin tissue freezes due to cold exposure. Can be superficial or deep.

- **Frostnip:** Redness of skin due to cold exposure.

- **FTD:** Frontotemporal Dementia

- **G-tube:** Feeding tube surgically inserted through the abdomen.

- **GAD:** Generalized Anxiety Disorder

- **Gastric:** Of/relating to the stomach.

- **Gastric lavage:** Pumping the stomach

- **Gastroenteritis:** Food poisoning.

- **GBS:** Guillain-Barre Syndrome

- **GCS:** Glasgow Coma Scale

- **Gestation:** Pregnancy, or the period of time between conception and birth.

- **GI:** Gastrointestinal

- **GERD:** Gastrointestinal Reflux Disease

- **GHB:** Gamma hydroxybutyrate

- **Glioblastoma:** An aggressive type of brain cancer.

- **Glucose:** A simple sugar. Necessary for all cellular processes.

- **Graft:** The surgical transplantation of healthy tissue (usually skin or blood vessels) over unhealthy.

- **Gravidity:** The number of times a woman has been pregnant

- **Great Vessels:** The large blood vessels leading to/from the heart: the superior and inferior vena cava, the aorta, the pulmonary arteries, and the pulmonary veins.

- **GSW:** Gunshot wound

- **Guarding:** Involuntary tensing of the abdomen.

- **Gurney:** Narrow, wheeled bed with rails and adjustable height.

- **Gustatory:** Relating to taste.

- **Gynecomastia:** Enlarged breast tissue, particularly in men.

H

- **H&P:** History and Physical

- **Hallucination:** Sensing (seeing/hearing/feeling/smelling/tasting) things that are not there.

- **Haloperidol:** Potent antipsychotic medication

- **HCAP:** Healthcare Acquired Pneumonia

- **Heat Exhaustion:** Fatigue, headache, nausea/vomiting, dizziness, and profuse sweating, caused by heat. Often exacerbated by exertion. Generally, not life-threatening.

- **Heat Stroke:** Life-threatening heat emergency characterized by hyperthermia and changes in mental status.

- **Heimlich Maneuver:** A maneuver used to dislodge a foreign body from the throat during choking.

- **Hematemesis:** Vomit blood.

- **Hematoma:** A collection of pooled blood

- **Hematochezia:** Bright red blood in the stool.

- **Hemoglobin AIC:** Marker indicating success of long-term blood glucose control

- **Hemorrhage:** Profuse blood loss

- **Hemoptysis:** Coughing up blood

- **Hemostat:** Surgical tool used to control bleeding. Looks like blunt scissors.

- **Hemothorax:** Blood in the chest cavity.

- **HER2:** Human Epidermal growth factor 2. A tumor marker for breast cancer.

- **Herniate:** When part of an organ is pushed out of its normal body cavity through a small hole.

- **HHNS:** Hyperosmolar Hyperglycemic Nonketotic Syndrome

- **High Altitude Cerebral Edema (HACE):** Fluid on the brain caused by altitude.

- **High Altitude Pulmonary Edema (HAPE):** Fluid on the lungs caused by altitude.

- **HIPAA:** Health Insurance Portability and Accountability Act

- **HOCM:** Hypertrophic Obstructive Cardiomyopathy

- **Hospitalist:** Doctor who primarily cares for patients in the hospital

- **House:** The hospital

- **HSV:** Herpes Simplex Virus

- **Humerus:** The bone of the upper arm.

- **Hyperglycemia:** High blood pressure

- **Hyperlipidemia:** High cholesterol

- **Hyperosmolarity:** Increased concentration of electrolytes in blood.

- **Hyperpigmentation:** Areas of increased pigmentation (darkening) of the skin.

- **Hypertension:** High blood pressure

- **Hypertensive emergency:** A high blood pressure emergency.

- **Hyperthermia:** Elevated body temperature (>104°F)

- **Hyperthyroid:** A condition of having too much thyroid hormone.

- **Hypoglycemia:** Low blood glucose

- **Hypogonadism:** Small testicles.

- **Hypotension:** Low blood pressure.

- **Hypothermia:** Low body temperature (<95°F)

- **Hypothyroid:** Too low thyroid hormone.

- **Hypovolemic:** Low volume of blood.

I

- **IBC:** Inflammatory Breast Cancer

- **ICH:** Intracerebral Hemorrhage

- **ICI:** Intracardiac injection. An injection straight into the heart

- **ICP:** Intracranial Pressure. The pressure of fluids on the brain inside the skull.

- **ICU:** Intensive Care Unit

- **IIH:** Idiopathic Intracranial Hypertension.

- **IM:** Intramuscular; administered into the muscle

- **Incontinence:** Inability to control, usually of urine or feces.

- **Infantile Amnesia:** The normal inability to remember very young childhood.

- **Infarction:** Tissue death due to lack of oxygen.

- **Infection:** The invasion of bodily tissue by a pathogen, such as bacteria, virus, or parasite.

- **Inflammation:** Redness, swelling, and heat in a portion of the body due to activation of the immune system.

- **Inflatable Pneumatic Device (IPC):** Inflatable cuffs worn around the calves used to prevent blood clots in hospitalized patients

- **INO:** Internuclear ophthalmoplegia

- In situ: Latin for in place.

- **Insulin:** Hormone that facilitates transfer of glucose from the blood into the cells.

- **Intubate:** Procedure to thread a thin plastic tube (endotracheal tube) into the lungs, allowing for external ventilation (i.e., from a BVM or a ventilator)

- **IOP:** Intensive Outpatient Program

- **Ischemia:** Not enough blood flow to the tissues.

- **IV:** Intravenous: administered into the veins

- **IVC:** Inferior Vena Cava

- **IVF:** In Vitro Fertilization

J

- **Jaundice:** Yellowing of the whites of the eyes and skin, due to liver disease.

L

- **L-#:** Lumbar vertebra and number. (i.e, L1 = first lumbar vertebra, L5 = fifth lumbar vertebra)

- **Laceration:** A cut, often with irregular or torn edges.

- **Larynx:** The voice box

- **Lethargic:** A mildly decreased state of consciousness, with diminished and/or slowed response to the environment.

- **LGBTQ+:** Lesbian, Gay, Bisexual, Transexual, Queer, and more.

- **Ligament:** Bands of tough, elastic tissue that connect bone-to-bone, providing support around the joints.

- **Lithium:** A mood-stabilizing medication used to treat bipolar disorder.

- **LLQ:** Left lower quadrant of the abdomen.

- **Log roll:** A technique used to maintain C-spine while rolling a patient onto their side.

- **Lungs:** Air-filled organs used in breathing.

- **LUQ:** Left upper quadrant of the abdomen.

M

- **Malnutrition:** Inadequate intake or insufficient absorption of calories, vitamins, and nutrients.

- **Mastitis:** Inflammation of the nipples

- **Maxillofacial surgeon:** Dentist specialized in surgical reconstruction of the face and jaw.

- **MCA:** Middle cerebral artery

- **MCS:** Minimally Conscious State

- **MCL:** Medial collateral ligament of the knee.

- **MD:** Medical Doctorate

- **MDD:** Major Depressive Disorder

- **Mees Lines:** Pale/white, horizontal lines in the fingernails that appear after arsenic poisoning.

- **Melena:** Black stool, due to digested blood.

- **Meninges:** The covering of the brain. Separated into three subtypes: dura mater, arachnoid mater, and pia mater.

- **MERS:** Middle East Respiratory Syndrome

- **MFM:** Maternal Fetal Medicine

- **MG:** Myasthenia Gravis

- **Mitral valve:** Heart valve located between the left atria and the left ventricle.

- **MRI:** Magnetic Resonance Imaging

- **MS:** Multiple Sclerosis

- **Multi-infarct dementia:** Another name for vascular dementia.

- **Multimodal Hallucinations:** Hallucinations that include more than one sense.

- **MVC:** Motor Vehicle Collision

- **Myelosuppression:** Decreased activity of the bone marrow and its ability to make new blood cells.

- **Myocardial Infarction:** The medical term for a heart attack.

N

- **Naloxone (Narcan):** A medication used to treat opioid overdose.

- **Nasal cannula:** Plastic tubing the delivers oxygen to the nose

- **Nasogastric Tube (NG tube):** Plastic tube threaded down a nostril into the stomach.

- **Necrotic:** Dead or dying tissue.

- **Neurodivergent:** Someone whose brains work in a way that isn't typical, such as people with Autism or ADHD.

- **Neurologic deficits:** Abnormal bodily functions due to injury to a specific part of the brain.

- **Neuron:** A type of cell that uses electricity to send and receive signals within the brain and spinal cord.

- **Neuropathy:** Damage/dysfunction of the nerves.

- **Nerve:** A type of cell that uses electricity to transmit signals between the brain/spinal cord and the rest of the body.

- **Neuromuscular Junction:** The molecular space between nerve and muscle cells, where communication between nerve and muscle occurs.

- **NG Tube:** Nasogastric tube

- **NICU:** Neonatal Intensive Care Unit

- **Nitroglycerin:** Medication used to relieve pain and increase blood flow to the heart during a myocardial infarction (heart attack).

- **Normotensive:** Normal blood pressure.

- **Nosocomial:** Hospital-acquired.

- **NP:** Nurse Practitioner

- **NPH:** Normal Pressure Hydrocephalus

- **NPO:** *nil per os.* Nothing by mouth.

- **NSAID:** Nonsteroidal anti-inflammatory medication, such as ibuprofen.

- **Nuchal rigidity:** Neck stiffness associated with bacterial meningitis.

- **Nulliparous:** A woman who has never given birth.

O

- **Obstetrician-Gynecologist:** A doctor specialized in treating the female reproductive system, including pregnancy and fertility.

- **Obtunded:** A severely decreased state of consciousness, with diminished and/or slowed response to the environment.

- **OCD:** Obsessive Compulsive Disorder

- **Oliguria:** Low urine production

- **Olfactory:** Relating to smell.

- **Opisthions:** An extreme spasming of the muscles causing the back to arch.

- **OR:** Operating Room

- **ORIF:** Open Reduction Internal Fixation. Surgical fracture repair.

- **Orthopnea:** Trouble breathing when lying down

- **Orthostatic hypotension:** Temporary drop in blood pressure caused by changes in position.

- **OT:** Occupational Therapy/Therapist

- **Ovaries:** The female organ responsible for producing ova

- **Ovum:** A human egg, produced by the ovary.

- **PA:** Physician Assistant

- **PACU:** Post-Anesthesia Care Unit

- **Palpitations:** A feeling that the heart is galloping or beating unevenly.

- **Paracentesis:** Removing fluid from a body cavity using a large needle.

- **Paraneoplastic Syndrome:** Constellation of signs and symptoms caused by the body's upregulated immune response due to a tumor. Common in small cell lung cancer.

- **Parity:** The number of living children a woman has.

- **Pap smear:** Screening test for cervical cancer

- **Papilledema:** Swelling of the nerve at the back of the eye.

- **Paresis:** Weakness

- **Paroxysmal:** Recurring in fits

- **Pathogen:** A bacteria, virus, fungus, or parasite that causes infection.

- **Pathognomonic:** Characteristic of a particular disease, injury, or condition.

- **PCA:** Posterior Cerebral Artery

- **PCI:** Percutaneous Intervention

- **PCP:** Phencyclidine, an illicit drug.

- **PE:** Pulmonary Embolism

- **PEA:** Pulseless Electrical Activity, meaning the heart's electricity is not generating a heartbeat.

- **Pediatrician:** A doctor specialized in caring for children.

- **Pericardium:** The fibrous sac that surrounds the heart

- **Pericarditis:** Inflammation of the pericardium.

- **Perforation:** A tear or hole in an organ.

- **PND:** Paroxysmal Nocturnal Dyspnea

- **PNS:** Peripheral nervous system—the nerves.

- **PEG tube:** Percutaneous Endoscopic Gastrostomy. Feeding tube surgically inserted through abdomen.

- **Petechiae:** Red/purple spots on skin caused by burst blood vessels.

- **PET Scan:** Positron Emission Tomography Scan.

- **Pleura:** The thin fibrous tissue surrounding the lungs.

- **Pleural space:** The space between the lung tissue and the pleura

- **Pleuritic chest pain:** Chest pain worse with breathing in

- **PHI:** Protected Health Information

- **Phonophobia:** Sensitivity to sound

- **Photophobia:** Sensitivity to light.

- **Physiatrist:** Doctor specializing in patients needing physical rehabilitation.

- **Pia mater:** The delicate tissue directly covering the brain.

- **PID:** Pelvic Inflammatory Disease. Usually caused by chlamydia or gonorrhea infection.

- **Piloerection:** Goosebumps

- **Placenta:** The organ that protects and feeds the fetus during pregnancy. Also called the afterbirth.

- **Placenta accrete:** When the placenta grows too deeply into the uterus.

- **Placenta previa:** When the placenta covers the cervix, causing bleeding.

- **PNES:** Psychogenic non-epileptic seizures. Formerly called "pseudo seizures."

- **Pneumothorax:** Collapsed lung.

- **PNS:** Peripheral Nervous System.

- **PO:** per os. Latin for "by mouth"

- **POC:** People/Person of color

- **Polydipsia:** Increased thirst

- **Polyuria:** Increased urination

- **Postdrome:** The last stage of a migraine

- **Postictal:** The state of impaired consciousness after a seizure.

- **Postpartum:** After delivery of a baby.

- **POV:** Point of view

- **PPA:** Primary Progressive Aphasia

- **PPD:** Purified Protein Derivative—test for tuberculosis.

- **PPE:** Personal Protective Equipment, such as gloves, face masks, and gowns.

- **Preeclampsia:** A condition of high blood pressure and evidence of kidney damage in a pregnant woman.

- **Prodrome:** An early indication of disease, such as migraine

- **Prognosis:** The likely outcome of a disease, injury, or condition.

- **Prolonged Mechanical Ventilation (PVM):** Needing to consistently be on a ventilator for more than three weeks.

- **Prone:** Lying face down.

- **Proned/Proning:** Placing a patient who is having trouble breathing in a face-down position to increase lung capacity

- **Proximal:** Closer to the center of the body.

- **Pseudodementia:** A reversible dementia caused by severe depression.

- **Pseudomonas:** Bacteria that tends to colonize burns. Smells sweet.

- **Psychiatrist:** Medical doctor (MD or DO) specialized in the treatment of mental illness

- **Psychologist:** Mental health providers (Master's or Ph.D. in Psychology) trained in psychotherapy and psychoanalysis.

- **PsyD:** Doctorate in Psychology

- **PT:** Physical Therapy/Therapist

- **PTA:** Posttraumatic Amnesia; a type of amnesia, usually anterograde, that forms after brain injury.

- **Ptosis:** Drooping eyelid

- **PTSD:** Post-Traumatic Stress Disorder

- **PUD:** Peptic ulcer disease.

- **Pulmonary arteries:** The arteries that carries blood from the heart to the lungs

- **Pulmonary edema:** Fluid in the lungs.

- **Pulmonary Hygiene:** Exercises/procedures used to keep the airways clear. Sometimes called *pulmonary toilet.*

- **Pulmonary veins:** The veins that carry blood from the lungs back to the heart.

- **Pulse oximeter:** Device used to measure blood oxygen levels

- **PVS:** Persistent Vegetative State

Q

- **Quadriplegia:** Paralysis of all four limbs. Also called tetraplegia.

- **QRS Complex:** The typical EKG heart rhythm pattern.

R

- **RA:** Rheumatoid Arthritis.

- **Radial artery:** The large artery in the wrist.

- **Radiate:** Pain traveling from one area of the body to another.

- **Radius:** The large bone in the lower arm.

- **RBCs:** Red Blood Cells

- **Refeeding Syndrome:** A dangerous syndrome characterized by a shift in electrolytes caused by the reintroduction of food after a period of starvation.

- **Refractory Status Epilepticus (RSE):** A seizure lasting more than 5 minutes that does not respond to medication. Indication for a therapeutic coma.

- **Regurgitation:** To bring up food from the stomach OR the insufficiency of a heart valve leading to backflow of blood.

- **Renal:** Of/relating to the kidneys

- **Retardation:** Slowed or slowing.

- **Retrograde amnesia:** Loss of previously formed memories.

- **Rhabdomyolysis:** Muscle breakdown

- **Rhythm Strip:** The result of an EKG: the heart's electrical rhythm, printed on white paper with red lines.

- **RICE:** Rest, Ice, Compression, Elevation

- **Rictus sardonicus:** A painful spasm of the muscles of the face causing the appearance of a grin.

- **Rigors:** Chills and shaking during a fever

- **Rigor mortis:** The stiffness of death

- **RLQ:** Right lower quadrant of the abdomen

- **Rounding:** The process of going around the hospital to check in on every patient

- **RSE:** Refractory Status Epilepticus. An unrelenting seizure that does not respond to medications.

- **RT:** Respiratory Therapist

- **RUQ:** Right upper quadrant of the abdomen.

S

- **S#:** Sacral vertebra and number. (i.e., S1 = first sacral vertebra)

- **SAD:** Seasonal Affective Disorder

- **SAH:** Subarachnoid hemorrhage

- **SARS:** Severe Acute Respiratory Syndrome

- **SBO:** Small bowel obstruction.

- **SCA:** Sudden Cardiac Arrest

- **Scalpel:** Sharp surgical instrument used to cut tissue

- **SCI:** Spinal Cord Injury

- **SCLC:** Small Cell Lung Cancer

- **Sclera:** The whites of the eye

- **Scrubs:** Loose medical clothing, often light green or pale blue, worn to protect the wearer against bodily fluids and minimize transmission of contaminants.

- **Seizure:** Electrical disturbance in the brain that may or may not cause convulsions.

- **Serum sickness:** Immune reaction to venom of snakes, spiders, etc.

- **SI:** Suicidal Ideation

- **Signs:** The objective indications of disease, illness, or injury (i.e., low blood pressure)

- **Skilled Nursing Facility (SNF):** Care facility providing high-level nursing care.

- **Skin graft:** Healthy skin surgically placed over lost/damaged skin.

- **SLE:** Systemic Lupus Erythematosus. Commonly called lupus.

- **SLP:** Speech-language Pathologist

- **Somatization:** When psychological distress is felt as physical symptoms.

- **Spasticity:** Abnormal muscle tightness, usually due to brain or spinal cord damage.

- **Spleen:** An easily injured organ in the abdomen responsible for producing infection-fighting white blood cells (WBCs) and filtering the blood.

- **Sprain:** Damage to the ligaments surrounding a joint.

- **Sputum:** The stuff you cough up (phlegm)

- **SSRI:** Selective Serotonin Reuptake Inhibitors. First-line treatment for depression and anxiety, among others.

- **Stable:** The condition is not getting worse.

- **Starvation:** A severe calorie deficiency. Has several stages.

- **Status epilepticus:** A seizure lasting more than 5 minutes

- **Stenosis:** Narrowing

- **Stethoscope:** Instrument used to listen to the heart, lungs, and abdomen.

- **STI:** Sexually Transmitted Infection (previously called STD)

Since not all infections lead to disease, STI is more accurate than STD.

- **Straight Catheter ("Straight Cath"):** A plastic tube inserted into the urethra to drain the bladder, then immediately removed.

- **Staphylococcus:** Class of bacteria notorious for causing abscesses and wound infections.

- **Stenosis:** Narrowing, particularly of a blood vessel

NATALIE DALE, MD

- **Streptococcus:** Class of bacteria notorious for causing abscesses and wound infections.

- **Stretcher:** Narrow, wheeled bed with collapsible legs. Used in the field.

- **Stupor:** Severely diminished consciousness; only minimally responsive to the environment.

- **Subconjunctival Hemorrhage:** Burst blood vessel in the eye.

- **Supine:** Lying face up.

- **Surgical Drain:** Plastic tubing, often connected to suction or suction bulb, meant to remove fluids or gas from the body.

- **Sutures:** Stitches.

- **SVC:** Superior Vena Cava

- **Symptoms:** The subjective feelings of disease, illness, or injury (i.e., a stomachache)

- **Syncope:** Temporary loss of consciousness

T

- **Tachycardia:** A fast heart rate.

- **Tachypnea:** A fast breathing rate.

- **TB:** Tuberculosis

- **TBI:** Traumatic Brain Injury

- **TED hose:** Compression stockings designed to prevent blood clots

- **Telemetry:** In-hospital constant monitoring of heart rhythm and vitals

- **TGA:** Transient Global Amnesia

- **Thorax:** Anatomic term for the chest.

- **Thoracic:** Relating to the thorax.

- **Thymus:** Small organ in the thorax where white blood cells mature.

- **TIA:** Transient Ischemic Attack

- **Tibia:** The large bone of the lower leg.

- **Tonic-Clonic seizure:** "Grand mal" seizure characterized by loss of consciousness and stiffening/jerking of all four limbs.

- **Trachea:** Organ that conducts air from the mouth down the neck and into the lungs.

- **Tracheostomy:** A surgical opening in the front of the neck used for patients requiring persistent ventilation.

- **Transect:** To cut through completely

- **Transdermal:** Administered through the skin.

- **Transmucosal:** Administered through the mucosa.

- **Trauma shears:** Heavy-duty scissors for cutting the clothes off victims.

- **Tricuspid valve:** The heart valve connecting the right atria to the right ventricle

- **Triptans:** Class of drugs used to treat migraines.

- **Troponins:** Proteins released into the blood by dying heart muscle.

- **TSS:** Toxic Shock Syndrome.

- **TTX:** Tetrodotoxin. A potent toxin found in pufferfish.

- **Type and screen:** Blood test to determine blood type

U

- **Ulna:** The thin, delicate bone in the lower arm.

- **Ultrasound:** Imaging study using soundwaves to generate a moving picture.

- **Urethra:** The anatomical tube leading from the bladder to the outside of the body.

- **Urologist:** A doctor specialized in the treatment of the bladder, urethra, testis, and certain kidney disorders.

- **Urticaria:** A red, raised, itchy rash. Also called hives or wheals.

- **UV:** Ultraviolet light.

V

- **VAP:** Ventilator Associated Pneumonia

- **Varices:** Enlarged veins, usually due to blood backup.

- **VBAC:** Vaginal Birth After C-section

- **Vein:** A blood vessel that returns blood to the heart.

- **Vena cava:** The large blood vessel (vein) that returns blood to the right atria of the heart.

  o **Inferior vena cava:** Drains blood from the lower half of the body into the heart

  o **Superior vena cava:** Drains blood from the upper half of the body into the heart

- **Ventilate:** To force air into the lungs. Can be done manually (with BVM or mouth-to-mouth) or with ventilator.

- **Ventilators:** Machines that deliver breaths to an intubated patient.

- **Ventricles:** The lower, muscular chambers of the heart

- **Ventricular Fibrillation:** Potentially deadly heart rhythm

- **Vital Signs:** Heart rate, breathing rate, blood pressure, and temperature. Weight and blood oxygenation also sometimes included.

W

- **WBCs:** White blood cells

- **WHO:** World Health Organization

- **Wound Debridement:** Surgical removal of dead tissue from a wound.

- **WPW:** Wolff-Parkinson White Syndrome

X

- **X-ray:** Study that uses radiation to generate a 2D image.

- **Xanax (Alprazolam):** Benzodiazepine medication used to treat anxiety.

Z

- **Zoonotic disease:** Disease that can be transferred from animals to humans

INDEX

Alcohol,

    induced amnesia, 319

    signs of chronic consumption, 227

    withdrawal seizures, 272

Alcoholic liver disease, 226-227

    alcoholic cirrhosis, 227

    alcoholic steatohepatitis, 226-227

    hepatic steatosis, 226

Allergy, 49

    allergic rhinitis, 49

    food allergies, 52-53

Alveoli, 8

ALS, see *amyotrophic lateral sclerosis*

Alzheimer's disease, 308-309

Aminata phalloides & Aminata bisporigera, 129

Amnesia,

    anterograde, 319

    autobiographical, 320

    dissociative, 320

    drug-induced, 320

    infantile, 319

    posttraumatic, 153, 161, 320-321

    retrograde amnesia, 319-320

    transient global amnesia, 321

Amnionitis, 103

Amputations, 200-201

    surgical, 200

    traumatic, 200-201

Amyotrophic lateral sclerosis (ALS), 245

Anaphylaxis, 50-52

Anaphylactic shock, 51-52

Anatomy of the,

    abdominal cavity, 36-37

Argon poisoning, 124-125

Arrhythmia, 23

Arsenic poisoning, 125

Arteries, 7

Aspirin overdose, 30

Asthma, 27, 240

Ataxia, 89-90, 126, 128, 249

Atria, 7-8

Atrial fibrillation, 44, 83, 240-241

Avulsion injuries, see *degloving injuries*

B

Bipolar disorder, 273-276

    bipolar depression, 273

    mania/hypomania, 273-275

    treatment, 275

    treatment adherence, 276

Benzodiazepines, 272, 328

Black lung disease (coal worker pneumoconiosis), 246

Blood donation, 341-342

Blood types, 340-341

Body mass index (BMI), 225

Botulinum toxin, 30

Bowel, 39

  obstruction, 39

  rest, 39

Brain

  bleeds, 156-158

  bruise, see *cerebral contusion*

  cancer, 294

  herniation, 95

  penetrating injuries, 158-159

  tumors, 264

Breast cancer,

　　　　NATALIE DALE, MD

with Lewy bodies, 310-311

vascular dementia, 309-310

Depression, see *major depressive disorder*

Diabetes, 229-239

    causes of, 229-230

    complications 237-239

    emergencies, 233-237

        diabetic ketoacidosis (DKA), 233-234)

        hyperosmolar hyperglycemic nonketotic syndrome (HHNS), 234-235

        hypoglycemia, 235-237

    treatment, 232-233

    types, 230-232

        gestational, 230

        insipidus, 230

        Type 1, 230-231

        Type 2, 231-232

Diaphragm, 8

    rupture, 180

Diffuse axonal injury, 155

Dislocations, 199

Diverticulitis, 41

DMSO, 133

Doctor specialties, 349-345

Dysphagia, 20

Dyspnea, 24

E

EKG see *electrocardiogram*

Eclampsia, 99-100

ECT, see *electroconvulsive therapy*

Echocardiogram, 32, 178

Ectopic pregnancy, 100

EEG see *electroencephalogram,*

Electrocardiogram (EKG/ECG), 11, 178

Graves' disease, 256-257

Gravidity & Parity, 98

Guillain-Barré syndrome, 32

H

Haloperidol, 329

Hanging, 146

Hallucination, 277, 305

Hashimoto's thyroiditis, 257

Headache, 260-265

    cluster, 263

    migraine, 261-263

    secondary causes, 264

    tension-type, 260-261

    thunderclap, 264

Heart attack, see *Myocardial infarction*

    Hollywood, 23

Heart disease, 11-14

Heart failure, see *Congestive heart failure*

Heart valve diseases, 243-244

Heartburn, see GERD

Heimlich maneuver, 28-29

Hemoptysis, 59, 178, 296

Hemothorax, 173-174

Herpes zoster, 21

High blood pressure, see Hypertension

High cholesterol, see Hyperlipidemia

HIV/AIDs, 34, 339

Holiday heart syndrome, 19

Hospitalist, 345

Hygiene hypothesis, 247-248

Hyperbaric oxygen therapy, 31

Hyperemesis gravidarum, 100

Hyperlipidemia, 223-224

L

M

N

motor, 24

Neutropenia, febrile, 68

Nitrous oxide, 330

Normal pressure hydrocephalus, 313-314

NSAIDs, 42

O

Obesity, 224-226

Obsessive compulsive disorder (OCD), 283-284

Obstetrical emergencies, 103-105

Obstetrician-gynecology doctors, 98

Opioids, 31

    overdose, 31

    sedation, 328

Organophosphate poisoning, 31

Optic neuritis, 249

P

Pancreatitis, 21, 42

Panic attacks, 270-272

Parkinson's disease, 338

Pelvic inflammatory disease, 337

Peptic ulcer disease, 42

Percutaneous intervention, 12

Perforated organs, 47

    esophageal, 142-143

    gastric, 185

    intestinal, 184-145

    tracheal, 142

Pericardial effusion, 14

Pericarditis, 14

Phobias, 272-273

    agoraphobia, 272

    social phobia, 272-273

    specific phobia, 273

S

Scalp injuries, 137-138

Scarlet fever, 61

Schizophrenia, 276-280

    Disorganized symptoms of, 278-279

    Negative symptoms of, 277-278

    Positive symptoms of, 276-277

    Treatment, 279

Second impact syndrome, 162

Sedating medications, 327-330

    intramuscular, 329

    oral, 328-329

Seizure, 74-82

    aura, 77-78

    complications, 80-81

    diagnosis and treatment, 79-80

    grand mal, see *tonic-clonic*

    nonepileptic, 81-82

    postictal state, 78-79

    status epilepticus, 81

    triggers, 75

    types, 75-76

        absence, 76

        atonic, 76

        myoclonic, 76

        tonic-clonic, 76-78

Semen analysis, 336

Sepsis, 27, 64

Shaken baby syndrome, 155

Shingles, see *Herpes zoster*

Shortness of breath, see *dyspnea*

Shoulder dystocia, 104

Skin grafts, 215

     NATALIE DALE, MD

T

WORKS CITED

1: CHEST PAIN

1. Groves, Elliot and Mladin, Vidovich. "Length of Stay after PCI." *American College of Cardiology*, 5 Aug. 2015. https://www.acc.org/latest-in-cardiology/articles/2019/08/02/13/57/length-of-stay-after-pci.

2. Nathan, Ashwin S., et al. "Association between 90-Minute Door-to-Balloon Time, Selective Exclusion of Myocardial Infarction Cases, and Access Site Choice." *Circulation: Cardiovascular Interventions*, vol. 13, no. 9, 2020, https://doi.org/10.1161/circinterventions.120.009179.

3. Lee, Sang Eun, et al. "Coronary Artery Bypass Graft versus Percutaneous Coronary Intervention in Acute Heart Failure." *Heart*, BMJ Publishing Group Ltd and British Cardiovascular Society, 1 Jan. 2020, www.http://heart.bmj.com/content/106/1/50.

4. Levy, David. "Aortic Dissection." *StatPearls [Internet].*, U.S. National Library of Medicine, 15 Dec. 2021, https://www.ncbi.nlm.nih.gov/books/NBK441963/.

5. "Study: Death Rate from Lung Clots Is on the Rise after Years of Decline." *National Heart Lung and Blood Institute*, U.S. Department of Health and Human Services, https://www.nhlbi.nih.gov/news/2020/study-death-rate-lung-clots-rise-after-years-decline.

6. Mol, Karen Anne, et al. "Non-Cardiac Chest Pain: Prognosis and Secondary Healthcare Utilisation." *Open Heart*, Archives of Disease in Childhood, 1 Oct. 2018, https://openheart.bmj.com/content/5/2/e000859.

7. Schumann, Jessica A. "Costochondritis." *StatPearls [Internet].*, U.S. National Library of Medicine, 10 July 2021, www.ncbi.nlm.nih.gov/books/NBK532931/.

8. Dusenberry, Maya. "'Everybody Was Telling Me There Was Nothing Wrong'." *BBC Future*, BBC, 29 May 2018, www.bbc.com/future/article/20180523-how-gender-bias-affects-your-healthcare.

1. "Choking: First Aid." *Mayo Clinic*, Mayo Foundation for Medical Education and Research, 14 Oct. 2020, https://www.mayoclinic.org/first-aid/first-aid-choking/basics/art-20056637

2. "Heimlich Maneuver on Self: Medlineplus Medical Encyclopedia." *MedlinePlus*, U.S. National Library of Medicine, https://medlineplus.gov/ency/article/001983.htm.

3. "Polio Elimination in the United States." *Centers for Disease Control and Prevention*, Centers for Disease Control and Prevention, 28 Sept. 2021, https://www.cdc.gov/polio/what-is-polio/polio-us.html.

4. Geocadin, Romergryko G, et al. "Management of Brain Injury after Resuscitation from Cardiac Arrest." *Neurologic Clinics*, U.S. National Library of Medicine, May 2008, www.ncbi.nlm.nih.gov/pmc/articles/PMC3074242/.

5. Patterson, Emma, et al. "The Efficacy and Usability of Suction-Based Airway Clearance Devices for Foreign Body Airway Obstruction: A Manikin Randomised Crossover Trial." *Resuscitation Plus*, Elsevier, 8 Jan. 2021, https://www.sciencedirect.com/science/article/pii/S2666520420300680.

3: ABDOMINAL PAIN

1. Kendall, John, and Maria Moreira. "Evaluation of the Adult with Abdominal Pain in the Emergency Department." *UpToDate*, 29 Dec. 2020, www.uptodate.com/contents/evaluation-of-the-adult-with-abdominal-pain-in-the-emergency-department.

2. "Appendicitis." *Mayo Clinic*, Mayo Foundation for Medical Education and Research, 7 Aug. 2021, www.mayoclinic.org/diseases-conditions/appendicitis/symptoms-causes/syc-20369543#:~:text=Although%20anyone%20can%20develop%20appendicitis,ages%20of%2010%20and%2030.

3. Cervellin, Gianfranco, et al. "Epidemiology and Outcomes of Acute Abdominal Pain in a Large Urban Emergency DEPARTMENT: Retrospective Analysis of 5,340 Cases." *Annals of Translational Medicine*, AME Publishing Company, Oct. 2016, www.ncbi.nlm.nih.gov/pmc/articles/PMC5075866/

4. Kendall, John, and Maria Moreira. "Evaluation of the Adult with Abdominal Pain in the Emergency Department." *UpToDate*, 29 Dec. 2020, www.uptodate.

com/contents/evaluation-of-the-adult-with-abdominal-pain-in-the-emergency-department.

5. Zafari, Maziar. "Myocardial Infarction - Prognosis." *Latest Medical News, Clinical Trials, Guidelines - Today on Medscape*, 5 Dec. 2020, www.medscape.com/answers/155919-15097/what-is-the-prognosis-of-acute-myocardial-infarction-mi-heart-.

6. Lohsiriwat, Varut. "Colonoscopic Perforation: Incidence, Risk Factors, Management and Outcome." *World Journal of Gastroenterology*, vol. 16, no. 4, 2010, p. 425., https://doi.org/10.3748/wjg.v16.i4.425.

7. Cervellin, Gianfranco, et al. "Epidemiology and Outcomes of Acute Abdominal Pain in a Large Urban Emergency Department: Retrospective Analysis of 5,340 Cases." *Annals of Translational Medicine*, AME Publishing Company, Oct. 2016, https://www.ncbi.nlm.nih.gov/pmc/articles/PMC5075866/#:~:text=Our%20study%20showed%20that%20AAP,diagnosis%20at%20the%20second%20visit.

8. Randal Bollinger, R., et al. "Biofilms in the Large Bowel Suggest an Apparent Function of the Human Vermiform Appendix." *Journal of Theoretical Biology*, vol. 249, no. 4, 2007, pp. 826—831., https://doi.org/10.1016/j.jtbi.2007.08.032.

4: ALLERGY & ANAPHYLAXIS

1. Willingham, Emily. "Why Did Mylan Hike Epipen Prices 400%? Because They Could." *Forbes*, Forbes Magazine, 25 Aug. 2016, www.forbes.com/sites/emilywillingham/2016/08/21/why-did-mylan-hike-epipen-prices-400-because-they-could/?sh=360f0c38280c.

2. Mustafa, Shahzad S. "Anaphylaxis." *Practice Essentials, Background, Pathophysiology*, Medscape, 18 May 2021, https://emedicine.medscape.com/article/135065-overview#a6.

5: FEVER

1. "Definitions of Symptoms for Reportable Illnesses." *Centers for Disease Control and Prevention*, Centers for Disease Control and Prevention, 30 June 2017, https://www.cdc.gov/quarantine/air/reporting-deaths-illness/definitions-symptoms-reportable-illnesses.html

2. "Top 20 Pneumonia Facts." *American Thoracic Society*, American Thoracic Society, 2019. https://www.thoracic.org/patients/patient-resources/resources/top-pneumonia-facts.pdf

3. Kalanuria, Atul Ashok, et al. "Ventilator-Associated Pneumonia in the ICU." *Critical Care (London, England)*, BioMed Central, 18 Mar. 2014. www.ncbi.nlm.nih.gov/pmc/articles/PMC4056625/.

4. "Ventilator-Associated Pneumonia: Getting to Zero...and Staying There." *Institute for Healthcare Improvement*, 2016, www.ihi.org/resources/Pages/ImprovementStories/VAPGettingtoZeroandStayingThere.aspx#:~:text=%E2%80%8BWith%20a%20mortality%20rate,need%20mechanical%20help%20to%20breathe.

5. "CDC - Malaria - Malaria Worldwide - Impact of Malaria." *Centers for Disease Control and Prevention*, Centers for Disease Control and Prevention, 16 Dec. 2021, https://www.cdc.gov/malaria/malaria_worldwide/impact.html.

6. "What Is the Prognosis of Encephalitis?" *Latest Medical News, Clinical Trials, Guidelines - Today on Medscape*, 23 Mar. 2020, www.medscape.com/answers/791896-104293/what-is-the-prognosis-of-encephalitis.

6: SYNCOPE & SEIZURES

1. Dale, Natalie. "Drugs." *Volume 1: Setting & Character*. Writer's Guide to Medicine. Ranunculus Press, December 2021.

2. "Epilepsy Auras." *Epilepsy Society*, 28 June 2021, epilepsysociety.org.uk/epilepsy-auras#:~:text=An%20'aura'%20is%20the%20term,into%20another%20type%20of%20seizure.

3. Pohlmann-Eden, Bernd, et al. "The First Seizure and Its Management in Adults and Children." *BMJ (Clinical Research Ed.)*, BMJ Publishing Group Ltd., 11 Feb. 2006, www.ncbi.nlm.nih.gov/pmc/articles/PMC1363913/.

4. Group, Northeast Regional Epilepsy. "Epilepsy Information." *Northeast Regional Epilepsy Group RSS*, www.epilepsygroup.com/epilepsy-information-sub2-detail5-59-19-94-79/epilepsy-seizure-driving-transportation-law-legal-state.htm.

5. Dale, Natalie. "Consciousness & Coma." *Volume 1: Setting & Character*. Writer's Guide to Medicine. Ranunculus Press, 2021.

6. Kammerman, S, and L Wasserman. "Seizure Disorders: Part 1. Classification and Diagnosis." *The Western Journal of Medicine*, BMJ Group, Aug. 2001, www.

ncbi.nlm.nih.gov/pmc/articles/PMC1071497/#:~:text=Tonic%2Dclonic%20
(grand%2Dmal)%20seizures%20occur%20in%2025,of%20generalized%20
seizure%20in%20adults.

7. Kammerman, S, and L Wasserman. "Seizure Disorders: Part 1. Classification
    and Diagnosis." *The Western Journal of Medicine*, BMJ Group, Aug. 2001, www.
    ncbi.nlm.nih.gov/pmc/articles/PMC1071497/#:~:text=Tonic%2Dclonic%20
    (grand%2Dmal)%20seizures%20occur%20in%2025,of%20generalized%20
    seizure%20in%20adults.

8. Rudolf, Gabrielle. "Childhood Absence Epilepsy." *Orphanet: Rare Diseases*, Nov.
    2015, www.orpha.net/consor/cgi-bin/OC_Exp.php?Lng=GB&Expert=64280.

7: STROKE

1. Fisher, Conrad. "Neurology." *USMLE Step 2 CK*, 2nd ed., Kaplan Medical, New
    York, NY, 2015, pp. 273—276. Master the Boards.

2. Smajlović, Dževdet. "Strokes in Young Adults: Epidemiology and Prevention."
    Vascular Health and Risk Management, Dove Medical Press, 24 Feb. 2015,
    https://www.ncbi.nlm.nih.gov/pmc/articles/PMC4348138/#:~:text=The%20
    large%20studies%20indicate%20that,100%2C000%2Fyear%20for%20
    intracerebral%20hemorrhage.

3. Carey, David P., and Leah T. Johnstone. "Quantifying Cerebral Asymmetries
    for Language in Dextrals and Adextrals with Random-Effects Meta Analysis."
    Frontiers, Frontiers, 1 Jan. 1AD, https://www.frontiersin.org/articles/10.3389/
    fpsyg.2014.01128/full.

4. Patel, Neel, and Scott Simon. "Intracerebral Hemorrhage." *AANS*, Ameri-
    can Association of Neurological Surgeons, 2020, https://www.aans.org/
    en/Patients/Neurosurgical-Conditions-and-Treatments/Intracerebral-
    Hemorrhage#:~:text=Intracerebral%20hemorrhage%20(bleeding%20into%20
    the,or%20abnormal%20development%20or%20trauma.

5. Russo, Allison, and Roxanne M Andrews. "Statistical Brief #51: Hospital Stays
    for Stroke and Other Cerebrovascular Diseases, 2005." *Healthcare Cost and
    Utilization Project*, Agency for Healthcare Research and Quality, May 2008,
    https://www.hcup-us.ahrq.gov/reports/statbriefs/sb51.pdf.

1. "Preterm Birth." *Centers for Disease Control and Prevention*, Centers for Disease Control and Prevention, 1 Nov. 2021, https://www.cdc.gov/reproductivehealth/maternalinfanthealth/pretermbirth.htm.

2. Dekker, Rebecca. "The Evidence on: Due Dates." *Evidence Based Birth*®, 25 Oct. 2021, https://evidencebasedbirth.com/evidence-on-due-dates/.

3. Winnie, Kirsten, and John Saultz. "Family Physicians Delivering Babies? It's Time to Decide." *Family Medicine*, vol. 53, no. 5, 2021, pp. 325—327., https://doi.org/10.22454/fammed.2021.782821.

4. "Miscarriage." *Mayo Clinic*, Mayo Foundation for Medical Education and Research, 16 July 2019, www.mayoclinic.org/diseases-conditions/pregnancy-loss-miscarriage/symptoms-causes/syc-20354298.

5. Iftikhar, Noreen. "Premature Baby Survival Rates." *Healthline*, Healthline Media, 29 May 2020, www.healthline.com/health/baby/premature-baby-survival-rate.

6. Le, Tao, et al. *First Aid for the USMLE Step 3*. 4th ed., McGraw-Hill Education, 2016.

7. John R Smith, MD. "Postpartum Hemorrhage." *Background, Problem, Epidemiology*, Medscape, 17 Oct. 2021, https://emedicine.medscape.com/article/275038-overview.

8. Venkatesh, Giriyappa, and Narasimhaiah G Manjunath. "Postpartum Blue Is Common in Socially and Economically Insecure Mothers." *Indian Journal of Community Medicine*, vol. 36, no. 3, 2011, p. 231., https://doi.org/10.4103/0970-0218.86527.

9: SUICIDE

1. Stack, S. "Media Coverage as a Risk Factor in Suicide." *Journal of Epidemiology & Community Health*, BMJ Publishing Group Ltd, 1 Apr. 2003, jech.bmj.com/content/57/4/238.

2. "Explore Suicide in the United States: 2021 Annual Report." *America's Health Rankings*, https://www.americashealthrankings.org/explore/annual/measure/Suicide/state/ALL.

3. Kuntz, Leah. "Pregnancy and Postpartum Suicide Risk: The New Numbers."

Psychiatric Times, Psychiatric Times, 25 Nov. 2020, www.psychiatrictimes.com/view/pregnancy-and-postpartum-suicide-risk-the-new-numbers.

4. "Suicide Statistics." *American Foundation for Suicide Prevention*, American Foundation for Suicide Prevention, 21 July 2021, afsp.org/suicide-statistics/.

5. Schrieber, Jennifer, and Larry Culpepper. "Suicidal Ideation and Behavior in Adults." *UpToDate*, 23 Sept. 2021, https://www.uptodate.com/contents/suicidal-ideation-and-behavior-in-adults.

6. Ng, Chung Wai Mark, et al. "Depression in Primary Care: Assessing Suicide Risk." *SMJ*, 2017, www.smj.org.sg/article/depression-primary-care-assessing-suicide-risk.

7. Brådvik, Louise. "Suicide Risk and Mental Disorders." *International Journal of Environmental Research and Public Health*, MDPI, 17 Sept. 2018, www.ncbi.nlm.nih.gov/pmc/articles/PMC6165520/.

8. "Planned and Impulsive Suicide Attempts." *Planned and Impulsive Suicide Attempts | Suicide Prevention Resource Center*, 6 Aug. 2021, www.sprc.org/news/planned-impulsive-suicide-attempts.

9. Çelik, Mustafa, et al. "Copycat Suicides without an Intention to Die after Watching TV Programs: Two Cases at Five Years of Age." *Noro Psikiyatri Arsivi*, Turkish Neuropsychiatric Society, Mar. 2016, www.ncbi.nlm.nih.gov/pmc/articles/PMC5353244/.

10. Kindelan, Katie, and Sabina Ghebremedhin. "2 California Families Claim '13 Reasons Why' Triggered Teens' Suicides." *ABC News*, ABC News Network, 28 June 2013, abcnews.go.com/US/california-families-claim-13-reasons-triggered-teens-suicides/story?id=48323640.

10: POISONING

1. Bradbury, Neil. *A Taste for Poison: Eleven Deadly Substances and the Killers Who Used Them*, HarperNorth, Manchester, 2022, pp. 156-157, 217—238.

2. Auwärter, V, et al. "Analytical Investigations in a Death Case by Suffocation in an Argon Atmosphere." *Forensic Science International*, vol. 143, no. 2-3, 2004, pp. 169—175., https://doi.org/10.1016/j.forsciint.2004.02.043.

3. Blumenberg, Adam. "Arsenic Toxicity." *Practice Essentials, Background, Pathophysiology*, Medscape, 11 Apr. 2022, https://emedicine.medscape.com/article/812953-overview.

4. Cavanaugh, Ray. "The Dangers of Dimethylmercury." *Chemistry World*, Chemistry World, 27 Jan. 2020, https://www.chemistryworld.com/opinion/the-dangers-of-dimethylmercury-/3010064.article.

5. "Nicotine Poisoning: Symptoms, Causes, Treatment & Prevention." *Cleveland Clinic*, 25 Oct. 2021, https://my.clevelandclinic.org/health/diseases/21582-nicotine-poisoning.

6. Horowitz, Zane B, and Michael J Moss. "Amatoxin Mushroom Toxicity - Statpearls - NCBI Bookshelf." *StatPearls*, NCBI Bookshelf, 11 Aug. 2021, https://www.ncbi.nlm.nih.gov/books/NBK431052/.

7. Horowitz, Zane B. "Mushroom Toxicity Workup: Approach Considerations, Laboratory Studies, Imaging Studies." *Mushroom Toxicity Workup: Approach Considerations, Laboratory Studies, Imaging Studies*, Medscape, 9 Nov. 2019, https://emedicine.medscape.com/article/167398-workup#c2.

8. "Rodenticides." *National Pesticide Information Center*, Mar. 2016, http://npic.orst.edu/factsheets/rodenticides.html.

9. Benzer, Theodore. "Tetrodotoxin Toxicity Clinical Presentation: History, Physical Examination." *Tetrodotoxin Toxicity Clinical Presentation: History, Physical Examination*, Medscape, 9 Aug. 2021, https://emedicine.medscape.com/article/818763-clinical#showall.

10. Janssen, Renée M., et al. "Two Cases of Cardiac Glycoside Poisoning from Accidental Foxglove Ingestion." *Canadian Medical Association Journal*, vol. 188, no. 10, 2016, pp. 747—750., https://doi.org/10.1503/cmaj.150676.

11. Hariharan, Uma. "Intestinal Oleander Poisoning and Critical Care Management: A Rare Case Report." *Anesthesia & Clinical Care*, vol. 3, no. 1, 2016, pp. 1—2., https://doi.org/10.24966/acc-8879/100018.

11: HEAD & NECK INJURIES

1. Kaiser, Robert. "The Dangers from Knife and Weapon Slashing." *Security Magazine RSS*, Security Magazine, 24 Jan. 2019, www.securitymagazine.com/articles/89752-the-danger-of-slashing.

2. Monahan, Kathleen et.al. "Neurological Implications of Nonfatal Strangulation and Intimate Partner Violence." *Future Medicine*. 22 Aug 2019. https://www.futuremedicine.com/doi/10.2217/fnl-2018-0031

3. "Facts of Victim Strangulation." *Strangulation Training Institute*, Alliance for Hope International, pai.wv.gov/events/Documents/Strangulation%20Packet%20LET2017.pdf.

4. Mukunth, Vasudevan. "Gruesome, Clumsy and Irreversible: The Science BEHIND 'HANGING by THE NECK'." *The Wire Science*, 20 Mar. 2020, science.thewire.in/the-sciences/nirbhaya-convicts-hanging-tihar-jail-cervical-fracture-long-drop-method/.

12: TRAUMATIC BRAIN INJURY

1. Young, Becky. "Diffuse Axonal Injury: Prognosis, Symptoms, and Treatment." *Healthline*, Healthline Media, 29 Sept. 2018, www.healthline.com/health/diffuse-axonal-injury#treatment.

2. Pellot, Joel E. "Cerebral Contusion." *StatPearls [Internet].*, U.S. National Library of Medicine, 7 Feb. 2021, www.ncbi.nlm.nih.gov/books/NBK562147/.

3. Rosyidi, Rohadi Muhammad, et al. "Toward Zero Mortality in Acute Epidural HEMATOMA: A Review in 268 Cases Problems and Challenges in the Developing Country." *Interdisciplinary Neurosurgery*, Elsevier, 10 Feb. 2019, www.sciencedirect.com/science/article/pii/S2214751918302871#:~:text=Based%20on%20the%20severity%2C%20the,one%20of%20the%20most%20lethal.

4. Magazine, Smithsonian. "Phineas Gage: Neuroscience's Most Famous Patient." *Smithsonian.com*, Smithsonian Institution, 1 Jan. 2010, https://www.smithsonianmag.com/history/phineas-gage-neurosciences-most-famous-patient-11390067/.

5. Villaret, Andrea Bolzoni, et al. "Intracerebral Bullet Removal through an Endoscopic TRANSNASAL CRANIECTOMY." *Surgical Neurology International*, Medknow Publications & Media Pvt Ltd, 2012, www.ncbi.nlm.nih.gov/pmc/articles/PMC3551493

6. Lau, Brian C., et al. "Which on-Field Signs/Symptoms Predict Protracted Recovery from Sport-Related Concussion among High School Football Players?" *The American Journal of Sports Medicine*, vol. 39, no. 11, 2011, pp. 2311—2318., https://doi.org/10.1177/0363546511410655.

7. Cantu, Robert C. "Posttraumatic Retrograde and Anterograde Amnesia: Pathophysiology and Implications in Grading and Safe Return to Play." *Journal of Athletic Training*, National Athletic Trainers' Association, Inc., Sept. 2001, www.ncbi.nlm.nih.gov/pmc/articles/PMC155413/.

8. Pachalska, Maria, et al. "A Case of 'Borrowed Identity Syndrome' after Severe Traumatic Brain Injury." *Medical Science Monitor: International Medical Journal of Experimental and Clinical Research*, International Scientific Literature, Inc., Feb. 2011, www.ncbi.nlm.nih.gov/pmc/articles/PMC3524703/.

9. Wong, Wilson. "'Move Ahead': GABBY Giffords Discusses Her Recovery and Reflects on 10-Year Anniversary Of near-Fatal SHOOTING." *NBCNews.com*, NBCUniversal News Group, 8 Jan. 2021, www.nbcnews.com/news/us-news/move-ahead-gabby-giffords-discusses-her-recovery-reflects-10-year-n1253474.

10. Abrams, Jonathan. "Phillip Adams Had Severe C.T.E. at the Time of Shootings." *The New York Times*, The New York Times, 14 Dec. 2021, https://www.nytimes.com/2021/12/14/sports/football/phillip-adams-cte-shootings.html#:~:text=A%20neuropathologist%20found%20an%20%E2%80%9Cunusually,in%20April%20before%20shooting%20himself.

13: SPINE & SPINAL CORD INJURIES

1. Fischer, Itzhak, et al. "Spinal Cord Concussion: Studying the Potential Risks of Repetitive Injury." *Neural Regeneration Research*, Medknow Publications & Media Pvt Ltd, Jan. 2016, www.ncbi.nlm.nih.gov/pmc/articles/PMC4774225/.

2. "When Damaged, the Adult Brain Repairs Itself by Going Back to the Beginning." *ScienceDaily*, ScienceDaily, 15 Apr. 2020, https://www.sciencedaily.com/releases/2020/04/200415133654.htm.

3. Doty, Pamela. "Cliff Jumping: Things to Know." *DVIDS*, US Army Corp of Engineers, 26 Aug. 2020, https://www.dvidshub.net/news/376879/cliff-jumping-things-know.

14: INJURIES TO THE CHEST

1. Page, David W. *Body Trauma: A Writer's Guide to Wounds and Injuries.* Behler Publications, 2007.

2. Cubasch, Herbert, and Elias Degiannis. "The Deadly Dozen of Chest Trauma." *Southern Medical Journal*, vol. 97, no. 7, July 2004, pp. 369—372., doi:10.1097/00007611-200407000-00011.

3. Porter-Woodruff, Jordan A. "Silent Killer: Everything You Need to Know about Aortic Dissection." *Silent Killer: Everything You Need to Know about*

Aortic Dissection - UChicago Medicine, UChicago Medicine, 12 Feb. 2018, www.uchicagomedicine.org/forefront/heart-and-vascular-articles/silent-killer-everything-you-need-to-know-about-aortic-dissection.

15: GUT WOUNDS

1. "Abdominal Injuries." *Electronic Library of Trauma Lectures* 2012, health.ucdavis.edu/cppn/documents/stn/speaker_notes/10_Speaker%20Notes_08338_STN-Abdominal%20Injuries.pdf.

2. Rodríguez-Hermosa, José Ignacio, et al. "Gastric Perforations from Abdominal Trauma." *Digestive Surgery*, Karger Publishers, 28 Mar. 2008, www.karger.com/Article/Abstract/121906.

3. Debi, Uma. "Pancreatic Trauma: A Concise Review." *World Journal of Gastroenterology*, vol. 19, no. 47, 2013, p. 9003., https://doi.org/10.3748/wjg.v19.i47.9003.

4. Cirocchi, Roberto, et al. "Damage Control Surgery for Abdominal Trauma." *The Cochrane Database of Systematic Reviews*, U.S. National Library of Medicine, 28 Mar. 2013, pubmed.ncbi.nlm.nih.gov/23543551/.

5. "Being Wounded." *Violence: A Writer's Guide*, by Rory Kane Miller, Wyrd Goat Press, 2012, pp. 225—233.

6. Joseph, Weinstein, et al. "Low Velocity Gunshot Wounds Result in Significant Contamination Regardless of Ballistic Characteristics." *American Journal of Orthopedics*, MD Edge, Jan. 2014, 5.cdn.mdedge.com/files/s3fs-public/Document/September-2017/043010014_01.pdf.

7. Andrews, Evan. "What Killed Harry Houdini?" *History.com*, A&E Television Networks, 31 Oct. 2016, https://www.history.com/news/what-killed-harry-houdini#:~:text=The%20official%20cause%20of%20Houdini's,their%20backstage%20encounter%20in%20Montreal.

8. Villaret, AndreaBolzoni, et al. "Intracerebral Bullet Removal through an Endoscopic Transnasal Craniectomy." *Surgical Neurology International*, vol. 3, no. 1, 2012, p. 155., https://doi.org/10.4103/2152-7806.104749.

16: INJURIES TO THE ARMS & LEGS

1. "How to Come Back Stronger and Faster after an Ankle Sprain." *Central Vermont*

Medical Center, 15 Nov. 2018, www.cvmc.org/blog/rehabilitation-therapy/how-come-back-stronger-and-faster-after-ankle-sprain#:~:text=Grade%201%20 sprains%20are%20light,ligament%20and%20possible%20bone%20fracture.

2. "70 Percent of ALL Traumatic Amputations Involve the Upper Limbs." *ISHN RSS*, ISHN, 4 May 2016, www.ishn.com/articles/103914-percent-of-all-traumatic-amputations-involve-the-upper-limbs.

3. Meenach, Dean. "How to Manage Traumatic Amputations and Uncontrolled Bleeding." *How To Manage Traumatic Amputations And Uncontrolled Bleeding | Bound Tree*, 30 Apr. 2014, www.boundtree.com/university/trauma/how-to-manage-traumatic-amputations-and-uncontrolled-bleeding.

4. Lekuya, Hervé Monka, et al. "Degloving Injuries with versus without Underlying Fracture in a Sub-Saharan AFRICAN Tertiary Hospital: A Prospective Observational Study." *Journal of Orthopaedic Surgery and Research*, BioMed Central, 5 Jan. 2018, www.ncbi.nlm.nih.gov/pmc/articles/PMC5756448/.

17: BURNS

1. Warby, Rachel. "Burn Classification." *StatPearls [Internet].*, U.S. National Library of Medicine, 5 Sept. 2020, www.ncbi.nlm.nih.gov/books/NBK539773/.

2. Bounds, Emily J. "Electrical Burns." *StatPearls [Internet].*, U.S. National Library of Medicine, 4 May 2021, www.ncbi.nlm.nih.gov/books/NBK519514/.

3. Zane, Richard D., and Joshua M. Kosowsky. *Pocket Emergency Medicine.* Wolters Kluwer, 2015.

4. Gupta, Kapil, et al. "Smoke Inhalation Injury: Etiopathogenesis, Diagnosis, and Management." *Indian Journal of Critical Care Medicine: Peer-Reviewed, Official Publication of Indian Society of Critical Care Medicine*, Medknow Publications & Media Pvt Ltd, Mar. 2018, www.ncbi.nlm.nih.gov/pmc/articles/PMC5879861/.

5. Slotnik, Daniel E. "Dax Cowart, Who Suffered for Patients' Rights, Dies at 71." *The New York Times*, The New York Times, 15 May 2019, www.nytimes.com/2019/05/15/obituaries/dax-cowart-dead.html.

6. Thompson, Kristy. "Fire Dynamics." *NIST*, 2 June 2021, www.nist.gov/el/fire-research-division-73300/firegov-fire-service/fire-dynamics.

7. Amin, Mohamed, et al. "Role of Fiberoptic Bronchoscopy in Management

of Smoke Inhalation Lung Injury." *Egyptian Journal of Chest Diseases and Tuberculosis*, vol. 64, no. 3, 2015, pp. 733—737., https://doi.org/10.1016/j.ejcdt.2015.03.015.

18: LIFESTYLE DISEASES

1. Levine, James A. "Poverty and Obesity in the U.S." *Diabetes*, vol. 60, no. 11, 2011, pp. 2667—2668., https://doi.org/10.2337/db11-1118.

2. Jackson, Whitney. "Alcohol-Related Liver Disease - Hepatic and Biliary Disorders." *Merck Manuals Professional Edition*, Merck Manuals, 18 Apr. 2022, https://www.merckmanuals.com/professional/hepatic-and-biliary-disorders/alcohol-related-liver-disease/alcohol-related-liver-disease.

3. Sabish, TA. "Lifestyle Diseases: Consequences, Characteristics, Causes and Control." *Journal of Cardiology & Current Research*, vol. 9, no. 3, 2017, https://doi.org/10.15406/jccr.2017.09.00326.

19: DIABETES

1. Agabegi, Steven S., et al. *Step-up to Medicine*. 3rd ed., Lippincott Williams & Wilkins, 2013.

2. Croke, Lisa M. "Type 2 Diabetes Mellitus: ACP Releases Updated Guidance Statement on A1C Targets for Pharmacologic Glycemic Control." *American Family Physician*, 1 Nov. 2018, https://www.aafp.org/afp/2018/1101/p613.html.

3. Croke, Lisa M. "Type 2 Diabetes Mellitus: ACP Releases Updated Guidance Statement on A1C Targets for Pharmacologic Glycemic Control." *American Family Physician*, 1 Nov. 2018, https://www.aafp.org/afp/2018/1101/p613.html.

4. "Diabetes and Heart Disease." *Johns Hopkins Medicine*, 19 Nov. 2019, https://www.hopkinsmedicine.org/health/conditions-and-diseases/diabetes/diabetes-and-heart-disease.

20: CHRONIC BREATHLESSNESS

1. "Understanding Changes in Life Expectancy." *Cystic Fibrosis Foundation*, https://www.cff.org/managing-cf/understanding-changes-life-expectancy.

2. Lorditch, Emilie. "No More Mucus." *MSU Today*, 23 Nov. 2021, https://msutoday.msu.edu/news/2021/no-more-mucus-trikafta.

21: AUTOIMMUNE DISEASES

1. Scudellari, Megan. "Cleaning up the Hygiene Hypothesis." *Proceedings of the National Academy of Sciences*, vol. 114, no. 7, 2017, pp. 1433—1436., https://doi.org/10.1073/pnas.1700688114.

2. Agabegi, Steven S, and Elizabeth D Agabegi. *Step-Up to Medicine*. 3rd ed., Lippincott Williams & Wilkins, 2013.

3. Souza, Ana, et al. "Multiple Sclerosis and Mobility-Related Assistive Technology: Systematic Review of Literature." *The Journal of Rehabilitation Research and Development*, vol. 47, no. 3, 2010, p. 213., https://doi.org/10.1682/jrrd.2009.07.0096.

4. Wendell, Linda C., and Joshua M. Levine. "Myasthenic Crisis." *The Neurohospitalist*, vol. 1, no. 1, 2011, pp. 16—22., https://doi.org/10.1177/1941875210382918.

5. Wallace, D.J., & Hahn, B.H. (2013). Dubois' lupus erythematosus and related syndromes. (8th ed.) Philadelphia, PA: Elsevier Saunders.

6. Somers, Emily C., et al. "Population-Based Incidence and Prevalence of Systemic Lupus Erythematosus: The Michigan Lupus Epidemiology and Surveillance Program." *Arthritis & Rheumatology*, vol. 66, no. 2, 2014, pp. 369—378., https://doi.org/10.1002/art.38238.

22: HEADACHE

1. Ji Lee, Mi, et al. "Increased Suicidality in Patients with Cluster Headache." *Cephalalgia*, vol. 39, no. 10, 2019, pp. 1249—1256., https://doi.org/10.1177/0333102419845660.

2. Blanda, Michelle. "Tension Headache." *Background, Pathophysiology, Etiology*, Medscape, 12 Jan. 2022, https://emedicine.medscape.com/article/792384-overview#a3.

1. Kupfer, David. *Diagnostic and Statistical Manual of Mental Disorders: DSM-5.* American Psychiatric Association Publishing, 2022.

2. Longo, Lance P., and Brian Johnson. "Addiction: Part I. Benzodiazepines-Side Effects, Abuse Risk and Alternatives." *American Family Physician*, 1 Apr. 2000, https://www.aafp.org/afp/2000/0401/p2121.html.

3. Horton, Lisa. "Why Bipolar Patients Don't Take Their Meds." *EurekAlert!*, 19 May 2021, https://www.eurekalert.org/news-releases/584317#:~:text=Nearly%20half%20of%20people%20with,taking%20their%20medication%20as%20prescribed.

4. Lim, Anastasia, et al. "Prevalence and Classification of Hallucinations in Multiple Sensory Modalities in Schizophrenia Spectrum Disorders." *Schizophrenia Research*, vol. 176, no. 2-3, 2016, pp. 493—499., https://doi.org/10.1016/j.schres.2016.06.010.

5. "The Brain as Explained by John Cleese." *YouTube*, 2010, https://www.youtube.com/watch?v=FQjgsQ5G8ug. Accessed 23 Mar. 2022.

6. Kimberlie Dean, Ph.D. "Risk of Being Subjected to Crime, Including Violent Crime, after Onset of Mental Illness." *JAMA Psychiatry*, JAMA Network, 1 July 2018, https://jamanetwork.com/journals/jamapsychiatry/fullarticle/2680807.

7. Latalova, Klara, et al. "Violent Victimization of Adult Patients with Severe Mental Illness: A: NDT." *Neuropsychiatric Disease and Treatment*, Dove Press, 9 Oct. 2014, https://www.dovepress.com/violent-victimization-of-adult-patients-with-severe-mental-illness-a-s-peer-reviewed-fulltext-article-NDT.

8. Deangelis, Tori. "Mental Illness and Violence: Debunking Myths, Addressing Realities." *Monitor on Psychology*, American Psychological Association, 1 Apr. 2021, https://www.apa.org/monitor/2021/04/ce-mental-illness.

9. Varshney, Mohit, et al. "Violence and Mental Illness: What Is the True Story?" *Journal of Epidemiology & Community Health*, BMJ Publishing Group Ltd, 1 Mar. 2016, https://jech.bmj.com/content/70/3/223.

10. Rueve, Marie, and Randon Welton. "Violence and Mental Illness." *Psychiatry*, vol. 5, no. 5, May 2008, pp. 34—48., https://doi.org/https://www.ncbi.nlm.nih.gov/pmc/articles/PMC2686644/.

1. "Cancer." *World Health Organization*, World Health Organization, 3 Mar. 2021, www.who.int/news-room/fact-sheets/detail/cancer.

2. "More Cancer Types - Seer Cancer Stat Facts." *SEER*, National Cancer Institute, seer.cancer.gov/statfacts/more.html.

3. "About Breast Cancer in Men." *Johns Hopkins Medicine*, www.hopkinsmedicine.org/health/conditions-and-diseases/breast-cancer/about-breast-cancer-in-men.

4. "Skin Cancer." *American Academy of Dermatology*, 1 June 2021, www.aad.org/media/stats-skin-cancer.

5. "Survival Rates for Selected Adult Brain and Spinal Cord Tumors." *American Cancer Society*, 5 May 2020, www.cancer.org/cancer/brain-spinal-cord-tumors-adults/detection-diagnosis-staging/survival-rates.html.

6. "Neuroblastoma (for Parents) - Nemours Kidshealth." Edited by Eric S. Sandler, *KidsHealth*, The Nemours Foundation, Jan. 2017, kidshealth.org/en/parents/neuroblastoma.html.

7. "Quick Brain Tumor Facts." *National Brain Tumor Society*, 22 Mar. 2021, braintumor.org/brain-tumor-information/brain-tumor-facts/.

8. "Leukemia - Acute Myeloid - Aml - Statistics." *Cancer.Net*, 21 Apr. 2021, www.cancer.net/cancer-types/leukemia-acute-myeloid-aml/statistics#:~:text=AML%20is%20the%20second%20most,of%20diagnosis%20is%20age%2068.

9. Agabegi, Steven S., et al. *Step-up to Medicine*. 3rd ed., Lippincott Williams & Wilkins, 2013.

10. Toro, Ross. "How Gender Reassignment Surgery Works (Infographic)." *LiveScience*, Purch, 26 Aug. 2013, www.livescience.com/39170-how-gender-reassignment-surgery-works-infographic.html.

11. Smith, Yolanda. "Radiation Therapy Dosage." *News*, 23 Mar. 2021, www.news-medical.net/health/Radiation-Therapy-Dosage.aspx.

12. "Understanding Radiation Therapy." *Cancer.Net*, 23 Sept. 2020, www.cancer.net/navigating-cancer-care/how-cancer-treated/radiation-therapy/understanding-radiation-therapy.

13. Nurse, Rachel. "I'm 22 with Stage 3 Cancer and This Is Why I Find the 'Sick Girl' Trope in Films so Misogynistic." *Glamour UK*, Glamour UK, 8 Feb. 2021, https://www.glamourmagazine.co.uk/article/sick-girl-trope.

1. Agabegi, Steven S., et al. *Step-up to Medicine*. Third ed., Wolters Kluwer, 2014. Pg. 215-217.

2. "Frontotemporal Dementia." *Alzheimer's Disease and Dementia*, Alzheimer's Association, 2021, www.alz.org/alzheimers-dementia/what-is-dementia/types-of-dementia/frontotemporal-dementia.

3. "Creutzfeld Jakob Disease." *NHS Choices*, NHS, 14 June 2018, www.nhs.uk/conditions/creutzfeldt-jakob-disease-cjd/.

4. Williams, Susan Schneider. "The Terrorist inside My Husband's Brain." *Neurology*, Wolters Kluwer Health, Inc. on Behalf of the American Academy of Neurology, 27 Sept. 2016, n.neurology.org/content/87/13/1308.

5. Reeves, Benjamin C., et al. "Glymphatic System Impairment in Alzheimer's Disease and Idiopathic Normal Pressure Hydrocephalus." *Trends in Molecular Medicine*, vol. 26, no. 3, 2020, pp. 285—295., https://doi.org/10.1016/j.molmed.2019.11.008.

FAQ WORKS CITED

1. Ciccarelli, Saundra K., and J. Noland White. "Dissociative Disorders." *Psychology: DSM 5*, Pearson, Boston, Mass, 2014, pp. 291—307.

2. "Fentanyl and Carfentanil." *Ottawa Public Health*, https://www.ottawapublichealth.ca/en/public-health-topics/fentanyl-and-carfentanil.aspx.

3. Einarsen, Cathrine Elisabeth, et al. "Moderate Traumatic Brain Injury: Clinical Characteristics and a Prognostic Model of 12-Month Outcome." *World Neurosurgery*, Elsevier, 31 Mar. 2018, https://www.sciencedirect.com/science/article/pii/S1878875018306582#:~:text=All%20Patients%20with%20Moderate%20TBI&text=The%20in%2Dhospital%20case%2Dfatality,injury%20(GOSE%20score%201).

4. "Moderate to Severe Traumatic Brain Injury Is a Lifelong Condition." *CDC. Gov*, https://www.cdc.gov/traumaticbraininjury/pdf/moderate_to_severe_tbi_lifelong-a.pdf.

5. Dhaliwal JS, Rosani A, Saadabadi A. Diazepam. [Updated 2021 Sep 14]. In: StatPearls [Internet]. Treasure Island (FL): StatPearls Publishing; 2022 Jan-. Available from: https://www.ncbi.nlm.nih.gov/books/NBK537022/

6. "'Date Rape' Drugs: What You Need to Know." *"Date Rape" Drugs: What You Need to Know | SUNY Geneseo,* https://www.geneseo.edu/health/date-rape-drugs#:~:text=Rohypnol%20is%20a%20drug%20that,a%204%2D6%20hour%20duration.

7. "Barbiturates." *Sutter Health,* https://www.sutterhealth.org/health/teens/drugs/barbiturates#:~:text=after%20intravenous%20use.-,%22Short%2Dacting%22%20and%20%22intermediate%2Dacting%22%20barbiturates,last%20up%20to%20six%20hours.

8. Scheppke, Kenneth A, et al. "Prehospital Use of I.M. Ketamine for Sedation of Violent and Agitated Patients." *The Western Journal of Emergency Medicine,* Department of Emergency Medicine, University of California, Irvine School of Medicine, Nov. 2014, https://www.ncbi.nlm.nih.gov/pmc/articles/PMC4251212/.

9. "Parenteral Benzodiazepines." *Core EM,* https://coreem.net/core/parenteral-benzodiazepines/.

10. Dunstan, Maja. "Scientific Scribbles." *Scientific Scribbles,* 22 Oct. 2016, https://blogs.unimelb.edu.au/sciencecommunication/2016/10/22/ether-the-first-anaesthetic/.

11. Arvidson, Bjorn. "NEG and NIOSH Basis for and Occupational Health Standard: Ethyl Ether." *US Department of Health and Human Services,* CDC, Feb. 1993, https://www.cdc.gov/niosh/docs/94-103/pdfs/94-103.pdf.

12. Foxall, K. "Chloroform Toxicological Overview." *Health Protection Agency,* 2007, https://assets.publishing.service.gov.uk/government/uploads/system/uploads/attachment_data/file/338535/Chloroform_Toxicological_Overview.pdf.

13. Payne, J. P. "The Criminal Use of Chloroform." *Anesthesia,* vol. 53, no. 7, 1998, pp. 685—690., https://doi.org/10.1046/j.1365-2044.1998.528-az0572.x.

14. "Infertility." *Centers for Disease Control and Prevention,* Centers for Disease Control and Prevention, 1 Mar. 2022, https://www.cdc.gov/reproductivehealth/infertility/index.htm#:~:text=Yes.,to%20term%20(impaired%20fecundity).

15. Gelbaya, Tarek A., et al. "Definition and Epidemiology of Unexplained Infertility." *Obstetrical & Gynecological Survey,* vol. 69, no. 2, 2014, pp. 109—115., https://doi.org/10.1097/ogx.0000000000000043.

16. "Oregon Secretary of State." *Oregon Secretary of State Administrative Rules,* https://secure.sos.state.or.us/oard/displayDivisionRules.action%3BJSESSIONID_OARD=FBnd3bo34wq3qP1LABNCNhlxdQyjItenmTt76m3LO0H2g9102V67%212024649768?selectedDivision=1027.

17. Tanaka, Kenichi. "Transfusion and Coagulation Therapy." *Pharmacology and Physiology for Anesthesia*, Science Direct, 2013, https://www.sciencedirect.com/topics/biochemistry-genetics-and-molecular-biology/acute-hemolytic-transfusion-reaction#:~:text=Acute%20hemolytic%20transfusion%20reactions%20are,hypotension%2C%20tachycardia%2C%20and%20hemoglobinuria.

18. Coss, Catherine. "Create Your Own Walking Blood Bank." *Wilderness Medicine Society Magazine*, Wilderness Medicine Society, 24 Mar. 2021, https://wms.org/magazine/1300/index.html#:~:text=A%20walking%20blood%20bank%20is,cells%2C%20plasma%2C%20and%20platelets.

19. Thompson, Patrick, and Geir Strandenes. "The History of Fluid Resuscitation for Bleeding." *Damage Control Resuscitation*, 2019, pp. 3—29., https://doi.org/10.1007/978-3-030-20820-2_1.

AFTERWORD

When I first came up with the idea of writing a "Writer's Guide to Medicine," I had no idea how much of an undertaking it would be. At first, I thought it would be a side project that I could work on when my fiction writing hit a wall.

Hah!

Medicine is way too broad a field—and way too important for writers—for me to condense it down into just one or two volumes. As much as I've already written in Volumes 1 & 2, I still have so much I want to share. What started out as a side project has snowballed into a multi-volume behemoth—and I couldn't be happier about it. Two volumes down, more to come!

If you loved this book, I would greatly appreciate it if you would write a little review on Amazon, Goodreads, B&N, or whichever other format you prefer. Authors like me rely on reviews to increase visibility and open doors to new audiences. Writing a review is one of the best and easiest ways you can help up-and-coming authors succeed. Even a few words can make a big difference. Thank you in advance!

For more on the progress of Volume 3, as well as information on upcoming lectures, freebies, bonus content, news, and events, please check out my website and subscribe to my newsletter! https://nataliedaleauthor.com/

Stay connected! *Volume 3: Mental Illness* is coming soon!

LIKE me on Facebook:
https://www.facebook.com/NatalieDaleAuthorMD

FOLLOW me on Instagram:
https://www.instagram.com/natalierose6627/

FOLLOW me on Twitter:
@DaleNatalie

ADD me on Goodreads:
https://www.goodreads.com/author/show/15282031.Natalie_Dale

ACKNOWLEDGMENTS

From the series' first inception to Volume 2's final copy edits, there are so many people who have helped make this book a reality.

First, a big thank you to my beta readers and critique group partners: Gary Baysinger, Warren Bull, Jessica Curtis, Mike Davis, Marilynne Eichinger, James Elstad, Warren Friedland, Lisa Hurley, Ann Johnson, Kalinda Little, Jim Martin, Jennie Miller, Dave Moore, Elli Ross, Austin Schock, and Jamie Smith. You not only helped me polish my writing but helped push me out of my comfort zone to get this book out into the world.

Second, to my doctor friends—Jacob Aaron and Alisha Crowley—who helped ensure I got all my medical facts correct. And to Nicolaas Vermeulen, PhD, for teaching me about household poisons. I will never look at a gardening center the same again.

Third, to all the professionals who helped make this book happen: my editor, Haley Paskalides, Streetlight Graphics for the beautiful formatting and cover design, and James Conroyd Martin for walking the world's most technologically incompetent Millennial through the process of publishing.

Finally, a big thanks to my family. To my parents, Jeannette Ellis and Russ Grattan, for their unending love and support. To my sister, Francine Grattan, for constantly reminding me to be inclusive of LGBTQ, neurodivergent, and BIPOC individuals. And finally, to my husband, my best friend, my alpha, beta, and zeta reader, Edward Dale.

So many thanks to everyone who helped me on this journey.

ABOUT THE AUTHOR

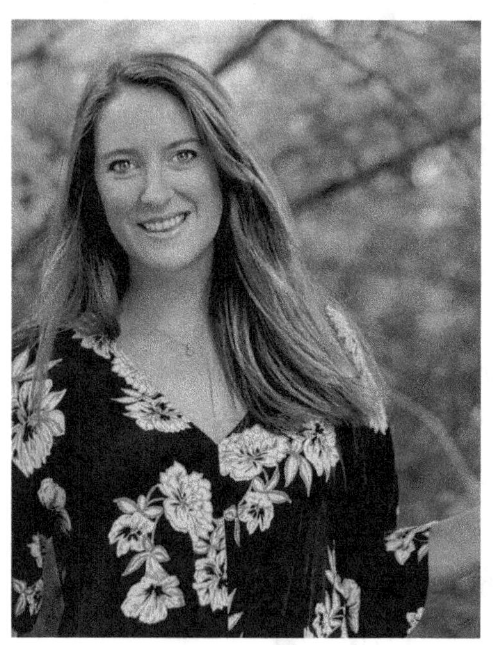

Natalie Dale, MD, is a writer and a non-practicing physician. After graduating Alpha Omega Alpha from the Chicago Medical School, she started residency in neurology at Oregon Health & Science University. Her essays and short stories have been published in *The Bump*, *National Alliance on Mental Illness*, *Writers Helping Writers*, *The Timberline Review*, *Wyldblood*, and the *ReAd, White & Blue Anthology*, among others. <u>Volume 1: Setting & Character</u> of her "Writer's Guide to Medicine" series was published by Ranunculus Press in 2021. She lives in Hillsboro, Oregon, with her husband, toothless cat, and neurotic rescue dog.

Want more great info? Check out my website and subscribe to my newsletter: **https://nataliedaleauthor.com/**

SNEAK PEEK AT VOLUME 3: MENTAL ILLNESS

CATATONIA

Catatonia is a complex medical condition associated with several different mental illnesses, including schizophrenia, depression, and bipolar disorder. Medical conditions, like stroke or Parkinson's disease, can also cause catatonia. It is characterized by a combination of psychiatric, language, and motor features.

- **Altered Level of Consciousness**

    o **Stupor:** Your character does not move or react to their environment, even though their eyes are open, and they are conscious. The presence of stupor indicates a severe form of catatonia.

    o **Agitation:** For no apparent reason, your character becomes agitated or excited.

- **Automatic Obedience:** Your character automatically obeys every instruction.

- **Imitation**

    o **Echolalia:** Imitating another person's speech; echoing a word.

    o **Echopraxia:** Imitating another's movements.

- **Language Changes**

    o **Mutism:** Your character doesn't speak or has trouble talking.

    o **Verbigeration:** Obsessive repetition of non-meaningful words.

    o **Word Salad:** Rapid-fire, incoherent speech (gibberish).

- **Movement Changes**

    o **Grimacing:** Unusual facial movements for no apparent reason.

    o **Stereotypy:** Repetitive, purposeless movements.

- o **Mannerisms:** Repetitive movements that initially had meaning, such as repeated saluting or grasping as if to shake a hand.

- **Postural Changes**

  - o **Waxy Flexibility:** Slight resistance to movement by the examiner.

  - o **Posturing:** Your character will strike a pose and stay there, perhaps for hours. An extreme version is **Catalepsy,** in which the limbs are rigid and remain in position even against force.

  - o **Negativism:** Your character will resist any attempts to move their body, reacting with the same amount of force given (i.e., if the examiner pushes harder, they push back with the same strength).

Your character doesn't have to exhibit all these symptoms; several, such as mutism and echolalia, are contradictory. If you want your character to be catatonic, you only need three of these symptoms. The most common signs of catatonia are stupor and mutism.

DON'T FORGET TO CHECK OUT
VOLUME 1: SETTING & CHARACTER

Available in e-book and paperback

Paperback Amazon:
https://www.amazon.com/Writers-Guide-Medicine-Setting-Character/
dp/B09NRRFS73

Ebook Amazon:
https://www.amazon.com/Writers-Guide-Medicine-Setting-Character-ebook/
dp/B09MZZL1SR